Global Cardiovascular Health

Editors

GERALD S. BLOOMFIELD
MELISSA S. BURROUGHS PEÑA

CARDIOLOGY CLINICS

www.cardiology.theclinics.com

Consulting Editors
JORDAN M. PRUTKIN
DAVID M. SHAVELLE
TERRENCE D. WELCH
AUDREY H. WU

February 2017 • Volume 35 • Number 1

ELSEVIER

1600 John F. Kennedy Boulevard • Suite 1800 • Philadelphia, Pennsylvania, 19103-2899

http://www.theclinics.com

CARDIOLOGY CLINICS Volume 35, Number 1
February 2017 ISSN 0733-8651, ISBN-13: 978-0-323-52834-4

Editor: Stacy Eastman
Developmental Editor: Alison Swety

Cardiology Clinics (ISSN 0733-8651) is published quarterly by Elsevier Inc., 360 Park Avenue South, New York, NY 10010-1710. Months of issue are February, May, August, and November. Business and Editorial Offices: 1600 John F. Kennedy Blvd., Ste. 1800, Philadelphia, PA 19103-2899. Customer Service Office: 3251 Riverport Lane, Maryland Heights, MO 63043. Periodicals post-age paid at New York, NY and additional mailing offices. Subscription prices are $326.00 per year for US individuals, $604.00 per year for US institutions, $100.00 per year for US students and residents, $398.00 per year for Canadian individuals, $758.00 per year for Canadian institutions, $464.00 per year for international individuals, $758.00 per year for international institutions and $220.00 per year for Canadian and international students/residents. To receive student/resident rate, orders must be accompanied by name of affiliated institution, data of term, and the *signature* of program/residency coordinator on institution letterhead. Orders will be billed at individual rate until proof of status is received. Foreign air speed delivery is included in all *Clinics* subscription prices. All prices are subject to change without notice. **POSTMASTER:** Send address changes to *Cardiology Clinics*, Elsevier Health Sciences Division, Subscription Customer Service, 3251 Riverport Lane, Maryland Heights, MO 63043. **Customer Service: 1-800-654-2452 (U.S. and Canada); 314-447-8871 (outside U.S. and Canada). Fax: 314-447-8029. E-mail: journalscustomerservice-usa@ elsevier.com (for print support); journalsonlinesupport-usa@elsevier.com (for online support).**

Reprints. For copies of 100 or more, of articles in this publication, please contact the Commercial Reprints Department, Elsevier Inc., 360 Park Avenue South, New York, NY 10010-1710. Tel.: 212-633-3874; Fax: 212-633-3820; E-mail: reprints@elsevier.com.

Cardiology Clinics is also published in Spanish by McGraw-Hill Interamericana Editores S. A., P.O. Box 5-237, 06500, Mexico D. F., Mexico; in Portuguese by Reichmann and Alfonso Editores Rio de Janeiro, Brazil; and in Greek by Dimitrios P. Lagos, 8 Pondon Street, GR115-28 Ilissia, Greece.

Cardiology Clinics is covered in *MEDLINE/PubMed (Index Medicus), Excerpta Medica, The Cumulative Index to Nursing and Allied Health Literature* (CINAHL).

Contributors

AUTHORS

MARWAH ABDALLA, MD, MPH
Assistant Professor, Center for Behavioral
Cardiovascular Health, Division of Cardiology,
Department of Medicine, Columbia University
Medical Center, New York, New York

WILSON ARUASA, MMED
Moi Teaching and Referral Hospital, Eldoret,
Kenya

FELIX A. BARASA, MMED
Moi Teaching and Referral Hospital, Eldoret,
Kenya

ANDREA BEATON, MD
Division of Cardiology, Children's National
Health System, Washington, DC

CATHERINE PASTORIUS BENZIGER, MD
Cardiology Fellow, Division of Cardiology,
University of Washington, Seattle, Washington

ANDREA BERATARRECHEA, MD, MSc
South American Center of Excellence for
Cardiovascular Health, Institute for Clinical
Effectiveness and Health Policy, Buenos Aires,
Argentina

MARIA LAZO-PORRAS, MD
CRONICAS Center of Excellence in Chronic
Diseases, Universidad Peruana Cayetano
Heredia, Lima, Peru

CLAUDIA LEUNG, BS
Feinberg School of Medicine, Northwestern
University, Chicago, Illinois

MARYA LIEBERMAN, PhD
Department of Chemistry and Biochemistry,
University of Notre Dame, Notre Dame, Indiana

FELIX LIMBANI, MPH
Centre for Health Policy, School of Public
Health, University of the Witwatersrand,
Johannesburg, South Africa

PETER LIU, MD
University of Ottawa, Ottawa, Ontario, Canada

PATRICIO LOPEZ-JARAMILLO, MD, PhD
Research Institute FOSCAL, Bucaramanga,
Colombia

IMRAN MANJI, BPharm
Affiliate Faculty, Department of Pharmacy
Practice, Purdue University College of
Pharmacy, West Lafayette, Indiana; Senior
Pharmacist, Department of Pharmacy, Moi
Teaching and Referral Hospital, Eldoret, Kenya

TARA McCREADY, PhD, MBA
Population Health Research Institute,
Hamilton, Ontario, Canada

WALTER MENDOZA, MD
United Nations Population Fund, Peru Country
Office, San Isidro, Lima, Peru

TIMOTHY MERCER, MD, MPH
Visiting Assistant Professor of Clinical
Medicine, Department of Medicine, Indiana
University School of Medicine, Indianapolis,
Indiana

J. JAIME MIRANDA, MD, MSc, PhD
School of Medicine, CRONICAS Center of
Excellence in Chronic Diseases, Universidad
Peruana Cayetano Heredia, Lima, Peru

ANA OLGA MOCUMBI, MD, PhD
Chronic and Non-Communicable Disease
Division, National Health Institutes and
Eduardo Mondlane University, Maputo,
Mozambique

SAILESH MOHAN, MD, MPH, PhD
Public Health Foundation of India, New Delhi,
India

DANIELA MOYANO, BSc
South American Center of Excellence for
Cardiovascular Health, Institute for Clinical
Effectiveness and Health Policy, Buenos Aires,
Argentina

**ARTHUR K. MUTYABA, MBChB, MMed,
FCP(SA)**
Division of Cardiology, Department of
Medicine, Groote Schuur Hospital, University
of Cape Town, Cape Town,
South Africa

BENSON NJUGUNA, BPharm
Affiliate Faculty, Department of Pharmacy
Practice, Purdue University College of
Pharmacy, West Lafayette, Indiana;
Pharmacist, Department of Pharmacy,
Moi Teaching and Referral Hospital, Eldoret,
Kenya

MPIKO NTSEKHE, MD, PhD, FACC
Division of Cardiology, Department of
Medicine, Groote Schuur Hospital, University
of Cape Town, Cape Town, South Africa

SHANTI NULU, MD, MPH
Section of Cardiovascular Medicine, Yale
School of Medicine, New Haven, Connecticut

OLUGBENGA OGEDEGBE, MD, MS, MPH
School of Medicine, New York University,
New York, New York

ELIJAH S. OGOLA, MMED
Department of Clinical Medicine, College of
Health Sciences, University of Nairobi, Nairobi,
Kenya

BRIAN OLDENBURG, PhD, MPsych
School of Population and Global Health,
University of Melbourne, Melbourne,
Australia

BRUCE OVBIAGELE, MD, MSc
Medical University of South Carolina,
Charleston, South Carolina

MAYOWA OWOLABI, MBBS, MSc, DrM
University of Ibadan, Ibadan, Nigeria

SONAK D. PASTAKIA, PharmD, BCPS, MPH
Department of Pharmacy Practice, Purdue
University College of Pharmacy, West
Lafayette, Indiana

DAVID PEIRIS, MBBS, PhD, MIPH
The George Institute for Global Health,
University of Sydney, Sydney,
Australia

ARTI PILLAY, PGDPH
Pacific Research Centre for the Prevention of
Obesity and Non-Communicable Diseases, Fiji
National University, Suva, Fiji

VILARMINA PONCE-LUCERO, BA
CRONICAS Center of Excellence in Chronic
Diseases, Universidad Peruana Cayetano
Heredia, Lima, Peru

DEVARSETTY PRAVEEN, MBBS, MD, PhD
The George Institute for Global Health,
Hyderabad, India

ANTONIO LUIZ PINHO RIBEIRO, MD, PhD
Professor, Division of Hospital das Clínicas and
School of Medicine, Department of Internal
Medicine and Cardiology, Universidade
Federal de Minas Gerais, Belo Horizonte,
Minas Gerais, Brazil

ALLMAN ROLLINS, MD
Department of Medicine, University of
California, San Francisco, San Francisco,
California

ADOLFO RUBINSTEIN, MD, MSc, PhD
South American Center of Excellence for
Cardiovascular Health, Institute for Clinical
Effectiveness and Health Policy, Buenos Aires,
Argentina

JON-DAVID SCHWALM, MD, MSc
Population Health Research Institute,
Hamilton, Ontario, Canada

WILSON K. SUGUT, MMED
Moi Teaching and Referral Hospital, Eldoret,
Kenya

AMANDA G. THRIFT, PhD
School of Clinical Sciences at Monash Health,
Monash University, Melbourne, Australia

SHELDON W. TOBE, MD, MScCH
University of Toronto, Toronto, Ontario,
Canada

DAN N. TRAN, PharmD
Department of Pharmacy Practice, Purdue
University College of Pharmacy, West
Lafayette, Indiana

KATHY TRIEU, MPH
The George Institute for Global Health,
University of Sydney, Sydney, Australia

RAJESH VEDANTHAN, MD, MPH
Zena and Michael A. Wiener Cardiovascular
Institute, Icahn School of Medicine at Mount
Sinai, New York, New York

ERIC J. VELAZQUEZ, MD
Department of Medicine, Duke Clinical
Research Institute, Duke Global Health
Institute, Duke University, Durham, North
Carolina

JACQUI WEBSTER, PhD
The George Institute for Global Health,
University of Sydney, Sydney, Australia

RUTH WEBSTER, PhD, MIPH
The George Institute for Global Health,
University of Sydney, Sydney, Australia

RUSS WHITE, MD, MPH, FACS(ECSA)
Tenwek Mission Hospital, Bomet, Kenya;
Alpert School of Medicine, Brown University,
Providence, Rhode Island

KAREN YEATES, MD, MPH
School of Medicine, Queens University,
Kingston, Ontario, Canada

KHALID YUSOFF, MBBS
Universiti Teknologi MARA, Selangor and UCSI
University, Kuala Lumpur, Malaysia

Contents

One of the major drivers of change in the practice of cardiology is population change. This article discusses the current debate about epidemiologic transition paired with other ongoing transitions with direct relevance to cardiovascular conditions. Challenges specific to patterns of risk factors over time; readiness for disease surveillance and meeting global targets; health system, prevention, and treatment efforts; and physiologic traits and human-environment interactions are identified. This article concludes that a focus on the most populated regions of the world will contribute substantially to protecting the large gains in global survival and life expectancy accrued over the last decades.

mHealth constitutes a promise for health care delivery in low- and middle-income countries (LMICs) where health care systems are unprepared to combat the threat of noncommunicable diseases (NCDs). This article assesses the impact of mHealth on NCD outcomes in LMICs. A systematic review identified controlled studies evaluating mHealth interventions that addressed NCDs in LMICs. From the 1274 abstracts retrieved, 108 articles were selected for full text review and 20 randomized controlled trials were included from 14 LMICs. One-way SMS was the most commonly used mobile function to deliver reminders, health education, and information. mHealth interventions in LMICs have positive but modest effects on chronic disease outcomes.

The initial infection of Chagas disease is typically asymptomatic, but approximately 30% of people will progress to a chronic cardiac form. Death is often sudden due to arrhythmias or progressive heart failure. Prevention through vector control programs and blood bank screening, along with strengthened surveillance systems and rapid information sharing, are key to decreasing disease burden globally. The epidemiology, diagnostic evaluation, diagnosis, and treatment of acute and chronic Chagas cardiac disease are discussed with focus on educating the primary care professionals and general cardiologists in nonendemic areas who have limited experience treating this disease.

As a subset of the growing epidemic of cardiovascular morbidity and mortality in low-income and middle-income countries (LMICs), the significant burdens of heart rhythm disorders also increase. Effective diagnostic and treatment modalities exist, but financial resources and expertise are limited. Cost-effective strategies exist to address most of these limitations, but many surmountable barriers need to be overcome to introduce and improve electrophysiologic care in LMICs. In this article, current and potential solutions are offered for the diagnostic and therapeutic challenges of managing bradyarrhythmias and tachyarrhythmias.

Over the last 2 decades human immunodeficiency virus (HIV) infection has become a chronic disease requiring long-term management. Aging, antiretroviral therapy, chronic inflammation, and several other factors contribute to the increased risk of cardiovascular disease in patients infected with HIV. In low-income and middle-income countries where antiretroviral therapy access is limited, cardiac disease is most commonly related to opportunistic infections and end-stage manifestations of HIV/acquired immunodeficiency syndrome, including HIV-associated cardiomyopathy, pericarditis, and pulmonary arterial hypertension. Cardiovascular screening, prevention, and risk factor management are important factors in the management of patients infected with HIV worldwide.

Environmental exposures in low- and middle-income countries lie at the intersection of increased economic development and the rising public health burden of cardiovascular disease. Increasing evidence suggests an association of exposure to ambient air pollution, household air pollution from biomass fuel, lead, arsenic, and cadmium with multiple cardiovascular disease outcomes, including hypertension, coronary heart disease, stroke, and cardiovascular mortality. Although populations in low- and middle-income countries are disproportionately exposed to environmental pollution, evidence linking these exposures to cardiovascular disease is derived from populations in high-income countries. More research is needed to further characterize the extent of environmental exposures.

Endomyocardial fibrosis (EMF) remains an important cause of restrictive cardiomyopathy worldwide. Patients cluster in specific geographic locations and are almost universally living in extreme poverty. Specific etiology remains elusive and is likely multifactorial. Untreated EMF has a very poor prognosis. Medical management can mitigate symptoms for a time but has no curative benefit. Early surgical interventions may improve survival but are not readily available in most EMF-endemic regions. Increased awareness, advocacy, and research are needed to further understand this neglected tropical cardiomyopathy and to improve survival of those affected.

Elevated blood pressure, a major risk factor for ischemic heart disease, heart failure, and stroke, is the leading global risk for mortality. Treatment and control rates are very low in low- and middle-income countries. There is an urgent need to address this problem. The Global Alliance for Chronic Diseases sponsored research projects focus on controlling hypertension, including community engagement, salt reduction, salt substitution, task redistribution, mHealth, and fixed-dose combination therapies. This article reviews the rationale for each approach and summarizes the experience of some of the research teams. The studies demonstrate innovative and practical methods for improving hypertension control.

Ambulatory blood pressure monitoring (ABPM) can assess out-of-clinic blood pressure. ABPM is an underutilized resource in low-income and middle-income countries but should be considered a complementary strategy to clinic blood pressure measurement for the diagnosis and management of hypertension. Potential uses for ABPM in low-income and middle-income countries include screening of high-risk individuals who have concurrent communicable diseases, such as HIV, and in task-shifting health care strategies.

Cardiovascular disease (CVD) is the leading cause of global mortality and is expected to reach 23 million deaths by 2030. Eighty percent of CVD deaths occur in low-income and middle-income countries (LMICs). Although CVD prevention and treatment guidelines are available, translating these into practice is hampered in LMICs by inadequate health care systems that limit access to lifesaving medications. In this article, we describe the deficiencies in the current LMIC supply chains that limit access to effective CVD medicines, and discuss existing solutions that are translatable to similar settings so as to address these deficiencies.

 Video content accompanies this article at http://www.cardiology.theclinics.com.

Owing to the high prevalence of tuberculosis (TB) and human immunodeficiency virus/AIDS, tuberculous heart disease remains an important problem in TB endemic areas. In this article, we reiterate salient aspects of the traditional understanding and approach to its management, and provide important updates on the pathophysiology, diagnosis, and treatment garnered over the past decade of focused clinical and basic science research. We emphasize that, if implemented widely, these improved evidence-based approaches to the disease can build on the early progress made in treating tuberculous heart disease and help further the goal of significantly reducing its historically high morbidity and mortality.

CARDIOLOGY CLINICS

THE CLINICS ARE AVAILABLE ONLINE!
Access your subscription at:
www.theclinics.com

CARDIOLOGY CLINICS

ISSUE OF RELATED INTEREST

Heart Failure Clinics October 2015 (Vol. 11, No. 4)
A Global Perspective/Health Inequity in Heart Failure
Pablo F. Castro, Naoki Sato, Robert J. Mentz, and Ovidiu Chioncel, Editors
Available at: http://www.heartfailure.theclinics.com

Preface
Five Reasons Why Global Health Matters to Cardiologists

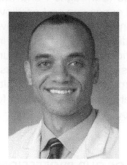

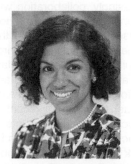

Gerald S. Bloomfield, MD, MPH, FACC, FASE, FAHA   Melissa S. Burroughs Peña, MD, MS

Editors

With less and less free time to ponder the grand questions in life, it can be a challenge for a practicing cardiologist to contemplate why global health matters. Yet, it is also undeniable that we live in a global environment. In 2014, over three billion people traveled internationally by air from 41,000 airports around the world, and by 2030, the number will increase to 5.9 billion.[1] Events happening in distant countries can now be broadcast directly to our televisions or phones in real time. How does this global interconnectedness impact our practice and profession? Here we offer five reasons global health matters, especially to cardiologists in high-income, or developed, countries.

PATIENTS TRAVEL

Cardiologists in developed countries need the skills to offer health advice to patients who have recently immigrated to developed countries. For example, 13% of all people living in the United States are foreign born, with California and New York having the highest portion of foreign-born residents. Familiarity with cardiovascular diseases (CVDs) endemic to other parts of the world prepares cardiologists to identify rare conditions. When was the last time you may have missed a case of Chagas disease (Benzinger CP, do Carmo GAL, Ribeiro ALP: Chagas cardiomyopathy: clinical presentation and management in the Americas, in this issue), or endomyocardial fibrosis (Beaton A, Mocumbi AO: Diagnosis and management of endomyocardial fibrosis, in this issue)? In addition, the Centers for Disease Control and Prevention receives approximately 125 reports each year of arriving travelers with active tuberculosis.[2] The potential morbidity from tuberculous pericarditis (Mutyaba AK, Ntsekhe M: Tuberculosis and the heart, in this issue) and other infectious cardiac diseases (eg, associated with HIV) (Bloomfield GS, Leung C: Cardiac disease associated with human immunodeficiency virus infection, in this issue) warrants attention to vectors that can cross borders. On the other hand, for cardiac patients traveling to developing countries, familiarity with the cardiac services in other countries can be useful in case of unforeseen circumstances (eg, Where could I have my device interrogated?) (Bestawros M: Electrophysiology in the developing world: challenges and opportunities, in this issue).

CULTURAL SENSITIVITY

Global health requires increased sensitivity to cross-cultural issues. Patients' explanatory models of disease often have cultural underpinnings, which in turn affect health care decisions and adherence to medications. Some underrepresented minority patients might distrust the health care system, possibly as a result of historical discrimination. The same may be true of recent immigrants. The role of kin in health care decision-making and disclosure can have cultural

Cardiol Clin 35 (2017) xiii–xv
http://dx.doi.org/10.1016/j.ccl.2016.10.001
0733-8651/17/© 2016 Published by Elsevier Inc.

foundations, which cardiologists should be prepared to consider.

DISCOVERY KNOWS NO BORDERS

No country has a monopoly on talent.[3] International collaboration has been a hallmark of cardiovascular clinical trails going back to the GISSI[4] and GUSTO studies.[5] Increasingly, collaboration with professionals from around the world informs how we derive evidence-based medicine. To do this well, investment must be made in global research training and capacity building (Barasa FA, Vedanthan R, Pastakia SD, et al: Approaches to sustainable capacity building for cardiovascular disease care in Kenya, in this issue). In turn, many recent innovations in cardiovascular care have roots in developing countries, including fixed-dose combination therapy and task redistribution to combat hypertension (Vedanthan R, Bernabe-Ortiz A, Herasme OI, et al: Innovative approaches to hypertension control in low- and middle-income countries, in this issue), the use of mobile phones to access rural populations and ensure that patients take their medicine (Beratarrechea A, Moyano D, Irazola V, et al: mHealth interventions to counter non-communicable diseases in developing countries: still an uncertain promise, in this issue) and ambulatory blood pressure monitoring for hypertension control (Abdalla M: Ambulatory blood pressure monitoring: a complimentary strategy for hypertension diagnosis and management in low and middle-income countries, in this issue). If we are intentional and receptive, we may find many potential solutions outside of our own borders.

SUTTON'S LAW

Willie Sutton, the bank robber, is often quoted as responding to the question, "Why did you rob banks?," by saying, "That's where the money is." Eighty percent of all deaths due to CVD occur in low- and middle-income countries. On an international level, interventions to combat CVD would potentially have the greatest impact in these countries (Mendoza W, Miranda JJ: Global shifts in cardiovascular disease, the epidemiologic transition and other contributing factors: toward a new practice of global health cardiology, in this issue). There are untenable international disparities in the burden of CVD and access to appropriate therapies (Tran DN, Njuguna B, Mercer T, et al: Ensuring patient-centered access to cardiovascular disease medicines in low- and middle-income countries through health-system strengthening, in this

issue). The persistent burden of rheumatic heart disease (Nulu S, Bukhman G, Kwan GF: Rheumatic heart disease: the unfinished global agenda, in this issue), infective endocarditis (Njuguna B, Gardner A, Karwa R, et al: Infective endocarditis in low- and middle-income countries, in this issue), and cardiotoxic environmental exposures in developing countries (Burroughs Peña MS, Rollins A: Environmental exposures and cardiovascular disease: a challenge for health and development in low- and middle-income countries, in this issue) should spur those in developed countries to act whenever possible. Action to address inequalities in the upstream determinants of health outcomes is always timely, and opportunities for the practicing cardiologist to engage are increasingly available.[6]

THE FUTURE OF OUR PROFESSION

The importance of global health to trainees cannot be overstated. This interest is driven by increased awareness of gross disparities between low-, middle-, and high-income countries. There are now many examples of cardiologists and fellows-in-training who have embraced global health as one of the main defining features of their practice and research.[7–10] Early clinical experiences in resource-limited settings usually derive a continuing return over one's career. The rewards span character development as well as clinical expertise. As Mark Twain said, "Travel is fatal to prejudice, bigotry, and narrow-mindedness, and many of our people need it sorely on these accounts. Broad wholesome, charitable views of men and things cannot be acquired by vegetating in one little corner of the earth all one's lifetime."

The fourteen articles in this issue of *Cardiology Clinics* offer a contemporary compendium of global health issues of high importance to the general cardiologist. Not only does global health impact our clinical practice and daily life but also globalization and interconnectedness will increasingly become the norm for how we train future generations.

Gerald S. Bloomfield, MD, MPH, FACC, FASE, FAHA
Duke Clinical Research Institute
Duke Global Health Institute
Department of Medicine
Duke University
2400 Pratt Street
Durham, NC 27705, USA

Melissa S. Burroughs Peña, MD, MS
Division of Cardiology
Department of Medicine
University of California
505 Parnassus Avenue
11th Floor, Room 1180D
San Francisco, CA 94143, USA

E-mail addresses:
gerald.bloomfield@duke.edu (G.S. Bloomfield)
Melissa.pena@ucsf.edu (M.S. Burroughs Peña)

REFERENCES

1. Mangili A, Vindenes T, Gendreau M. Infectious risks of air travel. Microbiol Spectr 2015;3:333–44.
2. Centers for Disease Control and Prevention (CDC). Public health interventions involving travelers with tuberculosis—U.S. ports of entry, 2007-2012. MMWR Morb Mortal Wkly Rep 2012;61:570–3.
3. Glass RI. What the United States has to gain from global health research. JAMA 2013;310:903–4.
4. Maggioni AP, Franzosi MG, Fresco C, et al. GISSI trials in acute myocardial infarction. Rationale, design, and results. Chest 1990;97:146S–50S.
5. The GUSTO Investigators. An international randomized trial comparing four thrombolytic strategies for acute myocardial infarction. The GUSTO investigators. N Engl J Med 1993;329:673–82.
6. Seals AA. ACC International outreach and the global cardiovascular community. J Am Coll Cardiol 2016; 67:3011–3.
7. Bloomfield GS, Huffman MD. Global chronic disease research training for fellows: perspectives, challenges, and opportunities. Circulation 2010;121:1365–70.
8. Abdalla M, Kovach N, Liu C, et al. The importance of global health experiences in the development of new cardiologists. J Am Coll Cardiol 2016;67(23):2789–97.
9. Patel A. Organizing a career in global cardiovascular health. J Am Coll Cardiol 2015;65:2144–6.
10. Binanay CA, Akwanalo CO, Aruasa W, et al. Building sustainable capacity for cardiovascular care at a public hospital in Western Kenya. J Am Coll Cardiol 2015;66:2550–60.

Global Shifts in Cardiovascular Disease, the Epidemiologic Transition, and Other Contributing Factors

Toward a New Practice of Global Health Cardiology

CrossMark

Walter Mendoza, MD[a], J. Jaime Miranda, MD, MSc, PhD[b,c],*

KEYWORDS

- Epidemiology • Demography • Health transitions • Developing countries • Cardiology
- Global health

KEY POINTS

- Developed countries had more than a century to double or triple their populations, whereas the same increases in population size in the developing world have occurred over decades.
- The epidemiologic transition theory Is not perfect but has improved the understanding of the changing dynamics of epidemiologic profiles.
- Changes in population structures and disease profiles, cardiovascular conditions, and their associated comorbidities will continue to challenge health care systems.
- A focus on the most populated regions of the world will contribute to protecting the large gains in global survival and life expectancy accrued over the last decades.
- From a low-income and middle-income country perspective, current challenges provide an opportunity to redefine the agenda of global health cardiology and global cardiovascular research.

Financial Conflicts of Interest: The authors have nothing to disclose.
Funding Sources: Dr J.J. Miranda acknowledges receiving current and past support from the Alliance for Health Policy and Systems Research (HQHSR1206660), Consejo Nacional de Ciencia, Tecnología e Innovación Tecnológica (CONCYTEC), DFID/MRC/Wellcome Global Health Trials (MR/M007405/1), Fogarty International Center (R21TW009982), Grand Challenges Canada (0335-04), International Development Research Center Canada (106887, 108167), Inter-American Institute for Global Change Research (IAI CRN3036), National Heart, Lung, and Blood Institute (5U01HL114180, HHSN268200900028C), National Institute of Mental Health (1U19MH098780), Swiss National Science Foundation (40P740-160366), UnitedHealth Foundation, Universidad Peruana Cayetano Heredia (Fondo Concursable No. 20205071009), and the Wellcome Trust (074833/Z/04/A, WT093541AIA, 103994/Z/14/Z).
Disclaimer: W. Mendoza is currently Program Analyst, Population and Development, at the United Nations Population Fund in Peru, which does not necessarily endorse this contribution.
[a] United Nations Population Fund, Peru Country Office, Av. Guardia Civil 1231, San Isidro, Lima 27, Peru; [b] School of Medicine, Universidad Peruana Cayetano Heredia, Av. Honorio Delgado 430, Urb. Ingeniería, San Martín de Porres, Lima 31, Peru; [c] CRONICAS Center of Excellence in Chronic Diseases, Universidad Peruana Cayetano Heredia, Av. Armendáriz 497, Miraflores, Lima 18, Peru
* Corresponding author. CRONICAS Center of Excellence in Chronic Diseases, Universidad Peruana Cayetano Heredia, Av. Armendáriz 497, Miraflores, Lima 18, Peru.
E-mail address: Jaime.Miranda@upch.pe

Cardiol Clin 35 (2017) 1–12
http://dx.doi.org/10.1016/j.ccl.2016.08.004
0733-8651/17/© 2016 Elsevier Inc. All rights reserved.

INTRODUCTION

As the world changes, the practice of cardiology, clinical cardiology, global health cardiology, and cardiology research will follow suit. One of the major drivers of change in the practice of cardiology, in both developed and developing countries, is population change, whose dynamics can be expressed by secular epidemiologic and demographic trends, with increasing survival and life expectancy across all age strata. These population changes, at the macro level, are not static or isolated but occur together with many other individual-level changes and adaptations, including, but not limited to, access to and usage of technological changes[1]; changes in health care delivery,[2,3] in medical training,[4] and in the practice of medicine[5]; or even changes within people; for example, changes in the height of populations over time,[6] as well as changes within individuals, such as the recently shown link between microbiota and stroke outcomes.[7] In this regard, over the last few years has become more common, and indeed necessary, to encourage interdisciplinary dialogues to better serve medical interventions at the individual and population levels.

A long trend in the mutual interaction of technologies, policies, and social movements; global demographic transition; and its epidemiologic correlates continues to increase population size across age groups, and since the early nineteenth century it has increased by 6 times. It is projected to further increase up to 10 times by the end of this century, and by then most countries will experience demographic aging. Life expectancy will continue to grow (it has doubled in last 2 centuries), whereas female fertility will continue to decline. By the early nineteenth century, 70% of women's adult life was dedicated to bearing children, a percentage that has now decreased to 14% because of lower fertility and longer and healthier living.[8]

Much of the transition in mortality and risk factors for noncommunicable diseases, including cardiovascular diseases, has been described in detail elsewhere,[9–17] but few have been addressed to a clinical audience, and in particular what do such transitions mean for low-income and middle-income settings. This article describes current debates and analyzes the pertinence and relevance of the epidemiologic transition, paired with the demographic transition and other ongoing transitions with direct relevance to cardiovascular conditions. In doing so, this article emphasizes the challenges of this transition for low-income and middle-income settings undergoing rapid epidemiologic shifts. In addition, this analysis of trends and context provides an entry point to delineate the need for a global health cardiology practice that aligns with the major challenges in the most populated regions of the world, which bear a growing burden of cardiovascular diseases and conditions.

THE EPIDEMIOLOGIC TRANSITION: ITS DEFINITION AND ITS PLACE IN HISTORY

The epidemiologic transition theory, or model, was coined in the early 1970s by Abdel Omran.[18] Published at a time when development debates were influenced by fears of the so-called demographic explosion, in Omran's[18] view the "key difference between epidemiologic transition and demographic transition theories was that the former unlike the latter allowed for multiple pathways to a low-mortality/low-fertility population regime."[19] In short, Omran's[18] theory identified the 3 phases of transition: pestilence and famine, receding pandemics, and degenerative and human created transition. These phases were later nuanced by Olshansky and Ault[20] who added a fourth stage: delayed degenerative or hybristic diseases (ie, influenced by individual behaviors and lifestyles).[21] In relation to cardiovascular disease, **Table 1** shows the classic stages of the epidemiologic transition. More recently, given the increase in body mass index worldwide,[22] some investigators propose a fifth stage in the transition: the age of obesity and inactivity.[23,24]

However, from a historical point of view, Omran[18] was not the first to link population changes to epidemiologic and mortality patterns. Alternative explanations of the epidemiologic changes in patterns of mortality were described a few decades before Omran's[18] views were published. Thomas McKeown described secular declines in England's mortality since the eighteenth century throughout the process of industrialization as a consequence of better nutrition and sanitation rather than of medical interventions.[25] In contrast, Omran's[18] thesis was more optimistic about the benefits of technology in the developing world, claiming that mortality decline depended more on developing interventions oriented toward supporting national and international programs of health service provision and environmental control.[25] Subsequent analyses, based on new methods and sources, revealed some flaws in the McKeown assumptions,[26] as has also happened to some of Omran[18] claims, in relation to the double burden or overlapping of both communicable and noncommunicable diseases.[27]

Importantly from a contextual point of view, such debates around patterns of mortality took place by the 1970s, after the dominance of a discourse

Table 1
Stages of the epidemiologic transition and its global status, by region

Stage	Description	Life Expectancy	Dominant Form of CVD	Percentage of Deaths Attributable to CVD	Percentage of the World's Population in This Stage	Regions Affected
Pestilence and famine	Predominance of malnutrition and infectious diseases	35	RHD cardiomyopathy caused by infection and malnutrition	5–10	11	Sub-Saharan Africa, parts of all regions, excluding high-income regions
Receding pandemics	Improved nutrition and public health lead to increase in chronic diseases, hypertension	50	Rheumatic valvular disease, IHD, hemorrhagic stroke	15–35	38	South Asia, southern east Asia and the Pacific, parts of Latin America and the Caribbean
Degenerative and human created	Increased fat and caloric intake, widespread tobacco use, chronic disease deaths exceed mortality from infections and malnutrition	60	IHD, stroke (ischemic and hemorrhagic)	>50	35	Europe and central Asia, northern east Asia and the Pacific, Latin America and the Caribbean, Middle East and North Africa, and urban parts of most low-income regions (eg, India)
Delayed degenerative diseases	CVD and cancer are leading causes of morbidity and mortality; prevention and treatment avoid death and delay onset; age-adjusted CVD declines	70	IHD, stroke (ischemic and hemorrhagic), CHF	<50	—	High-income countries, parts of Latin America, and the Caribbean

Abbreviations: CHF, congestive heart failure; CVD, cardiovascular disease; IHD, ischemic heart disease; RHD, rheumatic heart disease.
From Gaziano T, Reddy KS, Paccaud F, et al, editors. Disease control priorities in developing countries. 2nd edition. Washington, DC: World Bank and Oxford University Press. © World Bank. https://openknowledge.worldbank.org/handle/10986/7242 License CC BY 3.0 IGO.

around infectious diseases, by then allegedly soon to be globally controlled, and just some years before emerging and reemerging infectious diseases would recover momentum. In the last 2 decades the concept of the epidemiologic transition has gained even more attention, including its revisionist versions[28] stressing the relevance of the concept of societies, particularly for developing countries together with the World Bank, and its approaches to health economics,[29] showing concerns about the health of adults and chronic diseases. Far from being a perfect theory to explain transitions, Omran's[18] epidemiologic transition allowed for a conversation in terms of populations and specifically of population health. As suggested by others, "an expanded model of transition should account for the immense regional variation in disease burden, disparities in health systems, and the stacking of multiple kinds of epidemics within small areas and over short periods of time."[17]

NOT 1 BUT SEVERAL OVERLAPPING TRANSITIONS

The concept of transition, whether demographic or epidemiologic, is dynamic. From a global health point of view, one element merits attention: developed countries have had more time to double or triple their populations, usually more than 1 century, whereas the same increases in population size in the developing world have occurred over decades. Although most nations accommodate population growth, other transitions are directly relevant to cardiovascular health. Urbanization, nutrition and diet, food systems,[30] culture, and technology, interplay one with another to contribute to sustained increased survival in a long-term shift from low to high life expectancy.[31]

According to the demographic transition approach, in both the developing and developed world, the longevity transition merits attention.[32] As **Fig. 1** shows, the average remaining years to be lived at age 60 years will continue to increase, with a slight advantage for women compared with men. This longevity transition will have different impacts across heterogeneous societies depending on how they deal with mortality declines and growing morbidity. In so doing, health care delivery, its workforce, organization and infrastructure, ethics, economics, and health financing will be directly involved in shaping the future patterns of population morbidity and mortality.

In the late 1980s, Mexican researchers led by Frenk and colleagues[33] showed that in low-income and middle-income countries, along with the epidemiologic transition, there was a transition in the capacity of the health care system to deal with various conditions. In unequal and heterogeneous countries, such as those in Latin America, the paces of epidemiologic transition were

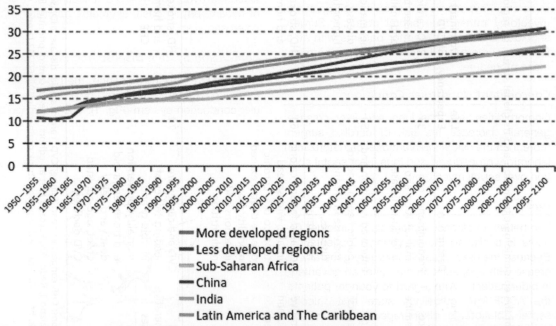

Fig. 1. Life expectancy at age 60 years, selected regions, 1950 to 2100. (*From* United Nations, Department of Economic and Social Affairs, Population Division. World population prospects: the 2015 revision, key findings and advance tables. 2015. Available at: http://esa.un.org/unpd/wpp/publications/files/key_findings_wpp_2015. pdf. Accessed May 4, 2016; with permission.)

different from those in developed countries, because simultaneously communicable diseases and poor nutritional and maternal conditions overlapped with noncommunicable diseases, both challenging health systems, a model they called the protracted-prolonged polarized model.[33] Making things even more complex, just 1 decade before Frenk and colleagues'[33] analysis, human immunodeficiency virus (HIV)/acquired immunodeficiency syndrome entailed a major unforeseen challenge to health systems and health prioritization, particularly for poor countries in sub-Saharan Africa.

CARDIOVASCULAR DISEASE MORTALITY AND RISK FACTORS FROM A LOW-INCOME AND MIDDLE-INCOME PERSPECTIVE

Much of the transition in terms of cardiovascular disease risk and mortality has been addressed in various recent reviews,[10–15] hence rather than repeating these findings this article discusses such trends with other major ongoing societal transitions and current challenges, especially for the practice of global health cardiology. More recently, for disability-related and mortality-related analyses, newer and more sophisticated methodological approaches have been developed, quantifying the changes in patterns of epidemiologic trends as they relate to sociodemographic conditions.[34] However, although the data are still limited, a different epidemiology of cardiovascular conditions is anticipated for the poorest populations.[35] As foreseen, cardiovascular conditions have played a chief role in driving a global increase in mortality, although this has mostly been caused by global aging and population growth.[11]

From a global health perspective, this scenario has achieved important high-level political pledges to tackle the impact of noncommunicable diseases,[36] particularly cardiovascular diseases.[37] In particular, cardiovascular premature mortality has recently been acknowledged as relevant to recent advances in health and development and has been included in the indicators set of the new sustainable development goals, but its projections for the next decade are not so optimistic.[30,38] The present environment requires the global health cardiology and preventive cardiology workforce and practitioners to be well acquainted with broader discourses and to understand the basics of time and place (ie, what transitions have occurred over time and where).

The mortality related to cardiovascular diseases is closely linked to changes over time in the profile of cardiovascular risk factors.[22,39–42] One of the seminal longitudinal studies, the Framingham Heart Study, was launched by the late 1940s[43] and contributed to the identification of major risk factors for the development of cardiovascular diseases,[44,45] such as high cholesterol levels and increased blood pressure, now known as common risk factors. In the same vein, high body mass index has been acknowledged as playing a major role in global disease burden in the last decades.[46] Therefore, understanding the patterns of common risk factors over time and across geographic regions is paramount for global health cardiology.

CHALLENGES FOR GLOBAL HEALTH CARDIOLOGY

In recent decades, a pattern of decreasing trends in cardiovascular disease mortality has been recorded and studied in high-income regions.[10,12] However, the dynamics of such trends are far from being completely known and understood in low-income and middle-income countries. The concept of the demographic transition calls for an understanding of the dynamics of changes in population age groups, because populations in general are becoming older. These changes are paired with the co-occurrence of multiple risk factors within the same individual, and within populations, which calls for a rethinking of current approaches to disease burden, especially so when health systems are largely designed for the provision of acute care[47]; for example, shifting an analysis of health patterns centered on mortality to one in which the focus is primarily on physical functioning, nonfatal morbidity, or disability. Importantly, morbidity is multidimensional by nature, introducing significant challenges related to health system performance, diagnostic technologies, and even cultural conditions such as the role of caregiving in societies. All of these have multiple implications and new data sources, methods, and metrics are to be expanded. In doing so, newer efforts to address these challenges will require reinforced values about data generation and data sharing,[48,49] and in this way a direct benefit for low-income and middle-income countries ought to be affirmed and protected.[50]

Low-income and middle-income countries carry at least three-quarters of the premature mortality caused by cardiovascular diseases.[51,52] To address this, international targets were set in 2011 to reduce the risk of premature noncommunicable disease deaths by 25% by 2025.[53] To address this larger goal, it has to be realized that what works in the developed world might not necessarily work nor should be mechanically implemented in low-income and middle-income countries. This realization has been shown in a series of modeling scenarios pursued for each geographic region.[54] The latest available report from the World Health Organization on noncommunicable diseases signals that only "42 countries had monitoring systems to report on the nine global targets [to achieve 25 by 25],"[55] thus clearly indicating the substantial gaps in disease surveillance. Together with the concomitant within-country disparities, these are even more evident at the subnational level. The paucity of data and key information from population-based studies on cardiovascular disease incidence, remission, medical care, and risk or protective factors[10,11] will limit the understanding of cardiovascular disease trends and dynamics in low-income and middle-income settings, and this is a major challenge for global health cardiology.

Challenges at the level of health systems are far more complex[56] and range from ensuring adequate strategies for primary, secondary, and tertiary prevention,[57,58] together with health care delivery services and systems that are affordable, accessible, culturally appropriate and of quality, to legal frameworks and policies. With life expectancy increasing, how to sustain ideal cardiovascular health across the lifespan[59] and for longer periods over the lifetimes of individuals, and populations, remains pivotal to accruing future larger gains in reducing morbidity and mortality. This need is more evident in low-income and middle-income countries characterized by contrasting settings with persistent inequality, where poverty contributes to and affects demographic and epidemiologic transitions.[35,60–62] For example, what primary prevention interventions might work, in the long run, in countries where obesity in the early years is increasingly common, as in emerging economies or in countries transitioning from low-income to middle-income status? Aging and increasing survival are expected to be a major driver of demographic and epidemiologic changes, so what are the most appropriate approaches to addressing comorbidity; not only cardiovascular but also other physical and mental chronic conditions? From an economic and development standpoint, acknowledging major underestimations in the costs associated with noncommunicable diseases at the household and national levels,[63,64] what are the costs of not making major decisions to address avoidable mortality and disability?

In addition, in the area of basic sciences and population health, further areas of interest are related to sex and gender differences in relation to mortality, disability, and distribution of risk factors in men and women. Two main drivers usually account for such discrepancies. First, women

have longer lifespans in practically all countries, although in some high-income countries such as the United Kingdom this female advantage in life expectancy is predicted to be reduced in the coming years.[65] Second, women tend to be worse off in receiving care for cardiovascular diseases,[66,67] usually linked to common gender-based discriminations, including access to prevention and treatment. However, a third factor that warrants attention for global health cardiology relates to the physiopathology of the heart's aging and its sex differences as a new field of research, a better understanding of which might suggest avenues to provide better treatment.[68] Besides aging, an important element of the women's health agenda directly related to noncommunicable diseases is preeclampsia, in which hypertension, obesity, and anemia affect the health of the mother.[69] In terms of the offspring, one of the outcomes of preeclampsia is a restriction of fetal growth, characterized by already well-described long-term consequences for increased risk of noncommunicable diseases, including cardiovascular and metabolic conditions.[70–72] Adding to the complexity of low-income and middle-income settings, the observed pathophysiologic changes are compounded with, and require broader expansions to explicitly assess, the human-environment interactions, particularly cardiovascular and metabolic adaptations to high-altitude settings.[73–77]

Without detailing the long list of potential challenges, the authors have expanded on Roth and colleagues'[17] knowledge gaps (**Table 2**), and present here some key aspects of (1) patterns of risk factors over time; (2) disease surveillance and meeting global targets; (3) health systems, prevention, and treatment efforts; and (4) physiologic traits and human-environment interactions. All of them, in addition to challenges to overcome, should be seen as opportunities to redefine the agenda of global health cardiology and global cardiovascular research. As Huffman and colleagues[78] argued, this will also require incorporating additional tools and skills such as implementation science, health systems research, and health policy research.

UNIFYING GLOBAL TRANSITIONS AND THE PRACTICE OF GLOBAL HEALTH CARDIOLOGY: WHY DOES THIS MATTER?

Despite the impressive achievements in cardiovascular diagnosis and treatment in the last decades in high-income settings, most of these achievements have yet to reach most of the people living in the global South. Information gaps, such as awareness about disease burden and

Table 2
Knowledge gaps and suggested next steps

Gaps in Knowledge	Suggested Next Steps
Mortality data remain absent or of limited quality in some countries, particularly in the poorest regions	• Further national investment in sample and comprehensive vital registration systems • Sharing of best practices for data collection and verbal autopsy • Efforts to improve ascertainment of death
Little is known about variation in cardiovascular risk factors and disease burden in some countries	• Expansion of household health examination surveys, with wider sharing of results • Broader collection of anthropometric and biomarker data, including blood pressure and glycosylated hemoglobin and cholesterol levels • Renewed efforts for population-based surveillance of CVD events, including myocardial infarction and stroke
Changes in cardiovascular mortality are more complex than suggested by a stepwise model of epidemiologic transition	• National health planning needs to consider a broad range of contextual factors, including local patterns of risk, policies that influence health, and current health system arrangements • Formal CVD costing studies in LMIC to address financial risk and health system efficiencies • Improved cross-cultural measures of disability related to CVD

Abbreviation: LMIC, low-income and middle-income countries.
From Roth GA, Huffman MD, Moran AE, et al. Global and regional patterns in cardiovascular mortality from 1990 to 2013. Circulation 2015;132(17):1676; with permission.

risk factor trends, are still present,[79] including underdiagnosis and misdiagnosis.[80] However, it was learned from the original conception of the epidemiologic transition, from larger global and regional health and development agendas, that long-term trends of change in population health cannot be overlooked. For example, there are currently millions of people living with HIV, which has now become a chronic condition whose cardiovascular effects might be neglected.[81]

Given that current transition trends will continue, the uniqueness of cardiovascular diseases might soon become outdated because of the narrow disease-specific approach compared with individuals living with comorbidities. Therefore, more collaborative, interdisciplinary, and integrative work (as observed with mental health, including the successful models of collaborative care to improve the management of depressive disorders[82–85]) will be the norm and will be demanded by patients and by health institutions, both public and private. How can cardiology, and global health cardiology, as a medical specialty prepare for such transition? How can health and social protection systems ensure that the increasing demands for cardiology and cardiac rehabilitation are

aligned within essential packages of health care provision, with acceptable conditions of quality and dignity? Globally, noncommunicable diseases have been linked to substantial impacts at the macroeconomic, health system, and household levels,[63,64,86,87] paired with important challenges to inform policy makers in low-income settings about the associated costs.[88] At the household level, stroke is one example of major financial hardship.[89] At the national level, the increase in hypertension in recent years in Mexico is projected to require an increase in financial requirements of 22% to 24%,[90,91] a scenario in which additional complexity is introduced if uninsured populations are considered.[92] Availability and affordability of medicines to those who need them has been reported in a large proportion of communities and households across upper middle-income, lower middle-income, and low-income countries.[93]

Furthermore, at the country level, because most of world population are and will remain facing a double disease burden of both infectious and noninfectious diseases, how can cardiology reshape and integrate its offerings within current well-established clinical practices? Also, a large share of primary prevention, which is much needed for cardiology outcomes, requires interactions with other nonclinical sectors beyond the clinical settings, and cannot be limited to patients now at retirement ages, but is needed by younger generations as well. All of these scenarios force the new cadre and workforce of global health cardiologists and practitioners to look beyond the prescription of pharmacologic drugs and devices and will force them to incorporate a wider range of practice and skills to inform their avenues for intervention.[30,94–96]

From a demographic and long-term perspective, because this might be considered the century of aging, interventions cannot be limited to patients who are currently elderly but must also be available for those who will reach senior years in the coming decades. How can current adolescents and youth be involved in the prevention, and even treatment, of noncommunicable diseases?[97,98] Challenges and opportunities are even greater when focusing cardiovascular prevention efforts in infancy.[99,100] There is strong evidence to support beneficial effects of child obesity prevention programs on body mass index, particularly for programs targeted to children aged 6 to 12 years.[99] An overview of systematic reviews of population-level interventions that had an environmental component directed to preventing or reducing obesity in children aged 5 to 18 years showed modest impact of a broad range of environmental strategies on anthropometric outcomes.[100] Most of the unhealthy or protective behaviors and living conditions are initiated and imprinted at these early ages, and the modern technology and information revolution may provide delivery channels to connect and make prevention opportunities available to these population groups.

From a health services perspective, a major challenge is how to continue sharing priorities between communicable and noncommunicable diseases,[101] while learning from those other countries where the epidemiologic profiles have already changed in the last decades. Other challenges include legitimate concerns about sustaining an adequate political commitment to mainstream cardiovascular diseases, particularly in the global South.[102]

Clinical practice, promotion, and prevention in cardiology cannot easily be limited or simplistically narrowed only to risk factors at the individual level during a one-to-one short-term clinical encounter. A minimal understanding of the wider contextual frameworks shaping a population's health and health outcomes enables clinical practitioners to better serve their patients. Such an understanding is an essential rather than a desirable skill.

Consequently, a population health approach is increasingly becoming a core component in the practice of cardiology.[103]

The question, then, is not why the practice of cardiology is changing but, on the contrary, what has happened to force and accommodate such change as the norm. This article signals major transitions that have occurred in recent decades, with an emphasis on low-income and middle-income countries. Generational changes, again at the individual and population levels, have rapidly occurred and become established. One of the obvious examples has been the rapid transition from the Barker hypothesis (low birth weight and worse cardiovascular profiles and mortality later in life) and the switch from undernutrition to overweight within a few decades. In the same time frame, in high-income countries, the benefits of prevention and improved health care have been documented, along with the known harmful effects of poor access to health care, and income inequalities.[104] Low-income and middle-income countries, together with practitioners of global health cardiology, have the opportunity to reshape the anticipated trends of cardiovascular diseases and curb their negative impacts. The demographic transition is introducing large segments of the world's population to aging. Having accomplished some major successes with the child survival agenda, especially in low-income and middle-income settings, these newer adults deserve not to repeat the same fate of mortality described in the original epidemiologic transitions. For this reason, it matters.

SUMMARY

The epidemiologic transition theory, since it was first proposed, gave an intellectual boost to understanding the changing dynamics of epidemiologic profiles. The epidemiologic transition provided a complement to the discourse of demographic change. Despite its criticisms and revisions, it is still a useful concept that influences public health debates, and has proved to be influential, particularly in changing societies. Most countries are facing the rapidly emerging needs of populations living longer lifespans, with cardiovascular conditions situated at the core of increasing disease burdens. In these scenarios of changes in population structures and disease profiles, cardiovascular conditions and their associated comorbidities will continue to challenge health care systems. Protecting large gains in global survival and achievements in life expectancy, accrued over recent decades in low-income and middle-income countries, requires a broad range of interventions. Fostering encounters and intersections, from human resources to health systems, from individual to population-wide, from health to nonhealth sectors, and benefiting from technological changes and human rights approaches, will provide a solid basis and framework to ensure long-term access to prevention services as well as health care. A renewed workforce in global health cardiology must swiftly adapt to these changing environments.

ACKNOWLEDGMENTS

The authors thank Antonio Bernabé-Ortiz, Rodrigo M Carrillo-Larco, María Lazo-Porras, and Shiva Raj Mishra for their feedback provided in earlier versions of this article.

REFERENCES

1. Fogel RW. Secular trends in physiological capital: implications for equity in health care. Perspect Biol Med 2003;46(3 Suppl):S24–38.
2. Berwick DM. Era 3 for medicine and health care. JAMA 2016;315(13):1329–30.
3. Bauchner H, Berwick D, Fontanarosa PB. Innovations in health care delivery and the future of medicine. JAMA 2016;315(1):30–1.
4. Miller BM, Moore DE Jr, Stead WW, et al. Beyond Flexner: a new model for continuous learning in the health professions. Acad Med 2010;85(2): 266–72.
5. Leppin AL, Montori VM, Gionfriddo MR. Minimally disruptive medicine: a pragmatically comprehensive model for delivering care to patients with multiple chronic conditions. Healthcare (Basel) 2015; 3(1):50–63.
6. NCD Risk Factor Collaboration (NCD-RisC). A century of trends in adult human height. eLife 2016;5:e13410.
7. Benakis C, Brea D, Caballero S, et al. Commensal microbiota affects ischemic stroke outcome by regulating intestinal γδ T cells. Nat Med 2016; 22(5):516–23.
8. Lee R. The demographic transition: three centuries of fundamental change. J Econ Perspect 2003; 17(4):167–90.
9. Ali MK, Jaacks LM, Kowalski AJ, et al. Noncommunicable diseases: three decades of global data show a mixture of increases and decreases in mortality rates. Health Aff 2015;34(9):1444–55.
10. Ezzati M, Obermeyer Z, Tzoulaki I, et al. Contributions of risk factors and medical care to cardiovascular mortality trends. Nat Rev Cardiol 2015;12(9): 508–30.
11. Roth GA, Forouzanfar MH, Moran AE, et al. Demographic and epidemiologic drivers of global cardiovascular mortality. N Engl J Med 2015; 372(14):1333–41.
12. O'Flaherty M, Buchan I, Capewell S. Contributions of treatment and lifestyle to declining CVD mortality: why have CVD mortality rates declined so much since the 1960s? Heart 2013;99(3): 159–62.
13. Danaei G, Singh GM, Paciorek CJ, et al. The global cardiovascular risk transition: associations of four metabolic risk factors with national income, urbanization, and Western diet in 1980 and 2008. Circulation 2013;127(14):1493–502, 1502.e1–8.
14. O'Flaherty M, Huffman MD, Capewell S. Declining trends in acute myocardial infarction attack and mortality rates, celebrating progress and ensuring future success. Heart 2015;101(17):1353–4.
15. Wilmot KA, O'Flaherty M, Capewell S, et al. Coronary heart disease mortality declines in the United States from 1979 through 2011: evidence for stagnation in young adults, especially women. Circulation 2015;132(11):997–1002.
16. Di Cesare M, Bennett JE, Best N, et al. The contributions of risk factor trends to cardiometabolic mortality decline in 26 industrialized countries. Int J Epidemiol 2013;42(3):838–48.
17. Roth GA, Huffman MD, Moran AE, et al. Global and regional patterns in cardiovascular mortality from 1990 to 2013. Circulation 2015;132(17):1667–78.
18. Omran AR. The epidemiologic transition. A theory of the epidemiology of population change. Milbank Mem Fund Q 1971;49(4):509–38.
19. Weisz G, Olszynko-Gryn J. The theory of epidemiologic transition: the origins of a citation classic. J Hist Med Allied Sci 2010;65(3):287–326.
20. Olshansky SJ, Ault AB. The fourth stage of the epidemiologic transition: the age of delayed degenerative diseases. Milbank Q 1986;64(3): 355–91.
21. Rogers RG, Hackenberg R. Extending epidemiologic transition theory: a new stage. Soc Biol 1987;34(3–4):234–43.
22. NCD Risk Factor Collaboration (NCD-RisC). Trends in adult body-mass index in 200 countries from 1975 to 2014: a pooled analysis of 1698 population-based measurement studies with 19·2 million participants. Lancet 2016;387(10026): 1377–96.
23. Gaziano TA, Prabhakaran D, Gaziano JM. Global burden of cardiovascular disease. In: Mann DL, Zipes DP, Libby P, et al, editors. Braunwald's heart disease: a textbook of cardiovascular medicine. 10th edition. Philadelphia: Elsevier; 2015. p. 1–20.
24. Gaziano JM. Fifth phase of the epidemiologic transition: the age of obesity and inactivity. JAMA 2010; 303(3):275–6.
25. Santosa A, Wall S, Fottrell E, et al. The development and experience of epidemiological transition

theory over four decades: a systematic review. Glob Health Action 2014;7:23574.

26. Szreter S. The importance of social intervention in Britain's mortality decline c. 1850-1914: a re-interpretation of the role of public health. Soc Hist Med 1988;1(1):1–38.

27. Carolina Martínez S, Carolina MS, Gustavo Leal F, et al. Epidemiological transition: model or illusion? A look at the problem of health in Mexico. Soc Sci Med 2003;57(3):539–50.

28. Caldwell JC. Health transition: the cultural, social and behavioural determinants of health in the third world. Soc Sci Med 1993;36(2):125–35.

29. Feachem RGA, Kjellstrom T, Murray CJL, et al, editors. The health of adults in the developing world. New York: Oxford University Press; 1992.

30. Hawkes C, Popkin BM. Can the sustainable development goals reduce the burden of nutrition-related non-communicable diseases without truly addressing major food system reforms? BMC Med 2015;13:143.

31. Riley JC. The timing and pace of health transitions around the world. Popul Dev Rev 2005;31(4): 741–64.

32. Eggleston KN, Fuchs VR. The new demographic transition: most gains in life expectancy now realized late in life. J Econ Perspect 2012;26(3): 137–56.

33. Frenk J, Bobadilla JL, Sepúlveda J, et al. Health transition in middle-income countries: new challenges for health care. Health Policy Plan 1989; 4(1):29–39.

34. GBD 2013 DALYs and HALE Collaborators, Murray CJ, Barber RM, Foreman KJ, et al. Global, regional, and national disability-adjusted life years (DALYs) for 306 diseases and injuries and healthy life expectancy (HALE) for 188 countries, 1990-2013: quantifying the epidemiological transition. Lancet 2015;386(10009):2145–91.

35. Kwan GF, Mayosi BM, Mocumbi AO, et al. Endemic cardiovascular diseases of the poorest billion. Circulation 2016;133(24):2561–75.

36. United Nations General Assembly. Resolution adopted by the General Assembly RES/66/2. Political declaration of the High-level Meeting of the General Assembly on the Prevention and Control of Non-communicable diseases. New York, January 24, 2012.

37. Smith SC Jr, Chen D, Collins A, et al. Moving from political declaration to action on reducing the global burden of cardiovascular diseases: a statement from the Global Cardiovascular Disease Taskforce. Circulation 2013;128(23):2546–8.

38. Ordunez P, Campbell NR. Beyond the opportunities of SDG 3: the risk for the NCDs agenda. Lancet Diabetes Endocrinol 2016;4(1):15–7.

39. Global Burden of Metabolic Risk Factors for Chronic Diseases Collaboration. Cardiovascular disease, chronic kidney disease, and diabetes mortality burden of cardiometabolic risk factors from 1980 to 2010: a comparative risk assessment. Lancet Diabetes Endocrinol 2014;2(8):634–47.

40. Farzadfar F, Finucane MM, Danaei G, et al. National, regional, and global trends in serum total cholesterol since 1980: systematic analysis of health examination surveys and epidemiological studies with 321 country-years and 3.0 million participants. Lancet 2011;377(9765): 578–86.

41. NCD Risk Factor Collaboration (NCD-RisC). Worldwide trends in diabetes since 1980: a pooled analysis of 751 population-based studies with 4.4 million participants. Lancet 2016;387(10027): 1513–30.

42. Danaei G, Finucane MM, Lin JK, et al. National, regional, and global trends in systolic blood pressure since 1980: systematic analysis of health examination surveys and epidemiological studies with 786 country-years and 5·4 million participants. Lancet 2011;377(9765):568–77.

43. O'Donnell CJ, Elosua R. Cardiovascular risk factors. Insights from Framingham Heart Study. Rev Esp Cardiol 2008;61(3):299–310 [in Spanish].

44. Mendis S. The contribution of the Framingham Heart Study to the prevention of cardiovascular disease: a global perspective. Prog Cardiovasc Dis 2010;53(1):10–4.

45. Bitton A, Gaziano TA. The Framingham Heart Study's impact on global risk assessment. Prog Cardiovasc Dis 2010;53(1):68–78.

46. Forouzanfar MH, Alexander L, Anderson HR, et al. Global, regional, and national comparative risk assessment of 79 behavioural, environmental and occupational, and metabolic risks or clusters of risks in 188 countries, 1990–2013: a systematic analysis for the Global Burden of Disease Study 2013. Lancet 2015;386(10010):2287–323.

47. Atun R. Transitioning health systems for multimorbidity. Lancet 2015;386(9995):721–2.

48. Davies J, Yudkin JS, Atun R. Liberating data: the crucial weapon in the fight against NCDs. Lancet Diabetes Endocrinol 2016;4(3):197–8.

49. Davies J, Yudkin JS, Atun R. Liberating data: the WHO response - authors' reply. Lancet Diabetes Endocrinol 2016;4(8):648–9.

50. Engelgau MM, Sampson UK, Rabadan-Diehl C, et al. Tackling NCD in LMIC: achievements and lessons learned from the NHLBI-UnitedHealth Global Health Centers of Excellence Program. Glob Heart 2016;11(1):5–15.

51. World Health Organization. Global status report on noncommunicable diseases 2014. Geneva: World Health Organization; 2014. p. 298.

52. Mendis S, Davis S, Norrving B. Organizational update: the world health organization global

status report on noncommunicable diseases 2014; one more landmark step in the combat against stroke and vascular disease. Stroke 2015;46(5):e121–2.

53. Pearce N, Ebrahim S, McKee M, et al. Global prevention and control of NCDs: limitations of the standard approach. J Public Health Policy 2015;36(4): 408–25.

54. Sacco RL, Roth GA, Reddy KS, et al. The heart of 25 by 25: achieving the goal of reducing global and regional premature deaths from cardiovascular diseases and stroke: a modeling study from the American Heart Association and World Heart Federation. Circulation 2016;133(23):e674–90.

55. Noncommunicable diseases prematurely take 16 million lives annually, WHO urges more action. Geneva: World Health Organization; 2015. Available at: http://www.who.int/mediacentre/news/releases/2015/noncommunicable-diseases/en/. Accessed July 30, 2016.

56. Robinson HM, Hort K. Non-communicable diseases and health systems reform in low-and-middle-income countries. Pac Health Dialog 2012;18(1):179–90.

57. Schwalm JD, McKee M, Huffman MD, et al. Resource effective strategies to prevent and treat cardiovascular disease. Circulation 2016;133(8): 742–55.

58. Ordunez P. Cardiac rehabilitation in low-resource settings and beyond: the art of the possible. Heart 2016;102(18):1425–6.

59. Lloyd-Jones DM, Hong Y, Labarthe D, et al. Defining and setting national goals for cardiovascular health promotion and disease reduction: the American Heart Association's strategic impact goal through 2020 and beyond. Circulation 2010; 121(4):586–613.

60. Sliwa K, Acquah L, Gersh BJ, et al. Impact of socioeconomic status, ethnicity, and urbanization on risk factor profiles of cardiovascular disease in Africa. Circulation 2016;133(12):1199–208.

61. Ribeiro ALP, Duncan BB, Brant LCC, et al. Cardiovascular health in Brazil: trends and perspectives. Circulation 2016;133(4):422–33.

62. Miranda JJ, Wells JCK, Smeeth L. Transitions in context: findings related to rural-to-urban migration and chronic non-communicable diseases in Peru. Rev Peru Med Exp Salud Publica 2012;29(3):366–72 [in Spanish].

63. Muka T, Imo D, Jaspers L, et al. The global impact of non-communicable diseases on healthcare spending and national income: a systematic review. Eur J Epidemiol 2015;30(4):251–77.

64. Jaspers L, Colpani V, Chaker L, et al. The global impact of non-communicable diseases on households and impoverishment: a systematic review. Eur J Epidemiol 2015;30(3):163–88.

65. Bennett JE, Li G, Foreman K, et al. The future of life expectancy and life expectancy inequalities in England and Wales: bayesian spatiotemporal forecasting. Lancet 2015;386(9989):163–70.

66. Pastorius Benziger C, Bernabe-Ortiz A, Miranda JJ, et al. Sex differences in health care-seeking behavior for acute coronary syndrome in a low income country, Peru. Crit Pathw Cardiol 2011;10(2):99–103.

67. Dracup K. The challenge of women and heart disease. Arch Intern Med 2007;167(22):2396.

68. Keller KM, Howlett SE. Sex differences in the biology and pathology of the aging heart. Can J Cardiol 2016;32(9):1065–73.

69. Bilano VL, Ota E, Ganchimeg T, et al. Risk factors of pre-eclampsia/eclampsia and its adverse outcomes in low- and middle-income countries: a WHO secondary analysis. PLoS One 2014;9(3): e91198.

70. Cooper C, Phillips D, Osmond C, et al. David James Purslove Barker: clinician, scientist and father of the "fetal origins hypothesis". J Dev Orig Health Dis 2014;5(3):161–3.

71. Charles MA, Delpierre C, Bréant B. Developmental origin of health and adult diseases (DOHaD): evolution of a concept over three decades. Med Sci (Paris) 2016;32(1):15–20 [in French].

72. Wells JCK, Pomeroy E, Walimbe SR, et al. The elevated susceptibility to diabetes in India: an evolutionary perspective. Front Public Health 2016;4:145.

73. Penaloza D, Arias-Stella J. The heart and pulmonary circulation at high altitudes: healthy highlanders and chronic mountain sickness. Circulation 2007;115(9):1132–46.

74. Hultgren HN. Effects of altitude upon cardiovascular diseases. J Wilderness Med 1992;3(3):301–8.

75. Caravita S, Faini A, Bilo G, et al. Blood pressure response to exercise in hypertensive subjects exposed to high altitude and treatment effects. J Am Coll Cardiol 2015;66(24):2806–7.

76. Bilo G, Villafuerte FC, Faini A, et al. Ambulatory blood pressure in untreated and treated hypertensive patients at high altitude: the high altitude cardiovascular research-andes study. Hypertension 2015;65(6):1266–72.

77. Miele CH, Schwartz AR, Gilman RH, et al. Increased cardiometabolic risk and worsening hypoxemia at high altitude. High Alt Med Biol 2016;17(2):93–100.

78. Huffman MD, Labarthe DR, Yusuf S. Global cardiovascular research training for implementation science, health systems research, and health policy research. J Am Coll Cardiol 2015;65(13): 1371–2.

79. Lerner AG, Bernabe-Ortiz A, Gilman RH, et al. The "rule of halves" does not apply in Peru: awareness,

treatment, and control of hypertension and dia-betes in rural, urban, and rural-to-urban migrants. Crit Pathw Cardiol 2013;12(2):53–8.

80. Nkoke C, Luchuo EB. Coronary heart disease in sub-Saharan Africa: still rare, misdiagnosed or underdiagnosed? Cardiovasc Diagn Ther 2016; 6(1):64–6.

81. Guaraldi G, Zona S, Menozzi M, et al. Cost of noninfectious comorbidities in patients with HIV. Clinicoecon Outcomes Res 2013;5:481–8.

82. Thota AB, Sipe TA, Byard GJ, et al. Collaborative care to improve the management of depressive disorders: a community guide systematic review and meta-analysis. Am J Prev Med 2012;42(5): 525–38.

83. Gilbody S, Whitty P, Grimshaw J, et al. Educational and organizational interventions to improve the management of depression in primary care: a systematic review. JAMA 2003;289(23):3145–51.

84. Woltmann E, Grogan-Kaylor A, Perron B, et al. Comparative effectiveness of collaborative chronic care models for mental health conditions across primary, specialty, and behavioral health care settings: systematic review and meta-analysis. Am J Psychiatry 2012;169(8):790–804.

85. Diez-Canseco F, Ipince A, Toyama M, et al. Integration of mental health and chronic non-communicable diseases in Peru: challenges and opportunities for primary care settings. Rev Peru Med Exp Salud Publica 2014;31(1):131–6 [in Spanish].

86. Kankeu HT, Saksena P, Xu K, et al. The financial burden from non-communicable diseases in low- and middle-income countries: a literature review. Health Res Policy Syst 2013;11:31.

87. Chaker L, Falla A, van der Lee SJ, et al. The global impact of non-communicable diseases on macro-economic productivity: a systematic review. Eur J Epidemiol 2015;30(5):357–95.

88. Brouwer ED, Watkins D, Olson Z, et al. Provider costs for prevention and treatment of cardiovascular and related conditions in low- and middle-income countries: a systematic review. BMC Public Health 2015;15:1183.

89. Heeley E, Anderson CS, Huang Y, et al. Role of health insurance in averting economic hardship in families after acute stroke in China. Stroke 2009; 40(6):2149–56.

90. Arredondo A, Zuñiga A. Epidemiological changes and financial consequences of hypertension in Latin America: implications for the health system and patients in Mexico. Cad Saude Publica 2012; 28(3):497–502.

91. Arredondo A, Duarte MB, Cuadra SM. Epidemiological and financial indicators of hypertension in older adults in Mexico: challenges for health planning and management in Latin America. Int J Health Plann Manage 2016. [Epub ahead of print].

92. Arredondo A, Aviles R. Costs and epidemiological changes of chronic diseases: implications and challenges for health systems. PLoS One 2015; 10(3):e0118611.

93. Khatib R, McKee M, Shannon H, et al. Availability and affordability of cardiovascular disease medicines and their effect on use in high-income, middle-income, and low-income countries: an analysis of the PURE study data. Lancet 2016; 387(10013):61–9.

94. Wells JCK. Obesity as malnutrition: the dimensions beyond energy balance. Eur J Clin Nutr 2013; 67(5):507–12.

95. Ezzati M, Riboli E. Behavioral and dietary risk factors for noncommunicable diseases. N Engl J Med 2013;369(10):954–64.

96. Stampfer MJ, Hu FB, Manson JE, et al. Primary prevention of coronary heart disease in women through diet and lifestyle. N Engl J Med 2000; 343(1):16–22.

97. Baker R, Taylor E, Essafi S, et al. Engaging young people in the prevention of noncommunicable diseases. Bull World Health Organ 2016;94(7):484.

98. Diez-Canseco F, Boeren Y, Quispe R, et al. Engagement of adolescents in a health communications program to prevent noncommunicable diseases: Multiplicadores Jóvenes, Lima, Peru, 2011. Prev Chronic Dis 2015;12:E28.

99. Waters E, de Silva-Sanigorski A, Hall BJ, et al. Interventions for preventing obesity in children. Cochrane Database Syst Rev 2011;(12):CD001871.

100. Cauchi D, Glonti K, Petticrew M, et al. Environmental components of childhood obesity prevention interventions: an overview of systematic reviews. Obes Rev 2016. [Epub ahead of print].

101. Piot P, Caldwell A, Lamptey P, et al. Addressing the growing burden of non-communicable disease by leveraging lessons from infectious disease management. J Glob Health 2016;6(1):010304.

102. Reubi D, Herrick C, Brown T. The politics of non-communicable diseases in the global South. Health Place 2016;39:179–87.

103. Williams KA Sr, Martin GR. New American College of Cardiology population health agenda to focus on primary prevention. J Am Coll Cardiol 2015;66(14): 1625–6.

104. Kim D, Kawachi I, Hoorn SV, et al. Is inequality at the heart of it? Cross-country associations of income inequality with cardiovascular diseases and risk factors. Soc Sci Med 2008;66(8):1719–32.

mHealth Interventions to Counter Noncommunicable Diseases in Developing Countries
Still an Uncertain Promise

Andrea Beratarrechea, MD, MSc*, Daniela Moyano, BSc,
Vilma Irazola, MD, MSc, Adolfo Rubinstein, MD, MSc, PhD

KEYWORDS

- Low- and middle-income countries • mHealth • Chronic disease

KEY POINTS

- High population coverage by the mobile telephone network increased the possibilities of mHealth interventions in LMICs.
- Short text messages are the most common type of mHealth intervention used in LMICs.
- Results from randomized controlled trials showed a positive but modest effect of mHealth on NCDs outcomes.

THE PROMISE OF mHEALTH

Low- and middle-income countries (LMICs) carry a disproportionate burden of chronic diseases.[1] Health systems in these countries are facing a critical shortage of health professionals and resources making health services for persons with chronic diseases unavailable or low quality, which results in decreased life expectancy and quality of life.[2]

Mobile health (mHealth) interventions constitute a promise for health care delivery especially in resource-constrained settings in developing countries where mobile technology has a high penetration. In fact, cell phones and plans are lowering their cost, and cell devices are getting easier to use and are offering now more functionalities (eg, multimedia messaging service, bluetooth, Internet

access, applications, GPS, camera and video) allowing the implementation of low-cost interventions.

In many places in LMICs, people have better access to mobile phones services than to basic services, such as water, electricity, sewerage, and sanitation.[3] In recent years, mHealth has yielded positive health outcomes because of improvements in the supply side of health care systems.[4] In terms of effectiveness, extensive reviews and meta-analyses in high-income countries have shown that mHealth increased access to medical services for vulnerable and hard-to-reach populations, enhanced communication flows and coordination among health care organizations, allowed timely data collection, improved education and training of health care workers, spread information

The authors have nothing to disclose.
South American Center of Excellence for Cardiovascular Health, Institute for Clinical Effectiveness and Health Policy, Ravignani 2024, Buenos Aires C1414CPV, Argentina
* Corresponding author. South American Center of Excellence for Cardiovascular Health, Institute for Clinical Effectiveness and Health Policy, Ravignani 2024, Buenos Aires C1414CPV, Argentina.
E-mail address: aberatarrechea@iecs.org.ar

Cardiol Clin 35 (2017) 13–30
http://dx.doi.org/10.1016/j.ccl.2016.08.009
0733-8651/17/© 2016 Elsevier Inc. All rights reserved.

among the community, and improved health care delivery.[5–12]

Mobile technologies represent a potential tool for improving health care services and clinical outcomes for chronic diseases, especially in the developing world. High population coverage by the mobile phone network, with 91.8% penetration, was reported in LMICs by the International Telecommunications Union in 2015; however, Internet coverage is still low and only 34.1% of the population is online, compared with 81.3% in the developed world.[13] In this regard, affordable smartphones and a growth of mobile broadband will increase access and the possibilities of mHealth interventions in LMICs.

However, there is still limited evidence of the effectiveness of mHealth in relation to its impact and long-term effects on prevention and control of chronic diseases in the developing world.[14] This article assesses the impact of mHealth on noncommunicable diseases (NCDs) in adults in LMICs. It differs from a previous published systematic review[14] because it includes other mHealth interventions, such as mobile applications and e-health registries, in addition to voice communication and text messages. The period covered is between 2012 and 2016.

EVIDENCE OF MHEALTH TO COUNTER NONCOMMUNICABLE DISEASES IN LOW- AND MIDDLE-INCOME COUNTRIES
Method

Search strategy
Systematic literature searches were performed from February to May 2016 using the following electronic bibliographic databases: Cochrane Central Register of Controlled Trials, MEDLINE, EMBASE, and the Latin American and Caribbean Health Science Literature Database according to MOOSE and PRISMA guidelines. Key words used in these searches included the following: telecommunication, cellular phone, cell phone, mobile phone, short text message, multimedia message, mobile applications, e-health registries, lifestyle, reminder system, risk reduction, patient education, self-management, patient compliance, primary prevention, outcome assessment, developing countries, underserved areas, and the specific LMIC.

Studies were included if they (1) were randomized controlled trials (RCTs) or systematic reviews and meta-analyses of RCTs with original data, conducted in an LMIC as defined by the World Bank published between January 2012 and April 2016[15]; (2) included subjects older than 18 years of age; (3) addressed the impact of mobile

interventions on a chronic disease (asthma, diabetes, hypertension, tobacco use, cardiovascular disease, chronic respiratory disease, and cancer); and (4) measured outcomes including morbidity, mortality, hospitalization rates, behavioral or lifestyle changes, process of care improvements, clinical outcomes, costs, and self-reported outcomes, such as patient, compliance, knowledge, self-efficacy and health-related quality of life. Only articles published in English language were included. Data were limited to published studies from the aforementioned databases.

Randomly assigned pairs of reviewers independently evaluated selected abstracts. Articles whose abstracts met the inclusion criteria were reviewed by a separate, randomly assigned pair of reviewers. If the article met the inclusion criteria, these reviewers extracted pertinent data and assessed methodologic quality using the Cochrane Risk of Bias Assessment Tool.[16] Discrepancies in article inclusion, data extraction, and bias assessment were solved by team consensus. Early Reviewer Organizer Software version 2.0 was used by reviewers' for full text evaluations of articles, data abstraction, and quality assessment.[17]

Results

We retrieved 1274 abstracts using the search terms and 108 articles were selected for full review, 36 of which were excluded because they were conducted in upper-income countries; did not address mHealth (n = 11); were not RCTs, systematic reviews, or meta-analyses (n = 24); did not focus on chronic disease (n = 2); were not published in English (n = 1); and (n = 14) were provisional abstracts (**Fig. 1**). Included studies (n = 20) came from 14 LMICs: Malaysia (n = 1); India (n = 5); China (n = 2); Iran (n = 3); Pakistan (n = 2); Philippines (n = 1); Thailand (n = 1); South Africa (n = 2); Mexico (n = 2); Honduras (n = 1); Argentina, Guatemala, and Peru (n = 1); and Bolivia (n = 1). We finally included 20 studies (see **Fig. 1**).

Most of the studies evaluated more than one outcome and included chronic diseases, such as asthma (n = 1), diabetes (n = 11), hypertension (n = 4), prehypertension (n = 1), and cardiovascular disease (n = 4) (**Table 1**).

Fifteen studies addressed clinical outcomes, which included intermediate outcomes or markers of disease severity, such as forced expiratory volume, blood pressure, body mass index, cholesterol, glycosylated hemoglobin, hospitalization, and adherence to medication.[18–32] Only one study addressed process of care measures, such as

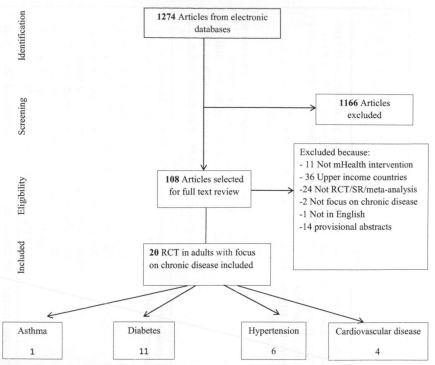

Fig. 1. Flow of information through the systematic review (SR).

follow-up for a definitive test in persons with an initial positive screening test as its main outcome.[33] Four studies examined patient compliance with diet, physical activity, and chronic medication[18,23,29,32]; four included, as an additional outcome, health-related quality of life measures[19,26,27,30]; and most evaluated changes in behaviors.[18,20,23–26,29–32,34–37] None of the evaluated studies included costs (see **Table 1**).

ASTHMA

Lv and colleagues[19] conducted a three-arm trial to evaluate in subjects with asthma whether daily short text messages about how to manage asthma in addition to in-person asthma education from a physician at the initial visit (SMS group) improved perceived control of asthma symptoms, forced expiratory volume in 1 second, and quality of life compared with receiving asthma education plus a free peak expiratory flow meter and training to use it (traditional group) or receiving asthma education at the initial visit (control group). The content of SMS included introduction to asthma, medication, asthma exacerbation triggers and strategies to avoid them, how to handle asthma acute attacks, and how to make an action plan. In this study, no differences were observed in the forced expiratory volume in 1 second among those who received the intervention but the SMS group

show improvements in the perceived asthma symptoms and in the quality of life. However, a high proportion of subjects withdrew from the study; only 71 (47.3%) completed the follow-up visit (30 in the SMS group, 27 in the traditional group, and 14 in the control group) representing a risk to study validity.

DIABETES

Most of the included studies focused on diabetes management and education. Only one study focused on diabetes prevention. Tamban and colleagues[23] evaluated whether the use of SMS improved adherence to management prescriptions and clinical outcomes in type 2 diabetes compared with standard care. In this study, no significant differences were found in terms of adherence to diet and physical activity but significant changes were observed in glycosilated hemoglobin (HbA_{1c}) in the intervention group compared with usual care.

Peimani and colleagues[24] compared in a three-arm RCT the effect of tailored SMS-based education and nontailored SMS-based education versus usual care to support and educate patients with type 2 diabetes in an outpatient diabetes clinic in Iran. In the tailored SMS-based education group, 75% of the SMS were customized to the two top barriers to adherence assessed during the

Table 1
Details of included studies

Study (Year)	Country	NCD	Study Design/Intervention	Outcomes
Lv et al,[19] 2012	China	Asthma	RCT. SMS about how to manage asthma every day + education control (n = 50) vs traditional group who received asthma information, a free PEF meter and training on its proper use (n = 50) vs CG who received only verbal asthma education information at the initial visit (n = 50). Follow-up 3 mo.	PCAQ-6 score (mean changes in the score) from baseline to 3 mo: SMS group 7.07 ± 4.44 vs 4.78 ± 5.77 traditional group and 3.00 ± 5.31 in CG, $P = .046$. Forced expiratory flow in 1 s (% predicted): no differences were detected between the groups. AQLQ(S) score (mean changes) from baseline to 3 mo: SMS 31.40 ± 30.42 vs traditional 16.52 ± 21.10 vs CF 4.21 ± 30.98, $P = .008$. The follow-up adherence rates were 60% in the SMS group, 54% in the traditional group, and 28% in CG; $P = .003$
Goodarzi et al,[20] 2012	Iran	Diabetes	RCT. Educational SMS (n = 50) vs usual care (n = 50) in clinical parameters among T2DP. Follow-up 4 mo.	At baseline HbA$_{1c}$ (%) 7.91 ± 1.24 in IG vs 7.83 ± 1.12 in CG, $P = $ NS; and at 4 mo HbA$_{1c}$ 7.02 ± 1.02 in IG vs 7.48 ± 1.26 in CG, $P = .024$. Cholesterol at baseline IG 180 ± 44.47 mg/dL vs CG 176.9 ± 31.15 mg/dL; and at 4 mo IG 165.95 ± 38.18 vs CG 187.2 ± 38.6, $P = .002$. Mean percentage of change in the score: Knowledge, IG 53.9% compared with CG 10.3%, $P<.001$; Practice, IG 38.5% compared with CG 10.4%, $P<.001$; and Self-efficacy, IG 13.19% compared with CG -3.10, $P<.001$.
Ramachandran et al,[22] 2013	India	Diabetes	RCT. Tailored SMS encouraging lifestyle change (n = 271) compared with standard lifestyle advice (n = 266) to reduce incident T2DP in men with impaired glucose tolerance. Follow-up 24 mo.	In the IG, 50 (18%) men developed T2DM over the 2 y compared with 73 (27%) men in the CG. Hazard ratio of 0.64 (95% CI, 0.45–0.92), $P = .015$. Number needed to treat to prevent one case of T2DM was 11 (95% CI, 6–55).

Tamban et al,[23] 2013	Philippines	Diabetes	RCT. SMS as an adjunct to the standard care (n = 52) vs standard care (n = 52) to improve adherence to diet and exercise and clinical parameters among T2DP. Follow-up 6 mo.	Adherence to diet and exercise was arbitrarily defined by the authors. Adherence to diet was defined as adhering to the dietary recommendation at least 4 d in a week and also eating 2–3 main meals in a day as recommended. Adherence to exercise was defined as adhering to the exercise recommendation of at least 5 d in a week and also having 30 min of exercise or more in a day. At 6 mo, significant differences were seen in mean number of meals/day, IG 2.61 ± 0.63 vs CG 2.29 ± 0.72 ($P = .018$) and mean number of minutes/exercise IG 37.40 ± 14.87 vs CG 31.44 ± 10.82 ($P = .021$), but not in the number of days patient complied with diet and exercise. At baseline HbA$_{1c}$ (%) IG 7.81 ± 1.40–6.99 ± 0.86 at 6 mo and in CG 7.86 ± 1.14–7.34 ± 0.90 at 6 mo, $P = .0452$.
Kumar et al,[33] 2015	India	Diabetes	RCT. Mobile reminders (n = 135) vs control (n = 133) on follow-up for definitive tests and screening yield for diabetes to outpatients in a primary care setting. Follow-up 3 working days.	85.7% of outpatients in IG returned for a definitive test vs 53.3% in CG. RR = 1.61 (95% CI, 1.35–1.91), $P<.001$. Number of patients who were diagnosed with diabetes in IG and CG arm were 27.1% and 14.8%, respectively. Number of patients who were diagnosed with prediabetes in IG and CG were 36.1% and 23%, respectively.

(continued on next page)

Table 1
(continued)

Study (Year)	Country	NCD	Study Design/Intervention	Outcomes
Peimani et al,[24] 2015	Iran	Diabetes	RCT. T-SMS (n = 50) vs non-T-SMS (n = 50) vs control (n = 50) on education of basic self-care skills among T2DP. Follow-up 3 mo.	HbA_{1c} and lipid profile were not affected by the intervention. A reduction in BMI was observed in both SMS groups, BMI at baseline 27.71 ± 5.29 in T-SMS and 27.14 ± 5.51 at 3 mo, BMI at baseline 27.40 ± 4.73 in non T-SMS and 26.90 ± 4.57 at 3 mo vs BMI at baseline 27.92 ± 4.97 in CG and 28.21 ± 5.15 at 3 mo, $P < .001$. FBS at baseline 172.44 ± 70.74 mg/dL in T-SMS and 152.54 ± 81.09 mg/dL at 3 mo, non T-SMS: FBS at baseline 169.54 ± 70.87 mg/dL and 147.82 ± 47.27 mg/dL at 3 mo. CG: FBS at baseline 166.94 ± 67.52 mg/dL and 165.32 ± 57.85 mg/dL at 3 mo, $P = .003$. Self-care inventory: at baseline 55.41 ± 10.54 in T-SMS and. 65.37 ± 10.26 at 3 mo, non-T-SMS at baseline 55.43 ± 10.67 and 65.79 ± 9.99 at 3 mo, CG at baseline 54.57 ± 9.13 and 49.98 ± 11.15 at 3 mo, $P < .001$. Diabetes self-care barriers: T-SMS at baseline 45.6 ± 11.06 and 31.42 ± 11.8 at 3 mo, non T-SMS at baseline 42.98 ± 10.20 and 29.24 ± 11.55 at 3 mo, CG at baseline 49.78 ± 10.62 and 57.56 ± 12.50 at 3 mo, $P < .001$. Diabetes management self-efficacy: T-SMS at baseline 57.40 ± 12.9 and 43.77 ± 11.50 at 3 mo, non T-SMS at baseline 53.63 ± 12.39 and 39.78 ± 8.67 at 3 mo vs CG at baseline 58.95 ± 11.86 vs 66.95 ± 11.38 at 3 mo, $P < .001$.

Wongrochananan et al,[26] 2015	Thailand	Diabetes	Cluster RCT. Interactive multimodality technology intervention in the intervention offices included email, SMS, and Web site with four main functions (self-regulation, self-monitoring and assessment, social support, and reminder system; linked to email and SMS) (n = 78) vs usual care (n = 48) in improving HbA_{1c} and self-management behaviors among T2DP patients. Follow-up 3 mo.	55 T2DP patients (70.5%) in the IG have a follow-up visit and 30 (62.5%) in the CG. A reduction in HbA_{1c} was observed, mean change in HbA_{1c} (%) in the IG: −0.28 (1.18) compared with +5.86 (1.00) in the CG, P = .001. No differences were observed in cholesterol, triglyceride, LDL-c, SBP, DBP, and BMI. No differences were found in diabetes self-efficacy and in diabetes quality of life but changes were observed in the self-care score. Mean change in the score in the IG +7.73 (11.86) compared with CG +1.84 (4.84), P <.05.
Shahid et al,[29] 2015	Pakistan	Diabetes	RCT. Mobile phone calls every 15 d (IG) (n = 220) vs usual care (CG) (n = 220) to improve HbA_{1c} and LDL-c among T2DP living in rural areas with poor glycemic control (HbA_{1c} ≥8%) and no chronic complications. Follow-up 4 mo.	Mean difference from baseline to 4 mo: HbA_{1c} (%) was −1.46 (0.07) in the IG vs −0.48 (0.04) in the CG at 4 mo, P<.001. LDL-c mean reduction was −23 (1.4) mg/dL in the IG compared with −9.04 (0.77) mg/dL in the CG, P<.001. Self-reported outcomes: adherence to a diet plan and the proportion of physically active patients have a greater increased in the IG at 4 mo compared with usual care.
Patnaik et al,[28,35] 2016	India	Diabetes	RCT. Intense lifestyle education using printed materials and computers + telephone calls + weekly SMS with educational tips (n = 50) vs control who received printed materials (n = 50) to decrease perceived stress among patients with diabetes. Follow-up 3 mo.	After 3 mo, total 55 patients (51%) (CG = 21; IG = 34) had a follow-up visit. No changes were observed between the groups in coronary heart disease risk factor and in clinical outcomes: BMI, waist-hip ratio, TC, FBS. Mean Cohen Perceived Stress Scale scores obtained were (18.9) at baseline for both groups. At 3-mo follow-up, the scores reduced to 17.05 in the IG and increased to 20.7 in the CG.

(continued on next page)

Table 1
(continued)

Study (Year)	Country	NCD	Study Design/Intervention	Outcomes
Anzaldo-Campos et al,[30] 2016	Mexico	Diabetes	RCT. PDI (n = 99) vs PD-TEI, which include a cell phone app + USB glucose meter (n = 102) vs CG (n = 100) among T2DP with poor glycemic control (HbA$_{1c}$ ≥8%). Follow-up 4 and 10 mo.	Mean difference from baseline to 10 mo: HbA$_{1c}$ (%) in PDI was -2.63 (3.73), −3.02 (2.83) in the PD-TEI, and −1.3 (3.29); $P<.001$. No differences were observed between PDI and PD-TEI. No changes were observed over time in TC, triglycerides, LDL-c, high-density lipoprotein cholesterol, and SBP, DBP. Self-reported outcomes: PDI and PD-TEI reported changes in the Diabetes Knowledge Questionnaire 24, 3.20 (3.28) and 3.24 (4.15) compared with CG 1.15 (4.05). No changes were observed in self-efficacy, depression, self-reported behaviors, and quality of life.
Piette et al,[21] 2012	Honduras and Mexico	Hypertension	RCT. Mobile monitoring and behavior-change calls plus home blood pressure monitoring and email alerts for health workers (n = 99) vs usual care (n = 101) on SBP among patients with hypertension. Follow-up 6 wk.	Mean difference in SBP was -4.2 mm Hg (95% CI, -9.1 to 0.7; $P = .09$) lower in the IG but not statistically significant. IG have fewer depressive symptoms in the Scale compared with CG mean difference -2.5 in the score 10-item Center for Epidemiologic Studies-Depression (95% CI, -4.1 to -0.8; $P = 0.04$). Improvements were observed in medication-related problems, perceived health status, and treatment satisfaction.

Rubinstein et al,[25] 2015	Argentina, Guatemala, and Peru	Prehypertension	RCT. mHealth counseling calls on lifestyle modification (reduction of dietary sodium intake, reduction of simple sugars and saturated fat intake, increase of fruit and vegetable intake, and promotion of physical activity) + SMS (n = 321) vs usual care (n = 316) in reducing blood pressure, body weight, and eating behaviors among prehypertensive patients. Follow-up 12 mo.	266 (84%) participants in the IG and 287 (89%) in the CG were assessed at 12 mo. The intervention did not result in a change in blood pressure compared with usual care. However, the study showed a significant net reduction in body weight (−0.66 kg; P = .04) and intake of high-fat and high-sugar foods/number of servings (−0.75; P = .008) in the IG vs the CG. Participants in IG who received more than 75% of the calls (≥9 calls) had a much higher reduction of their body weight −4.85 kg (95% CI, −8.21 to −1.48) and waist circumference −3.31 cm (95% CI, −5.95 to −0.67) and greater improvement in some eating behaviors.
Bobrow et al,[27] 2016	South Africa	Hypertension	RCT. SMS information-only (n = 457) vs SMS + interactive adherence support system (n = 458) vs usual care (n = 457) in maintaining and improving treatment adherence and blood pressure control among patients with hypertension. Follow-up 12 mo.	Mean adjusted difference in SBP at 12 mo for the SMS information-only compared with usual care was −2.2 mm Hg (95% CI, −4.4 to −0.04; P =.046) and for the SMS interactive compared with usual care was −1.6 mm Hg (95% CI, −3.7 to 0.6; P = .16). The adjusted OR for controlled blood pressure (<140/90 mm Hg) at 12 mo was 1.4 (95% CI, 1.0–1.9; P = .04) and 1.4 (95% CI 1.0–1.9; P = .04) for SMS information and SMS interactive, respectively, compared with usual care. The adjusted OR for improved availability of dispensed medicine was 1.86 (95% CI, 1.39–2.49; P<.0001) for SMS information compared with usual care and 1.60 (95% CI, 1.20–2.16; P = .002) for SMS interactive with usual care. EuroQol 5-D, Self-Report Questionnaire score, attendance at clinic appointments, retention in clinical care, treatment and clinic satisfaction, hypertension knowledge, self-reported adherence, hospital admissions, and differences in medication changes did not differ between groups.

(continued on next page)

Table 1
(continued)

Study (Year)	Country	NCD	Study Design/Intervention	Outcomes
Hacking et al,[36] 2016	South Africa	Hypertension	RCT. SMS information (n = 109) vs control (n = 114) to improve health knowledge and self-reported health-related behaviors among patients with hypertension. Follow-up 17 wk.	69.7% in IG and 61.4% in CG had a follow-up visit. Knowledge: no significant changes were observed. Positive self-reported behavior change was reported by participants in the SMS intervention.
Piette et al,[37] 2016	Bolivia	Hypertension and diabetes	RCT. Standard m-health (tailored IVR calls) (n = 27) vs m-health + CP (tailored IVR calls + feedback to the care partner through IVR summaries and suggestions for supporting the patient's self-care) (n = 45) in completion of IVR calls and in health self-report among patients with hypertension and diabetes. Follow-up 4 mo.	mHealth + CP patients completed significantly more IVR calls than standard mHealth patients (62.0% vs 44.9%; *P*<.047) mHealth + CP patients were significantly more likely than standard mHealth patients to report excellent health during their IVR calls (adjusted OR, 2.60; 95% CI, 1.07–6.32).
Khonsari et al,[18] 2014	Malaysia	CVD	RCT. SMS-based reminders on medication adherence (n = 31) vs usual care (n = 31) for medication adherence among patients after hospital discharge following acute coronary syndrome. Follow-up 8 wk postdischarge.	97% of the patients had a follow-up visit. MMAS-8 was measured at 8 wk postdischarge: high adherence (score of 8) IG 64.5% vs 12.9% for CG, medium adherence (score of 6 to <8) IG 19.4% vs 29% for CG, and low adherence (scores of <6) IG 16.1% vs 58.1% for CG. RR of being low adherent among CG was 4.09 (95% CI, 1.82–9.18) compared with IG, *P*<.0001. No statistically significant changes in New York Heart Association classification, death, and hospital readmissions rate were observed between study groups.

	Country	Disease	Design/Intervention	Results
Kamal et al,[32] 2015	Pakistan	CVD	RCT. SMS with reminders customized to their individual prescription + SMS with health information (n = 100) vs SMS with health information (n = 100) vs usual care (n = 100) for medication adherence in patients with >1 mo since last episode of stroke. Follow-up 2 mo.	Mean MMAS-8 score was measured at baseline IG 6.6 (0.7) vs 6.6 (0.16) in CG and at 2 mo in IG 7.4 (0.93) vs 6.7 (1.32), $P<.01$. No major effect was observed on SBP after the intervention. Mean DBP in IG was −2.6 mm Hg (95% CI, −5.5 to 0.15) lower compared with CG.
Boroumand et al,[34] 2015	Iran	CVD	RCT. SMS + follow-up telephone calls related to cardiac self-efficacy assessment (n = 35) vs telephone calls not related to cardiac self-efficacy assessment (n = 35) among participants hospitalized with coronary artery disease. Follow-up 4 mo.	Mean cardiac self-efficacy score: IG at baseline 30.5 compared with at 3 mo 53.1 and 59.1 at 4 mo; in CG the mean score obtained was 29.9 at baseline compared with 30.7 at 3 mo and 30.1 at 4 mo; $P<.001$.
Tian et al,[31] 2015	China and India	High risk of CVD	Cluster RCT. 23 villages (n = 1095 high-risk CVD participants) were assigned to CHWs monthly visits + smartphone for CHWs with an electronic decision support system with prompts to deliver the intervention + performance feedback and incentives or usual care, 24 villages (n = 991 high-risk CVD participants). Follow-up 12 mo.	Net pre-post difference in the proportion of patient-reported antihypertensive medication between the two groups was of 25.5%, $P<.001$. SBP reduction in the mean SBP between the groups (−2.7 mm Hg; $P = .04$). Net pre-post difference in the use of aspirin 17.1% ($P<.001$) and receiving monthly follow-up, 16% ($P<.001$). No differences were observed in tobacco use and salt awareness.

Abbreviations: AQLQ(s), Standard Asthma-Specific Quality of Life Questionnaire; BMI, body mass index; CG, control group; CHW, community health worker; CI, confidence interval; CP, care partners; CVD, cardiovascular disease; DBP, diastolic blood pressure; FBS, fasting blood sugar; HbA$_{1c}$, glycosylated hemoglobin; IG, intervention group; IVR, interactive voice response; LDL-c, low-density lipoprotein cholesterol; MMAS-8, Morisky Medication Adherence Scales−8 item; non-T-SMS, nontailored SMS-based education; OR, odds ratio; PCQ-6, perceived control asthma questionnaire; PD-TEI, Project Dulce technology-enhanced intervention; PDI, Project Dulce–only intervention; RR, relative risk; SBP, systolic blood pressure; T2DP, type 2 diabetes patients; TC, total cholesterol; T-SMS, tailored SMS-based education.

baseline visit using the Diabetes Self-Care Barriers assessment scale for older adults. In the nontailored SMS-based education group, random messages were sent. In both groups, participants received seven SMS per week during 3 months. No significant changes were observed in HbA_{1c} and lipid profile. However, a reduction of mean body mass index and fasting blood glucose were observed in both intervention groups.

Goodarzi and colleagues[20] evaluated at 3 months the impact of one-way educational messages (SMS) with information about exercise, diet, medication, and self-monitoring blood glucose levels on improving HbA_{1c}, lipid profile and knowledge, attitude, practice, and self-efficacy toward diabetes. Results showed an improvement in HbA_{1c} and cholesterol levels and in knowledge practice toward diabetes and self-efficacy in the intervention group.

Shahid and colleagues[29] compared in a two-arm RCT the effect of mobile phone calls on HbA_{1c} and low-density lipoprotein cholesterol values compared with usual care at 4 months in patients with type 2 diabetes with poor glycemic control and no chronic complications living in rural areas of Pakistan. The intervention included mobile phone calls every 15 days were patients were asked about self blood glucose monitoring, medication intake, healthy eating, and physical activity and received feedback from the investigator. Reductions were observed in HbA_{1c}, low-density lipoprotein cholesterol, and systolic blood pressure (SBP) in both groups; however, more pronounced reductions were found in the intervention group. Anzaldo-Campos and coworkers[30] evaluated the effect of a diabetes care and education program led by trained clinicians, nurses, and peers with mobile tools (Project Dulce technology-enhanced intervention/PD-TEI) and without them (Project Dulce/PDI) compared with usual clinical care on clinical and self-reported outcomes in patients with type 2 diabetes in Mexico. Patients with type 2 diabetes in the PD-TEI group received a cell phone where they have accessed to educational videos and materials and received interactive surveys (once a day during the first month and twice a week the second month) with questions regarding glucose measurements, carbohydrate intake, physical activity, and medication adherence. Providers also received alerts when patients reported out of range glucose values or missed their appointments. Clinical outcomes and self-reported outcomes were assessed at baseline, 4 months, and 10 months. Improvements in HbA_{1c} and in diabetes knowledge were reported in the intervention groups compared with usual care but no differences were observed between PD-TEI and PDI.

Two studies assessed the effect of mobile interventions to encourage lifestyle changes.[22,35] Ramachandran and colleagues[22] evaluated in Indian men with impaired glucose tolerance whether tailored SMS encouraging lifestyle changes reduced the incidence of type 2 diabetes at 24 months. The mobile phone message content was based on the transtheoretical model of behavioral change, which was assessed at baseline and at follow-up visits.[38] The investigators also took into account participants' preferences regarding timing and frequency of messaging to tailored SMS. Results of this study showed a significant reduction in the incidence of type 2 diabetes in the group who received tailored messages (18%) compared with the group who received standard lifestyle advice (27%), hazard ratio of 0.64 (95% confidence interval, 0.45–0.92; $P = .015$).

Patnaik and colleagues[28,35] evaluated the effect of a multicomponent intervention to reduce coronary heart disease risk factors and perceived stress among patients with diabetes. The intervention group received printed materials, telephone counseling calls every 3 weeks, and weekly SMS with lifestyle messages about healthy diet, physical activity, adherence to medication, and tips to manage stress during 3 months. Forty-five percent of the patients did not have a follow-up visit at 3 months and reported results were obtained from 21 patients in the control group (42%) and from 34 patients in the intervention group (68%). Substantial losses to follow-up were observed in both groups, with a greater tendency to loose subjects in the control group, which might affect the validity of the study.

Despite frequent diabetes screening and appropriate targeting of patients with high-risk, follow-up of those with abnormal results is uncommon and the yield of screening is low.[39] Kumar and colleagues[33] evaluated the effect of mobile reminder to improve screening yield during opportunistic screening for diabetes in outpatients attending primary care centers in India. This study showed positive results with improvement in follow-up for definitive test and outpatients in the intervention arm had 1.6 times more chances of returning for definitive test than control subjects.

A cluster randomized trial led by Wongrochananan and colleagues[26] evaluated whether a multicomponent intervention that included an mHealth component (SMS) improved HbA_{1c} and self-management behaviors at 3 months, compared with usual care. The intervention included emailing, SMS, and a Web site that addressed self-regulation, self-monitoring and assessment, social support, and a reminder system linked to the patient's email and mobile phone. Subjects enrolled were encouraged to log onto the Web site and set their personal goals for improving self-management behaviors. SMS and emails were sent to help them comply with the planned activities. Although the intervention showed improvements in HbA_{1c} levels and quality of life, the main limitation was its incomplete compliance with study procedures, and high drop-out rates.

HYPERTENSION

Four of the included studies focused on hypertension management and one on hypertension prevention. Piette and colleagues[21] assessed whether a multifaceted intervention that included a mobile intervention through automated calls for patients with hypertension plus home blood pressure monitoring and alerts via email for health care workers improved SBP. Patients with hypertension received automated calls during 6 weeks reminding them to measure blood pressure regularly and asking them about their SBP values, medication adherence, and salt intake. The system processed these responses and generated alerts when the patient reported that at least half of the time in the prior week he/she had had high SBP values or had been rarely or never taking their blood pressure medication. No effect was found on SBP; however, some improvements were observed in medication-related problems (eg, experiencing medication side effects, being confused by the complexity of the regimen, not being sure that the medication is important to get better) and in perceived health status.

Bobrow and colleagues[27] evaluated whether adherence support delivered via SMS with information only (one-way SMS) versus interactive text messaging (two-way SMS) improved treatment adherence and blood pressure control among patients with hypertension. In the group that received information only, SMS were one-way and encouraged patients to take their hypertensive medication, provided education about hypertension and its management, and reminders for scheduled appointments and prescription drugs refill at the clinic. In addition, in the interactive text messaging group, participants received the same messages plus a free service to reply to messages. Both interventions produced modest reductions on SBP. Medication changes, clinical appointments, hypertension knowledge, and self-reported adherence did not differ between the two groups.

Other studies assessed the effect of mHealth on self-reported health among hypertensives.[36,37] Piette and colleagues[37] evaluated the effect of tailored interactive voice response (IVR) calls to patients with hypertension plus an automated feedback to a care partner with summaries and suggestions for supporting the patient's self-care compared with noninteractive IVR calls in patients with hypertension. This study included patients with diabetes and hypertension and self-reported health was assessed at 4 months. Participants whose care partners received feedback were more likely to report excellent health than those who received IVR only.

Hacking and colleagues[36] used SMS to improve knowledge and self-reported health behaviors. Positive self-reported behavior change was reported but no improvement in knowledge was observed. A limitation of this study was its incomplete compliance with the follow-up interview.

Another study conducted by Rubinstein and colleagues[25] in Latin America evaluated the effect of mobile counseling plus tailored SMS to promote adoption of healthy lifestyles (healthy eating and physical activity) compared with usual care among prehypertensive subjects. Counseling calls were conducted on a monthly basis by nutritionists and the content of the calls and of the SMS focused on lifestyle modification. One-way SMS were sent on a weekly basis and content was based on the transtheoretical model of behavioral change, which was assessed in every monthly call.[38] Target behaviors treated in the calls were reduction of sodium intake, reduction of high fat and high sugar intake, increase in fruit and vegetable intake, and promotion of physical activity. The intervention did not result in a reduction of blood pressure values at 12 months; however, participants in the intervention group had a significant although modest reduction in weight and reported lower intake of high-fat and high-sugar foods.

CARDIOVASCULAR DISEASE

Two studies were conducted in patients with coronary artery disease, one in patients with stroke, and one in persons with high cardiovascular risk.[18,31,32,34] Two of them included SMS-based reminders to improve medication adherence.[18,32] In the study conducted by Kamal and colleagues[32] SMS were customized according to the patients' medical information and drug profile and sent during 8 weeks. Reminders were customized to the patient's prescription and participants were asked to respond stating if they were taking medication. In addition, two health information SMS were sent weekly.

Khonsari and colleagues[18] included patients who were discharged from hospital after an acute coronary syndrome. Patients received SMS reminders before every medication intake and also messages reminding patients to come to the hospital and have their prescribed medication refilled. Both studies showed improvement in the eight-item Morisky Medication Adherence Scale compared with usual care at 2 months of follow-up.[40]

Cardiac self-efficacy is related to adoption of healthy behaviors in patients with coronary disease. Boroumand and Moeini[34] evaluated the effect at 4 months of tailored SMS plus telephone calls versus telephone calls among patients hospitalized with coronary heart disease. In the intervention group, telephone calls were made twice a week during the first month and once a week during the second and third months. During telephone calls, cardiac self-efficacy was assessed and included such domains as maintenance of performance, management of disease symptoms, and regulation of cardiac risk factors.[41] The information provided was used to tailor SMS. Six messages per week, a total of 72 SMS, were sent during the study period. Results showed improvement in self-efficacy score in patients with coronary heart disease.

Tian and colleagues[31] evaluated in a cluster randomized trial the effect of a multicomponent intervention delivered by community health workers (CHWs) to improve cardiovascular management in persons with high cardiovascular risk living in rural villages in China and India. CHWs conducted monthly follow-up visits with the assistance of a mobile application that include an electronic decision support system to guide the implementation of two therapeutic lifestyle modifications (smoking cessation and salt reduction) and the appropriate prescription of hypertensive medication and aspirin. CHWs in the intervention group also received performance feedback and a financial incentive. Forty-seven villages were included, 23 in the intervention group with 1095 high cardiovascular risk participants and 24 villages with 991 participants in the control group. The net pre-post difference in the proportion of patient-reported antihypertensive medication was the main outcome.

In China, the intervention group had 24.4% higher net increase in the proportion of patient-reported antihypertensive medication compared with the control group and in India this net increase was 26.6%, both statistically significant. Use of aspirin was also more frequent in the intervention group at the end of the follow-up. A reduction in the SBP was observed in the intervention group with a mean difference pre-post between both arms of −2.7 mm Hg ($P = .04$). No changes were seen in tobacco use and in salt awareness.

DISCUSSION

According to the World Bank Classification, half of the studies included in this review correspond to upper-middle-income countries and half to LMICs. To date, low-income countries are not represented.

Labrique and colleagues[42] have developed a framework for 12 common mHealth and information and communication technology (ICT) applications that serve to map and catalog mHealth services and identify gaps to innovation, solutions, and implementation activity. The most represented domain in the reviewed articles was client education and behavior change in communication. In the included studies, mHealth was used as a channel to deliver education, increase patients' and care partners' knowledge, modify attitudes, and improve health-seeking behaviors and health-related lifestyle decisions. Three studies included an electronic decision support system for health workers as an additional component of the intervention. In two studies, the system generated alerts for health workers when it was detected that patients were not taking their chronic medication or were not under control,[21,30] and in another study the system generated prompts and guided CHWs to deliver lifestyle interventions and support the appropriate prescription of medication in persons with high cardiovascular risk during monthly visits[31]

Electronic data capture using mobile devices with easy user interfaces and offline data store have been implemented in many developed countries; however, no RCT have been conducted to evaluate if this mHealth intervention improves NCDs management.

One-way SMS was the most common used mobile function to deliver health education and health information. Only two studies used the IVR function.[21,37] This mobile function is easy to use and serves as a channel to deliver health information, especially in people with low health literacy levels.[43]

The impact of the proposed mHealth interventions on clinical outcomes was modest. One out of four included studies related to hypertension and prehypertension showed a small positive effect in blood pressure values.[27] Two of the four studies found modest reductions in weight; one was conducted in subjects with diabetes and was focused on diabetes education and the other implemented lifestyle modification strategies through mobile counseling calls and tailored SMS in prehypertensive patients.[24,25]

Five out of six studies showed a modest reduction in HbA_{1c} values compared with usual care.[20,23,26,29,30] As regards medication adherence, two out of three studies showed improvement in the Morisky Medication Adherence Scales.[18,32] Finally, five studies evaluated the long-term impact of mHealth to prevent or control NCDs.[22,25,27,30,31] Five studies reported loss to follow-up of more than 20% undermining of the reported results.[19,26,28,35,36]

There is an important gap between the scientific production of research and public health priorities in LMICs. In this sense, diabetes was the most represented chronic disease with the 11 studies. We found five studies addressing hypertension despite its much higher disease burden in our countries.[44] No mHealth studies on cancer screening or management were identified from LMICs.

Evidence-based information to guide policymakers is scarce in our countries and research does not fully match LMICs health priorities. Potential to inform policy makers depends on the level of evidence, adequacy among publications, burden of diseases covered, presence of recommendations, or actionable messages and information for adoption and scaling-up.

In regard to the quality of the evidence reported in the reviewed articles, we only included individual randomized controlled trials, randomized cluster trials, systematic reviews, and meta-analysis in our search strategy to strengthen the quality of the evidence; however, eight of the included studies had a small sample size.[18-20,23,24,34,35,37] Furthermore, the analysis of some of the studies was not based on an intention-to-treat approach, leading to biased results that may have overestimated the effects of the mHealth interventions. Only two studies included insightful messages and information that might be useful for scaling-up these interventions.[22,27]

Evidence is still scarce regarding the effectiveness of different types of mHealth interventions to counter chronic diseases. The implementation of other mHealth interventions and ICT applications (eg, for data collection and reporting, electronic decision support, electronic health records) depends on access to other mobile functions, such as multimedia messaging service, videos, and apps, which are available in smartphones and depend on access to mobile broadband.

In LMICs, there are several limitations regarding technology use and implementation of mHealth interventions, which include but are not limited to technological literacy, health workers' resistance to new technology, different patterns of cell phone usage among underserved populations, shared or lack of mobile phones for personal use, lost or stolen phones, limited connectivity, limited infrastructure, access to smartphones, and lack of standardized data security protocols to ensure interoperability and to maximize the full capabilities of mHealth and ICT applications.[45]

mHealth studies conducted require methodologic rigor to provide high quality of evidence and influence practice and policies. The strength of the evidence depends on the study design, the methodologic quality and the statistical precision, the magnitude of the measured effects, and the relevance of these effects to the implementation context.[46,47] Many mHealth studies in LMICs fail to apply rigorous criteria in this review.

Research regarding adoption and ownership of mHealth is still needed. Few studies reported process indicators related to delivery of the intervention and reach of the target population. Rubinstein and colleagues[25] reported process indicators regarding delivery of the intervention (dose, reach, and implementation fidelity), such as the number of participants who were reached by the nutritionist, mean number of counseling calls received, and median number of attempts to contact a participant. It also showed SMS sent, SMS received, and attrition rate of participants. Bobrow and coworkers[27] also reported the number of messages sent, SMS that had a failed delivery response, and technical errors related to the delivery of SMS.

As per cost-effectiveness, no studies were found. This constitutes an underresearched area because cost-effectiveness evaluations of these interventions are critical to inform and guide policy makers' investments.

When interpreting the results of this study, some limitations should be taken into consideration. Our review was restricted to studies with rigorous design, such as RCT, meta-analysis, or systematic reviews of clinical trials. This strategy may have excluded studies with less strong designs. However, because the evidence of beneficial effects is at best modest, the inclusion of quasiexperimental studies more prone to different type of biases could have overestimated their true effects.

Another limitation was the exclusion of gray literature in the search strategy. Although the chance of finding an RCT not indexed in the most common electronic databases is low, this possibility cannot be excluded.

Although in this review the number of RCTs using mHealth to address chronic diseases in LMIC has been duplicated compared with a previous systematic review,[14] at least half of the studies found have small sample size or were proof of concept trials, which makes it difficult to extrapolate the study results to larger LMIC populations.

SUMMARY

We found few studies addressing the impact of mHealth interventions on chronic disease outcomes in LMICs. mHealth was found to have positive impact on processes of care and clinical outcomes. Yet, the effect was modest. In addition, the evidence is still scarce with respect to the effectiveness of different types of mobile interventions to reduce chronic diseases. Further research is needed to assess the effectiveness and cost-effectiveness of mHealth strategies, particularly to address hypertension, cancer, and chronic respiratory diseases.

REFERENCES

1. Wild S, Roglic G, Green A, et al. Global prevalence of diabetes: estimates for the year 2000 and projections for 2030. Diabetes Care 2004;27(5):1047–53.
2. Berendes S, Heywood P, Oliver S, et al. Quality of private and public ambulatory health care in low and middle income countries: systematic review of comparative studies. PLoS Med 2011;8(4): e1000433.
3. Association GSM. The mobile economy 2014. London: GSMA Intelligence; 2014.
4. Thirumurthy H, Lester RT. M-health for health behaviour change in resource-limited settings: applications to HIV care and beyond. Bull World Health Organ 2012;90(5):390–2.
5. Cole-Lewis H, Kershaw T. Text messaging as a tool for behavior change in disease prevention and management. Epidemiol Rev 2010;32:56–69.
6. Krishna S, Boren SA, Balas EA. Healthcare via cell phones: a systematic review. Telemed J E Health 2009;15(3):231–40.
7. Fjeldsoe BS, Marshall AL, Miller YD. Behavior change interventions delivered by mobile telephone short-message service. Am J Prev Med 2009;36(2): 165–73.
8. Whittaker R, Borland R, Bullen C, et al. Mobile phone-based interventions for smoking cessation. Cochrane Database Syst Rev 2009;(4):CD006611.
9. Horvath T, Azman H, Kennedy GE, et al. Mobile phone text messaging for promoting adherence to antiretroviral therapy in patients with HIV infection. Cochrane Database Syst Rev 2012;(3):CD009756.
10. Free C, Phillips G, Galli L, et al. The effectiveness of mobile-health technology-based health behaviour change or disease management interventions for

health care consumers: a systematic review. PLoS Med 2013;10(1):e1001362.
11. Free C, Phillips G, Watson L, et al. The effectiveness of mobile-health technologies to improve health care service delivery processes: a systematic review and meta-analysis. PLoS Med 2013;10(1): e1001363.
12. Aranda-Jan CB, Mohutsiwa-Dibe N, Loukanova S. Systematic review on what works, what does not work and why of implementation of mobile health (mHealth) projects in Africa. BMC Public Health 2014;14:188.
13. Union IT. Global ICT developments. ICT Facts & Figures 2015. Available at: https://www.itu.int/en/ITU-D/Statistics/Documents/facts/ICTFactsFigures2015.pdf. Accessed May 2016.
14. Beratarrechea A, Lee AG, Willner JM, et al. The impact of mobile health interventions on chronic disease outcomes in developing countries: a systematic review. Telemed J E Health 2014;20(1):75–82.
15. World Bank Country and Lending Groups. 2016. Available at: https://datahelpdesk.worldbank.org/knowledgebase/articles/906519. Accessed January 2016.
16. Higgins JPT, Green S, editors. Cochrane handbook for systematic reviews of interventions Version 5.1.0. London (United Kingdom): The Cochrane collaboration; 2011. Available at: www.handbook.cochrane.org. Accessed June 15, 2016.
17. Ciapponi A, Glujovsky D, Bardach A, et al. EROS: a new software for early stage of systematic reviews [abstract]. Value Health 2011;14(7):A564.
18. Khonsari S, Subramanian P, Chinna K, et al. Effect of a reminder system using an automated short message service on medication adherence following acute coronary syndrome. Eur J Cardiovasc Nurs 2015;14(2):170–9.
19. Lv Y, Zhao H, Liang Z, et al. A mobile phone short message service improves perceived control of asthma: a randomized controlled trial. Telemed J E Health 2012;18(6):420–6.
20. Goodarzi M, Ebrahimzadeh I, Rabi A, et al. Impact of distance education via mobile phone text messaging on knowledge, attitude, practice and self efficacy of patients with type 2 diabetes mellitus in Iran. J Diabetes Metab Disord 2012;11(1):10.
21. Piette JD, Datwani H, Gaudioso S, et al. Hypertension management using mobile technology and home blood pressure monitoring: results of a randomized trial in two low/middle-income countries. Telemed J E Health 2012;18(8):613–20.
22. Ramachandran A, Snehalatha C, Ram J, et al. Effectiveness of mobile phone messaging in prevention of type 2 diabetes by lifestyle modification in men in India: a prospective, parallel-group, randomised controlled trial. Lancet Diabetes Endocrinol 2013; 1(3):191–8.

23. Tamban CA, Thiele Isip-Tan I, Jimeno C. Use of short message services (SMS) for the management of type 2 diabetes mellitus: a randomized controlled trial. Journal of the ASEAN Federation of Endocrine Societies 2013;28(2):143–9. Available at: http://www.asean-endocrinejournal.org/index.php/JAFES/article/view/68. Accessed October 26, 2016.

24. Peimani M, Rambod C, Omidvar M, et al. Effectiveness of short message service-based intervention (SMS) on self-care in type 2 diabetes: a feasibility study. Prim Care Diabetes 2015;10(4):251–8.

25. Rubinstein A, Miranda JJ, Beratarrechea A, et al. Effectiveness of an mHealth intervention to improve the cardiometabolic profile of people with prehypertension in low-resource urban settings in Latin America: a randomised controlled trial. Lancet Diabetes Endocrinol 2016;4(1):52–63.

26. Wongrochananan S, Tuicomepee A, Buranarach M, et al. The effectiveness of interactive multi-modality intervention on self-management support of type 2 diabetic patients in Thailand: a cluster-randomized controlled trial. Int J Diabetes Developing Countries 2015;35(2):230–6.

27. Bobrow K, Farmer AJ, Springer D, et al. Mobile phone text messages to support treatment adherence in adults with high blood pressure (SMS-Text adherence support [StAR]): a single-blind, randomized trial. Circulation 2016;133(6):592–600.

28. Patnaik L, Joshi A, Sahu T. Mobile based intervention for reduction of coronary heart disease risk factors among patients with diabetes mellitus attending a tertiary care hospital of India. J Cardiovasc Dis Res 2014;5(4):28–36.

29. Shahid M, Mahar SA, Shaikh S, et al. Mobile phone intervention to improve diabetes care in rural areas of Pakistan: a randomized controlled trial. J Coll Physicians Surg Pak 2015;25(3):166–71.

30. Anzaldo-Campos MC, Contreras S, Vargas-Ojeda A, et al. Dulce wireless Tijuana: a randomized control trial evaluating the impact of project Dulce and short-term mobile technology on glycemic control in a family medicine clinic in Northern Mexico. Diabetes Technol Ther 2016;18(4):240–51.

31. Tian M, Ajay VS, Dunzhu D, et al. A cluster-randomized, controlled trial of a simplified multifaceted management program for individuals at high cardiovascular risk (SimCard trial) in rural Tibet, China, and Haryana, India. Circulation 2015;132(9):815–24.

32. Kamal AK, Shaikh Q, Pasha O, et al. A randomized controlled behavioral intervention trial to improve medication adherence in adult stroke patients with prescription tailored Short Messaging Service (SMS)-SMS4 Stroke study. BMC Neurol 2015;15:212.

33. Kumar S, Shewade HD, Vasudevan K, et al. Effect of mobile reminders on screening yield during opportunistic screening for type 2 diabetes mellitus in a primary health care setting: a randomized trial. Prev Med Rep 2015;2:640–4.

34. Boroumand S, Moeini M. The effect of a text message and telephone follow-up program on cardiac self-efficacy of patients with coronary artery disease: a randomized controlled trial. Iranian J Nurs Midwifery Res 2016;21(2):171–6.

35. Patnaik L, Joshi A, Sahu T. Mobile phone-based education and counseling to reduce stress among patients with diabetes mellitus attending a tertiary care hospital of India. Int J Prev Med 2015;6:37.

36. Hacking D, Haricharan HJ, Brittain K, et al. Hypertension health promotion via text messaging at a community health center in South Africa: a mixed methods study. JMIR Mhealth Uhealth 2016;4(1):e22.

37. Piette JD, Marinec N, Janda K, et al. Structured caregiver feedback enhances engagement and impact of mobile health support: a randomized trial in a lower-middle-income country. Telemed J E Health 2016;22(4):261–8.

38. Prochaska JO, Di Clemente CC. Stages and processes of self-change of smoking: toward an integrative model of change. J Consult Clin Psychol 1983;51(3):390–5.

39. Ealovega MW, Tabaei BP, Brandle M, et al. Opportunistic screening for diabetes in routine clinical practice. Diabetes Care 2004;27(1):9–12.

40. Morisky DE, Ang A, Krousel-Wood M, et al. Predictive validity of a medication adherence measure in an outpatient setting. J Clin Hypertens 2008;10(5):348–54.

41. Sullivan MD, LaCroix AZ, Russo J, et al. Self-efficacy and self-reported functional status in coronary heart disease: a six-month prospective study. Psychosom Med 1998;60(4):473–8.

42. Labrique AB, Vasudevan L, Kochi E, et al. mHealth innovations as health system strengthening tools: 12 common applications and a visual framework. Glob Health Sci Pract 2013;1(2):160–71.

43. Piette JD, Rosland AM, Marinec NS, et al. Engagement with automated patient monitoring and self-management support calls: experience with a thousand chronically ill patients. Med Care 2013;51(3):216–23.

44. Irazola VE, Gutierrez L, Bloomfield G, et al. Hypertension prevalence, awareness, treatment, and control in selected LMIC communities: results from the NHLBI/UHG network of centers of excellence for chronic diseases. Glob Heart 2016;11(1):47–59.

45. Nelson LA, Zamora-Kapoor A. Challenges in conducting mHealth research with underserved

populations: lessons learned. J Telemed Telecare 2016;22(7):436–40.

46. Rychetnik L, Frommer M, Hawe P, et al. Criteria for evaluating evidence on public health interventions. J Epidemiol Community Health 2002;56(2):119–27.

47. National Health and Medical Research. Council, NHMRC How to use the evidence: assessment and application of scientific evidence. Canberra (Australia): Commonwealth of Australia, AusInfo; 2000.

Chagas Cardiomyopathy
Clinical Presentation and Management in the Americas

Catherine Pastorius Benziger, MD[a],
Gabriel Assis Lopes do Carmo, MD, PhD[b],
Antonio Luiz Pinho Ribeiro, MD, PhD[c],*

KEYWORDS

- Chagas disease • Neglected diseases • Cardiomyopathy • Epidemiology • Trypanocidal agents

KEY POINTS

- The diagnosis and treatment of Chagas disease require specific knowledge about the acute and chronic forms of the disease.
- The initial Chagas infection is typically asymptomatic but after a decade or longer, approximately 30% of people will progress to a chronic cardiac form of Chagas cardiomyopathy with symptoms including heart failure, arrhythmias, and thromboembolism.
- Death is often premature and sudden due to arrhythmias or progressive heart failure.
- Prevention of infection through vector control programs, along with strengthened surveillance systems and rapid information sharing, are key to addressing the continued challenges of Chagas disease control globally.

Individuals, not rarely, die in their youth with an apparently healthy condition and no signs of heart disease. Many of them die while in their job, without any reasonable explanation; others die in a moment of greater physical effort, fatigue or any incident capable of exhausting the energy of the poor myocardium.

—Carlos Chagas, 1922.

INTRODUCTION

Chagas disease (American Trypanosomiasis) was first described by Carlos Chagas in 1909 during a Malaria outbreak in Lassance, State of Minas Gerais, Brazil. In his first report, he identified the etiologic agent, the parasite *Trypanosoma cruzi*, the triatomine insect vector, as well as the disease cycle, a unique discovery by one individual in the history of medicine.[1] Starting in the sixteenth century, increased anthropomotic pressure due to agricultural and livestock activities transformed the natural environment and created transport of vectors and zoonotic foci and spread of infection. By the early twentieth century, Chagas disease was a rural and periurban neglected tropical disease, closely related to poverty. However, due to mass rural-to-urban migration, and increased

Disclosures: The authors have nothing to disclose.
[a] Division of Cardiology, University of Washington, 1959 Northeast Pacific Street, Seattle, WA 98195, USA;
[b] Hospital das Clínicas and School of Medicine, Universidade Federal de Minas Gerais, Av. Prof. Alfredo Balena, 190 - sala 246, Belo Horizonte Cep:30130-100, Minas Gerais, Brazil; [c] Division of Hospital das Clínicas and School of Medicine, Department of Internal Medicine and Cardiology, Universidade Federal de Minas Gerais, Rua Campanha, 98/101, Carmo, Belo Horizonte, Cep:30310-770, Minas Gerais, Brazil
* Corresponding author. Hospital das Clinicas and School of Medicine, UFMG, Rua Campanha, 98/101, Carmo, Belo Horizonte, Minas Gerais, Brazil.
E-mail address: alpr1963br@gmail.com

cardiology.theclinics.com

urbanization and intercontinental population movement, Chagas disease has recently gained attention due to the "globalization" of the disease.[2–5]

Chronic Chagas cardiomyopathy is the leading cause of nonischemic cardiomyopathy in Latin America and affects 20% to 40% of infected patients. The most ominous manifestations of the disease are related to heart failure, arrhythmias, heart blocks, and thromboembolism. In this article, we review the epidemiology, pathogenesis, presentation, and clinical management of Chagas disease.

EPIDEMIOLOGY

Chagas disease is a disease of poverty. It is on the World Health Organization's (WHO) list of 17 neglected tropical diseases because it shares similar characteristics, such as particular geographic dispersion affecting populations with poor socioeconomic status; high morbidity and consequent mortality with significant socioeconomic impact; biomedical and psychosocial barriers to diagnosis, treatment, and control; and limited availability of resources and political priority. It is endemic to continental Latin America because it is primarily transmitted through bites from the nocturnal "kissing bug," insects from the family Reduviidae, subfamily Triatominae, which is found in the region (**Fig. 1**). The vector defecates after sucking blood at night and the infection is transmitted through the parasite-

contaminated feces/urine through a break in the skin, mouth, or eye. It has no gender predominance but local variations exist depending on different routes of transmission. *T cruzi* also can be transmitted through blood transfusions, organ transplantation, laboratory accidents, and vertical transmission during childbirth. More recently, oral (foodborne) transmission has emerged as a new route in the Amazon region, where areas that were not considered endemic had outbreaks of acute Chagas disease. Epidemiologic studies suggest that oral transmission was responsible, likely due to local foods that were infected by feces of triatomine bugs, which subsequently infected the oral mucosa of the new reservoir hosts.[6]

The prevalence of the disease has been decreasing in the past decades, mostly due to successful vector and blood transfusion control programs in several Latin American countries.[7] These programs include systematic spraying with residual insecticide, house improvements, home hygiene, blood donor screening and information, education, and community activities to increase awareness. In 1985, the WHO estimated almost 18 million people were infected,[8,9] but in the updated 2015 WHO report, an estimated 5.7 million people were infected in 21 Latin American countries.[10] The Pan American Health Organization's country-level seroprevalence estimates for 2005 range from less than 1 per 10,000 (0.01%) in Panama to nearly 7% in Bolivia. The areas with the highest prevalence (up to 30% in certain

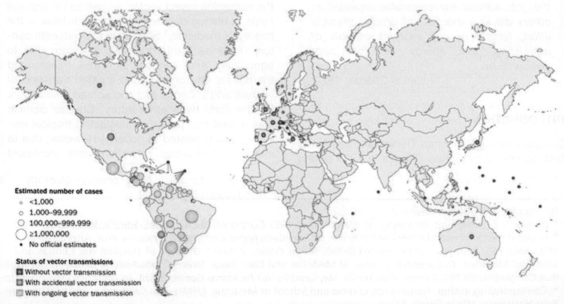

Fig. 1. WHO estimates of vector transmission between 2006 and 2009 of *Trypanosoma cruzi*. (*From* Ribeiro AL, Nunes MP, Teixeira MM, et al. Diagnosis and management of Chagas disease and cardiomyopathy. Nat Rev Cardiol 2012;9(10):578; with permission.)

communities) are in the Gran Chaco region, which includes central and south Bolivia, northern Argentina, and western Paraguay. Brazil, southern Peru, Ecuador, Nicaragua, El Salvador, and southern Mexico are also highly endemic (see **Fig. 1**). Bolivia has the highest prevalence and incidence rates, but Argentina, Brazil, and Colombia have the most people living with Chagas cardiomyopathy due to their larger population size. Argentina, Paraguay, and Bolivia have the highest seroprevalence of T cruzi in blood donors (prevalence between 2% and 3%). Congenital transmission is highest in Mexico (1788 cases in 2010) and Argentina (1457 cases in 2010).[10] Due to improvements in vector control, congenital transmission is higher than vectoral transmission in Argentina. Uruguay and Chile successfully eliminated vectoral transmission in the late 1990s and have no significant secondary mode of transmission, so risk of Chagas disease is essentially zero in these countries.

The occurrence of Chagas disease used to be restricted to specific locations in Central and South America. However, recent globalization and increase in air travel and immigration have expanded the disease to North America, Europe, Australia, and Japan.[11] In the United States, an estimated 300,000 people are affected, according to the US Centers for Disease Control and Prevention.[12]

The burden of Chagas disease is challenging to determine, as it requires estimating the prevalence of the infection, the prevalence of each of its sequelae among those with the infection, and the number of deaths attributable to the infection.[13] The 2013 Global Burden of Disease study estimated that Chagas disease was responsible for approximately 10,600 deaths (95% uncertainty interval (UI): 4200–33,000), a decrease from approximately 12,700 (95% UI: 5200–39,400) in 1990, with new cases declining annually from more than 700,000 in 1990 to 41,200 in 2013. Chagas disease accounts for 338,500 (95% UI: 183,800–846,400) disability-adjusted life years (DALYs)[14,15]; however, 4.2% of these Chagas-related DALYs and 21.7% of the Chagas-related health care costs now occur outside of Latin America.[16] Chagas disease is directly related to poverty as the presence of triatomine bugs is associated with the health risk of poor housing. It has the greatest socioeconomic impact of any parasite in Latin America. The economic impact including lost productivity is an estimated cost of US$ 1.2 billion annually, in addition to the medical costs for treating infected individuals who develop severe cardiac or digestive pathology, which are several times this amount.[9]

PATHOGENESIS

The pathogenesis of Chagas heart disease involves a complex interaction of different processes (**Fig. 2**),[17] related to tissue damage due to parasite persistence, inflammation, autoimmunity, fibrosis, dysautonomia, and microvascular changes.[18,19] After the acute, febrile phase, the T cruzi parasite hides in target tissues (namely the cardiac and digestive system muscles) and enters the chronic phase, almost always without clinical manifestations. However, a low-grade inflammation persists during the chronic phase related to the persistence of the parasite nests.

Myocardial damage due to persistence of the parasite is considered the most important mechanism in the development of Chagas cardiomyopathy.[20–22] Although necessary for the control of parasite proliferation, inflammation results in tissue damage leading to myocardial fibrosis and cardiac remodeling, and ultimately leading to Chagas cardiomyopathy.[18,23,24]

The progression of the disease is not uniform and immunoregulatory cytokines are critical for orchestrating the immune system's response, thus influencing disease development or quiescence.[25] Those with a more robust anti-inflammatory cytokine profile, represented by high expression of interleukin-10, typically remain in the indeterminate form indefinitely; whereas, those with an inflammatory profile, represented by high production of interferon-gamma and tumor necrosis factor-alpha, typically evolve more rapidly to the cardiac form.[25] Furthermore, autoimmunity may play a significant role in the pathogenesis of cardiomyopathy, as several reports have described autoantibodies and self-reactive T cells that were activated by T cruzi antigens both in patients and in animal models.[26] Autoimmunity can be triggered by 1 of 3 possible mechanisms: sensitization in the inflammatory environment after antigen exposure in damaged tissues, molecular mimicry, and polyclonal activation.[19]

Besides the immune system activation, additional mechanisms may play a role in the pathogenesis of Chagas disease. Dysautonomia is a typical feature of the disease and was confirmed by pathologic studies, which show cardiac neuronal depopulation,[27] and by functional studies evidenced by impaired parasympathetic response to pharmacologic and noninvasive maneuvers, such as handgrip and Valsalva maneuvers.[19,28] The pathogenic significance of vagal dysfunction is mostly elusive, but it seems to be related to a higher risk of sudden death observed in these patients.[29] Sympathetic denervation also can occur

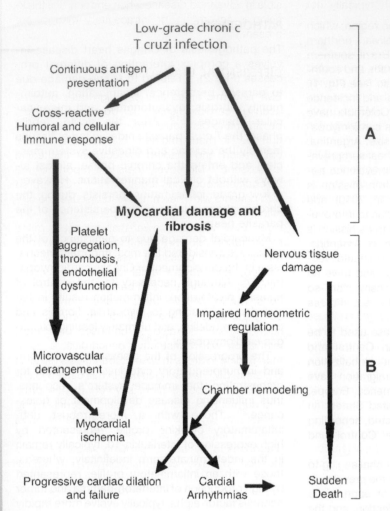

Low-grade chronic
T cruzi infection

Continuous antigen
presentation

Cross-reactive
Humoral and cellular
Immune response

Myocardial damage and fibrosis

Platelet
aggregation,
thrombosis,
endothelial
dysfunction

Nervous tissue
damage

Microvascular
derangement

Impaired homeometric
regulation

Chamber remodeling

Myocardial
ischemia

Progressive cardiac dilation
and failure

Cardial
Arrhythmias

Sudden
Death

A

B

Fig. 2. Schematic view of the patho-genesis of chronic Chagas disease. (*From* Marin-Neto JA, Cunha-Neto E, Maciel BC, et al. Pathogenesis of chronic Chagas heart disease. Circulation 2007;115:1119; with permission.)

and may participate in triggering malignant ventricular arrhythmias.[30]

Chagas disease also predisposes to microvascular dysfunction because of loss of protective endothelial factors, increased levels of prothrombotic components, and abnormal vascular reactivity due to dysautonomia.[19] Both functional and structural abnormalities may occur in the vasculature and may potentiate and amplify the chronic inflammation in the myocardial tissues.[31]

CLINICAL ASPECTS OF CHAGAS DISEASE

Chagas disease presents classically as 2 different phases: acute and chronic. Each phase has different clinical characteristics, diagnostic criteria, and treatment. The most common symptoms in the various Chagas disease phases are listed in **Table 1**.

Acute Phase

The acute phase, most frequent in children, generally occurs after 7 to 10 days of parasite inoculation and can last 6 to 8 weeks.[32,33] Recognition of the disease is achieved in only 1% to 2% of patients.[32] The main symptoms are fever and malaise in up to 5% of people, but sweating, muscular pain, anorexia, and, sometimes, vomiting and diarrhea, also can be present.[33,34] The main findings on physical examination are hepatosplenomegaly and signs of meningoencephalitis and heart failure, secondary to acute myocarditis.[33,34] Up to 8% of cases of vectoral transmission present with signs of parasite inoculation, called Chagoma. The most common, eyelid edema, is called Romaña's sign. Up to 10% of patients with recognized disease die in the acute phase, especially children, due to acute myocarditis.[32,33]

Table 1
Clinical phase of Chagas disease and typical symptoms

Phase	Symptoms
Acute	Variable, asymptomatic to nonspecific symptoms (fever, lymphadenopathy, hepatosplenomegaly, anemia, anorexia, diarrhea), Chagoma, myocarditis, meningoencephalitis
Chronic, indeterminant	Asymptomatic
Chronic, cardiac	Dilated cardiomyopathy, heart failure, arrhythmias, thromboembolism
Chronic, gastrointestinal	Megaesophagus, megacolon, dysphagia, odynophagia, constipation, and abdominal pain
Chronic, mixed cardiac, and gastrointestinal	Combination of the cardiac and gastrointestinal manifestations listed previously
Chronic, neurologic	Often secondary to Chagas cardiomyopathy with thromboembolic cerebrovascular events
Chronic, reactivation	Immunosuppressed (human immunodeficiency virus, leukemia, immunosuppressive medications); transplant patients often have subcutaneous nodules

However, more commonly this phase is asymptomatic.[33]

During the acute phase, the host body is exposed to a high level of parasitemia, which is detectable on laboratory tests, whereas serologic tests for *T cruzi* antibodies are often negative. Other nonspecific laboratory findings are leukocytosis with pronounced lymphocytosis, increased erythrocyte sedimentation rate, and abnormal liver function tests.

In acute cases transmitted by the oral route, there is lack of Chagoma and patients present with a febrile syndrome and myalgias, leg and facial edema, abdominal pain, hepatosplenomegaly, dyspnea, palpitations, and hemorrhagic jaundice. Differential diagnosis is broad and includes other infectious etiologies, such as dengue, hepatitis, Hantavirus infection, or severe leptospirosis.[6]

Chagas disease reactivation can occur after immunosuppression, especially after cardiac transplantation. The symptoms are similar to acute vectoral infection but the differential diagnosis includes other opportunistic infections and organ rejection.

Acute Chagas myocarditis has a similar presentation to other etiologies of myocarditis, including infectious agents, cardiotoxins, and radiation. Diagnosis can be made by detection of the parasite in myocardial biopsy of those exposed to a typical endemic setting and a high clinical suspicion. Cardiac test findings are nonspecific but denote the presence of myocarditis if present with electrocardiogram findings of low voltage,

bundle branch block, diffuse ST-T wave changes, or prolonged PR interval or more advanced atrioventricular block.[34,35] Sinus tachycardia is often present and attributable to fever alone. Arrhythmias, such as atrial fibrillation, ventricular premature beats and ventricular tachycardia (VT) are uncommon in the acute phase. Most electrocardiographic findings resolve within 1 year. Chest radiograph demonstrates an enlarged cardiac silhouette (cardiac-to-thoracic width ratio >50%), usually due to the presence of a pericardial effusion.[34,35] Echocardiography demonstrates a pericardial effusion with normal or near normal left and right ventricular function. Mitral and/or tricuspid regurgitation secondary to acute myocarditis are frequently present and often resolve with treatment of Chagas disease. Endomyocardial biopsy is generally not required to establish the diagnosis, but may confirm the diagnosis of Chagas myocarditis if intracellular *T cruzi* amastigote nests are identified as opposed to acute cellular rejection in those with heart transplantation (**Fig. 3**). Often only inflammatory changes with or without fibrosis are seen. Symptoms generally resolve over a period of 1 to 3 months.

Chronic Indeterminate Form

The chronic phase is initially called indeterminate, as the parasite remains hidden in the target tissues. Different clinical forms may be observed, including cardiac form without ventricular dysfunction, cardiac form with ventricular

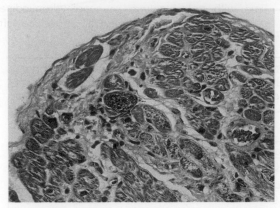

Fig. 3. Myocardial amastigote nest in a heart transplant patient with Chagas disease. (hematoxylin-eosin, original magnification ×40.) (*Courtesy of* Dr Paula Carmo, MD, Belo Horizonte, Minas Gerais, Brazil.)

dysfunction, gastrointestinal form, clinically manifested as megacolon or megaesophagus, and mixed cardiac and gastrointestinal.[33]

The indeterminate form was defined in 1985 as a positive Chagas laboratory test with serologic or parasite detection, but no clinical symptoms, signs, or abnormalities on a 12-lead electrocardiogram or radiographic evidence of cardiac or gastrointestinal involvement.[32,33,36] Although several other examinations, such as exercise treadmill test, 24-hour Holter monitor, myocardial scintigraphy, nuclear magnetic resonance, tests of autonomic evaluation, and even echocardiography, can show abnormalities, the 2011 Latin American guidelines on Chagas

disease ratified the previous definition, because long-term prognosis is similar to the general population.[33,37–45] A barium enema test is not required in those with indeterminate disease without constipation.

There are no formal guidelines for monitoring those in the indeterminate form but a repeat electrocardiogram every 1 to 2 years and repeat chest radiograph every 3 to 5 years is reasonable, because 2% to 5% of patients evolve to symptomatic disease each year.[32,46,47] An echocardiographic assessment every 3 to 5 years, or when a there is change in symptoms or electrocardiogram tracing, is recommended because the appearance of new electrocardiographic alterations is associated with a significant decrease (of 5% or more) in left ventricle ejection fraction.[48]

Chronic Determinate Forms

Patients with Chagas disease who develop clinical symptoms are divided into 3 groups: cardiac, digestive, and cardiodigestive forms. After 5 to 30 years, approximately 20% to 40% of patients with the indeterminate form will develop chronic Chagas cardiomyopathy and an additional 15% will develop chronic gastrointestinal disease.

The cardiac form of Chagas can present with or without ventricular failure. Previous nomenclature of arrhythmic or congestive forms are no longer used[33] and are currently classified according to international recommendations based on ventricular dysfunction (**Table 2**).[33] Chronic infection is confirmed with serologic tests and detection of immunoglobulin (Ig)G anti–*T cruzi* antibodies.

Table 2
Chagas disease classification according to ventricular dysfunction

Acute Phase		Chronic Phase			
	Indeterminate form	Cardiac form without ventricular failure	Cardiac form with ventricular failure		
	A	B1	B2	C	D
Acute Chagas disease	Positive Chagas serology, but no structural heart disease or symptoms of HF	Structural heart disease (ECG or echocardiography) without ventricular dysfunction and no signs or symptoms, actual or previous, of HF	Structural heart disease with global ventricular dysfunction, but no signs or symptoms, actual or previous, of HF	Ventricular dysfunction and signs or symptoms, actual or previous, of HF	Refractory heart failure, even at rest, despite optimal medical treatment and need of specialized interventions

Abbreviations: ECG, electrocardiogram; HF, heart failure.

Adapted from Andrade JP, Marin-Neto JA, Paola AA, et al. I Latin American guidelines for the diagnosis and treatment of Chagas cardiomyopathy. Arq Bras Cardiol 2011;96(6):436; with permission.

Symptoms include those of heart failure (dyspnea on exertion, fatigue, and edema), arrhythmias (palpitations, dizziness, weakness, and syncope), thromboembolism (systemic and pulmonary), and chest pain syndrome (angina).[49] Biventricular failure is often the first clinical manifestation; however, stroke or cardiac arrhythmia, including sudden death, also can occur.[32,50] The physical examination often demonstrates a loud holosystolic murmur of mitral and/or tricuspid regurgitation, wide splitting of the second heart sound due to right bundle branch block, and prominent diffuse apical thrust. Examination findings of right heart failure (elevated jugular venous pressure, peripheral edema, ascites, and hepatomegaly) are more pronounced than left-sided failure (dyspnea and pulmonary rales). Symptoms of chronic gastrointestinal disease sequelae include megaesophagus and megacolon manifestations, such as dysphagia, odynophagia, constipation, and abdominal pain.

Chest radiograph often shows cardiomegaly with or without pulmonary congestion pattern. The most common electrocardiographic findings are right bundle branch block (RBBB) and/or left anterior fascicular block (LAFB), which can occur early in the course of the disease (**Fig. 4**).[51] All types of atrial and ventricular arrhythmias may occur, including sinus node dysfunction, first-degree, second-degree, and third-degree atrioventricular block, and complex ventricular arrhythmias. Other frequent electrocardiographic

findings are abnormal Q waves, low QRS voltage, various degrees of atrioventricular block, diffuse ST-T changes; and QT interval prolongation.[51–53] In advanced disease, atrial fibrillation may be observed.[34,54] Although VT can arise from both ventricles, scar from fibrosis of the left ventricle is the main source of scar-related reentry VT and the inferolateral wall, in particular, is the most site of sustained VT on endocardial mapping.[55]

If a patient has either cardiac signs or symptoms, or the electrocardiogram or chest radiograph has abnormalities consistent with Chagas disease, the next step is transthoracic echocardiography and 24-hour ambulatory electrocardiographic (Holter) monitoring. A Holter monitor may help identify atrial and ventricular arrhythmias, as well as heart block. Echocardiographic findings vary from normal to severely impaired left and right ventricular systolic function. In early stages, mild segmental wall-motion abnormalities may be predictors of subsequent dysfunction. The most common wall-motion abnormality is in the inferolateral wall, which is the predominant source for macroreentrant VT. Moderate to severe mitral and/or tricuspid regurgitation are often present in chronic Chagas disease with more advanced stages and are secondary to ventricular dilation.[45]

Left ventricular apical aneurysm is common, whereas right ventricular aneurysm is much less common (**Fig. 5**). Ventricular mural thrombi form in the dilated cardiac chambers, particularly in left ventricular apical aneurysms, and can cause

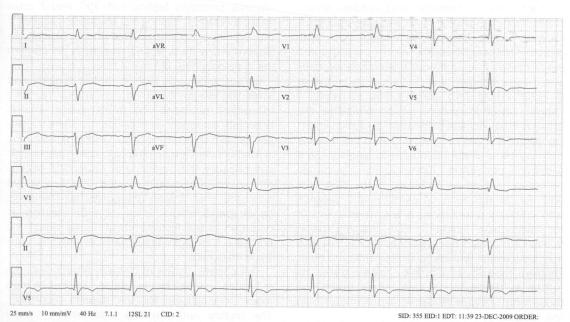

25 mm/s   10 mm/mV   40 Hz   7.1.1   12SL 21   CID: 2   SID: 355 EID:1 EDT: 11:39 23-DEC-2009 ORDER:

Fig. 4. Electrocardiogram of a patient with chronic Chagas disease showing the typical findings of an RBBB with LAFB.

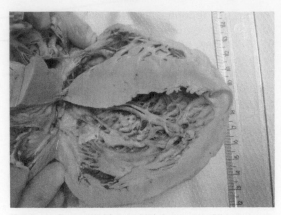

Fig. 5. Left ventricular apical aneurysm in an autopsied heart. (*Courtesy of* Dr Paula Carmo, MD, and Dr Stanley Araújo, MD, Belo Horizonte, Minas Gerais, Brazil.)

systemic emboli. Mural thrombi are equally frequent in the left and right chambers, but death is more common by emboli in the pulmonary circulation that can arise from either venous or right heart thrombi. Emboli also form in the atrial appendages in patients with atrial fibrillation. Chagas disease has a risk of stroke between 0.6% and 2.7% per year and seems to be an independent risk factor, with rates higher than other cardiomyopathies.[56–58] Apical aneurysms also can be seen in the apical variant of hypertrophic cardiomyopathy, which also would have apical hypertrophy that is not typically seen in Chagas disease, and is important to differentiate.

Chest pain is common and cardiac stress testing may be helpful to differentiate epicardial coronary artery disease from chest pain syndrome. However, baseline electrocardiographic abnormalities frequently make interpretation difficult. Stress imaging with radionuclide perfusion or echocardiographic imaging may be helpful if baseline electrocardiographic abnormalities are present. Radionuclide myocardial perfusion imaging using PET has not been studied in this disease but may be a useful alternative to single photon emission computed tomographic myocardial perfusion imaging as it can aid in the diagnosis and risk stratification of symptomatic patients with coronary artery disease and assessment of left ventricular function. PET imaging using fluorine-18 labeled deoxyglucose (FDG-PET) also may be a useful tool and complementary to other imaging modalities. Cardiac catheterization is helpful to diagnose coronary artery disease in those with unstable ischemic symptoms or high risk factors.

Cardiac MRI is helpful for assessment of left and right ventricular size and function if echocardiographic assessment is suboptimal, as well as to determine the presence and extent of myocardial fibrosis by late gadolinium enhancement. Extent of myocardial scar as detected by late gadolinium enhancement on cardiac MRI is correlated with New York Heart Association (NYHA) functional class and degree of electrocardiographic abnormalities and arrhythmias.[59]

Electrophysiology testing is warranted for assessment of sinus node dysfunction and atrioventricular conduction, as well as to induce VT when the origin of symptoms remains uncertain after noninvasive evaluation, especially in case of syncope.

As with the indeterminate phase, there are no formal guidelines for ongoing monitoring, especially given the heterogeneity in this clinical disease. It is reasonable to obtain an annual electrocardiogram, chest radiograph, and echocardiogram or as per guidelines depending on severity of disease and the patient's symptoms.

DIAGNOSIS

The diagnosis of acute Chagas disease is made by the detection of the parasite in blood samples or by seroconversion. Enzyme-linked immunosorbent assay (ELISA), indirect immunofluorescence (IIF), indirect hemagglutination (IHA) test, and parasite polymerase chain reaction (PCR) are the most widely available tests. There are also rapid diagnostic tests that can directly detect the causative parasite, *T cruzi*.[60] In the chronic phase, the parasitemia burden is lower and diagnosis often requires serologic testing with IgG anti–*T cruzi* antibody testing. Making the diagnosis requires 2 positive laboratory tests and if the results are discordant, a third test is necessary to confirm the diagnosis (**Fig. 6**).

Seroprevalence is high in certain regions and screening pregnant women for *T cruzi* is required to control mother-to-child transmission. This is especially important in nonendemic areas if a patient is from an endemic area. Testing of newborns in mothers who are serologically confirmed is difficult because the presence of anti-IgG *T cruzi* is often of maternal origin and the detection of IgM does not provide satisfactory results. Therefore, direct parasitologic tests or PCR testing is preferred in the first month of life to detect the parasite. Serologic tests can be ordered after 9 months of life.

The chronic nature of Chagas disease with an extended asymptomatic phase requires a high index of suspicion for the definite diagnosis. The history and physical examination should focus on 2 parts: the epidemiologic risk of infection by *T cruzi* and the symptoms of cardiac or

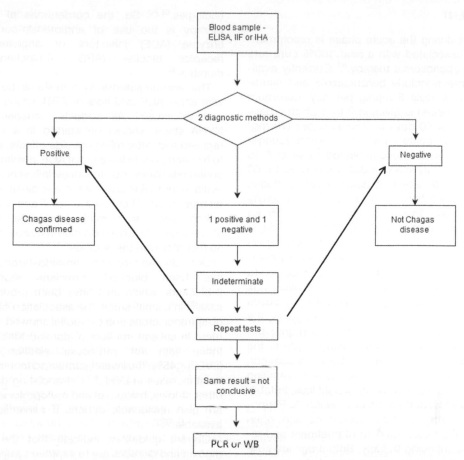

Fig. 6. Laboratory diagnostic algorithm of Chagas disease. ELISA, enzyme-linked immunosorbent assay; IIF, indirect immunofluorescence; IHA, indirect hemagglutination assay; PCR, polymerase chain reaction; WB, Western blot. (*Adapted from* Andrade JP, Marin-Neto JA, Paola AA, et al. I Latin American guidelines for the diagnosis and treatment of Chagas cardiomyopathy. Arq Bras Cardiol 2011;96(6):436; with permission.)

gastrointestinal organ involvement. The epidemiologic questions include asking about the patient's country of origin, including department or region, urban or rural residence, and if the patient ever lived in an adobe house. In addition, questions include asking about any prior knowledge of Chagas disease in the area or areas in which the patient has lived, maternal history of Chagas disease, and prior blood transfusion or transplant recipient in an endemic country.

To detect underlying heart disease, ask the patient about his or her symptoms as they relate to heart rhythm disturbances (palpitations, syncope), heart failure, venous and systemic thromboembolism (pulmonary or systemic embolism, usually cerebrovascular disease), and microvascular events (chest pain). Questions regarding gastrointestinal involvement include esophageal disorder symptoms (dysphagia, regurgitation, sore throat, night cough, drooling, parotid hypertrophy) and gastrointestinal symptoms (dyspepsia, heartburn, bloating, epigastric pain) and colonic symptoms (constipation). The physical examination should consist of height, weight, blood pressure, heart rate, detailed cardiovascular examination and thorough abdominal examination. In nonendemic countries, testing for *T cruzi* is recommended for adults originating in continental Latin America or who have made long stays (at least 1 month) to endemic regions, almost exclusively in rural areas, and have either a highly suggestive epidemiologic history, are currently pregnant or immunosuppressed, or have symptoms or signs suggestive of Chagas disease. The definite diagnosis of chronic Chagas disease requires serologic confirmation, as depicted in **Fig. 6.** ELISA and IFA with sensitivity > 99.5% and specificity from 97 to 98%. IHA tests have a sensitivity of 97 to 98% and specificity of 99%.[33]

TREATMENT

Treatment during the acute phase is recommended and associated with a near 100% cure rate with antitrypanosomal therapy.[61] Currently available regimens include benznidazole and nifurtimox. Benznidazole 5 mg/kg per day (maximum 300 mg/24 hours) is given in 2 to 3 divided daily oral doses for 60 days in chronic cases (10 mg/kg per day in acute cases). In children younger than 12 years, the recommended dose is 8 to 10 mg/kg per day in 3 to 4 daily oral doses for 60 days. The side effect of benznidazole includes mild gastrointestinal distress but it is generally well tolerated. Thus, patients weighing 65 kg receive the maximum 300 mg daily for 60 days. The most serious adverse reaction is skin hypersensitivity with the appearance of pruritic erythematous rash and can be severe, leading to discontinuation of therapy. The dose of nifurtimox is 8 to 10 mg/kg per day in 3 to 4 daily oral doses for 60 days. In children ages 11 to 16 years, the recommended dose is 12.5 to 15.0 mg/kg per day and in children younger than 11 years, the dose is 15 to 20 mg/kg per day. The most common side effects include anorexia, nausea, vomiting and abdominal pain, diarrhea, weight loss, irritability, drowsiness, and psychiatric disorders. Peripheral neuropathy is dose dependent and often occurs in the second month of treatment and requires discontinuing therapy. Both drugs are contraindicated in pregnant women and require delay in treatment until delivery. They are also contraindicated in patients with severe liver or kidney failure. Use of alcohol during treatment should be avoided. Due to side effects, only 50% to 60% of adult patients complete the entire treatment course.

Cure rates decrease in the chronic phase and, although the goal is to prevent the development of the clinical symptoms, persistence of parasitemia is a key factor in progression of disease. Preliminary observational studies suggested that antitrypanosomal therapy may have an impact in the prognosis of patients.[62–64] This information has led to the recommendation of treatment for specific situations of chronic Chagas disease by current guidelines.[33] However, although antitrypanosomal therapy leads to a reduction in parasitemia, there was no reduction in cardiac complications or death after a mean follow-up of 5.4 years, according to the large, randomized controlled trial, BENEFIT.[65]

Because of the lack of adequate studies, treatment choices for chronic Chagas cardiomyopathy are derived mainly from studies that included patients with nonischemic heart failure of other etiologies.[66,67] So, the cornerstone of medical therapy is the use of angiotensin-converting-enzyme (ACE) inhibitors or angiotensin II-receptor blocker (ARB), β-blockers, and diuretics.[68]

The renin-angiotensin system should be blocked with either ACE inhibitors or ARB, which are safe and effective.[69] All patients, independent of NYHA stage, should be started in a low-dose regimen and, after ruling out side effects, progress to higher doses. In the case of ACE inhibitor or ARB contraindications, due to kidney failure or hyperkalemia, hydralazine plus isosorbide dinitrate should be prescribed.[70] For NYHA class III and IV patients, spironolactone or eplerenone is indicated, because studies have shown a reduction in morbidity as well as mortality with these drugs.[71–73]

Once the renin-angiotensin-aldosterone system has been blocked, clinicians must start β-blockers, which also have been proven to be safe.[69] In a small study, the association of enalapril, spironolactone and carvedilol showed improvement in several markers of cardiac function. For those with left ventricular ejection fraction (LVEF) ≤45%, the investigators also found a significant increase in LVEF.[69] Extrapolating data from other studies, bisoprolol and metoprolol succinate are also reasonable options if carvedilol is not available.[33]

Current guidelines indicate that the use of digoxin and diuretics are to improve symptoms after maximal titration of medical therapy with an ACE inhibitor or ARB, blockade of aldosterone and β-blockers, because these agents have not been shown to decrease mortality in previous studies of patients with heart failure (not specifically studied in Chagas patients).[33]

For patients whom medical therapy has failed, referral to a center capable of performing heart transplantation is indicated. Although Chagas disease poses a worse prognosis when compared with other cardiomyopathies, after heart transplantation, patients have a better outcome.[74]

In an attempt to prevent cardioembolic stroke in Chagas disease, Sousa and colleagues[75] developed a score system to guide anticoagulation or aspirin use in this population. However, the small number of events and other limitations precludes the indiscriminate use of this score. Pharmacologic treatment for prevention of thromboembolism should follow the current guidelines on anticoagulation.

The widespread use of antiarrhythmics to prevent ventricular arrhythmias is generally not indicated, due to the paucity of information about the potential benefit.[68] Before prescribing antiarrhythmics, clinicians must be sure the patient is already on the maximum dose of β-blockers, if there are no contraindications. This may prevent premature ventricular beats, as well as other ventricular or atrial arrhythmias. The most used antiarrhythmic drug in Chagas disease is amiodarone. Despite its side effects on thyroid, skin, and lung, amiodarone reduces the number of shocks triggered by implanted cardioverter defibrillators (ICD).[76]

The use of ICDs for primary prevention in patients with ejection fraction ≤35% has never been tested in patients with Chagas disease. Lack of financial and health system resources, especially in Latin America, makes it nearly impossible to offer a primary prevention ICD to this subgroup of patients with Chagas disease. There is reasonable evidence that ICD should be used for secondary prevention[68,77,78] in patients with sustained VT or were resuscitated from sudden cardiac death, or with syncope due to inducible VT. Patients with Chagas disease who received an ICD are more prone to receive (appropriate) shocks and may benefit from the routine use of amiodarone[68,77] to decrease the frequency of shocks. Cases refractory to antiarrhythmic therapy may need to be treated by invasive ablation techniques.

The treatment of bradyarrhythmias with pacemaker placement and resynchronization therapy in Chagas disease should follow currently available guidelines.

PREVENTION

Despite the enormous benefit of preventive therapy on the control of many neglected tropical diseases, unfortunately it does not work for Chagas disease. The most effective approaches are vector control programs in endemic areas, which require retaining political interest, public health resources, and financial commitments, as well as active surveillance and control programs. For nonvectoral transmission, maintaining universal screening for blood donors and organ transplantation donors and recipients is an important opportunity to be able to provide care for those with positive results. Last, strategies to screen pregnant woman who are at increased risk of T cruzi infection, as well as screen neonates and any affected neonate's siblings are important strategies to reduce (and eliminate) disease transmission in areas in which vectoral transmission is low.[79,80]

Using pesticides developed for vector control, Chagas eradication has been effectively achieved in many areas in Latin America, such as much of Chile, Uruguay, and Brazil. However, it requires strong public health infrastructure and policies to implement adequate programs in the remaining countries of South and Central America. In certain rural areas of Argentina, Paraguay, Mexico, and Bolivia, inadequate housing and poor vector control remain a big problem. Thus, the disease continues to affect people living in extreme poverty who lack access to adequate health care and treatment. Insufficient prevention propagates the vicious cycle of ill health and subsequent poverty in these areas.

PROGNOSIS

Deaths are rare in the acute phase and most deaths attributable to Chagas disease result from downstream cardiovascular sequelae. Sudden death accounts for approximately 55% to 65% of deaths in patients with chronic Chagas and is likely underestimated due to underreporting, particularly in rural areas.[13] It is more common in those with severe underlying heart disease and is precipitated by intense exercise. The main causes are VT or ventricular fibrillation, complete atrioventricular block, or asystole.[77] Progressive heart failure accounts for 25% to 30% of deaths, and stroke in 10% to 15%.

The Rassi score is a risk score for predicting mortality and was developed in 424 patients with Chagas cardiomyopathy and validated in a separate cohort. It includes 6 independent predictors of mortality, and each predictor was assigned a point value (**Table 3**).[81,82] Several other predictors of adverse outcomes in Chagas disease are described. The most important are presented in **Table 4**. An algorithm has been proposed to guide mortality risk assessment (**Fig. 7**).

Table 3 Rassi score for predicting mortality in Chagas disease	
Risk Factor	**Points**
NYHA class III or IV	5
Cardiomegaly on chest radiograph	5
Segmental or global WMA[a]	3
Nonsustained VT[b]	3
Low QRS voltage[c]	2
Male sex	2

Patients were classified as low risk (score 0-6 points), intermediate (score 7-11 points) and high (score 12-20 points), with a mortality of 10%, 44% and 84% in 10 years of follow-up study, respectively.

Abbreviations: NYHA, New York Heart Association; VT, ventricular tachycardia; WMA, wall-motion abnormality.

[a] WMA is evaluated with echocardiogram.
[b] Nonsustained VT diagnosed on 24-hour ambulatory Holter.
[c] Low QRS voltage (<0.5 mV) on electrocardiogram.

Table 4
Predictors of adverse outcomes in Chagas disease

Author, Year	End Points	Prognostic Factors
Salles et al,[83] 2003	All-cause mortality	Age, heart rate, Q waves, QT dispersion, cardiomegaly, LVSD
Basquiera et al,[84] 2003	Cardiac death, presence of new ECG or echocardiogram abnormalities	Presence of parasitic DNA, male sex
Viotti et al,[85] 2004	New ECG abnormalities, change in clinical group or death	Change in clinical group, LVSD, LVEF
Viotti et al,[86] 2005	Disease progression or death	Age, LVSD, intraventricular conduction disorders, sustained VT, benznidazole treatment
Benchimol Barbosa et al,[87] 2007	Cardiac death or documented episodes of VT	Apical aneurysm, isolated premature ventricular beats >614 per 24 h, LVEF <62%
Cardinalli-Neto et al,[88] 2007	All-cause mortality	Number of shocks per patient with ICD by day 30
Ribeiro et al,[89] 2008	Cardiovascular death	LVEF, nonsustained VT, prolonged filtered QRS duration (signal-averaged ECG)
Theodoropoulos et al,[90] 2008	All-cause mortality	No β-blocker use, digoxin use, low serum sodium levels, LVEF, NYHA functional class
Nunes et al,[91] 2009	Death or cardiac transplantation	NYHA functional class, LVEF, right ventricular function, left atrial volume, E/e' ratio
Gonçalves et al,[92] 2010	All-cause mortality	Aged ≥39 years, black ethnicity, right bundle branch block and left anterior hemiblock, left bundle branch block, premature ventricular contractions
Lima-Costa et al,[93] 2010	All-cause mortality	Levels of B-type natriuretic peptide, ECG (Minnesota code) major abnormalities
Pedrosa et al,[94] 2011	Cardiovascular death	Exercise-induced ventricular arrhythmia, cardiomegaly on chest radiograph
Ribeiro et al,[95] 2011	Cardiovascular death	Repolarization variability, LVEF, nonsustained ventricular tachycardia, QRS duration >133 ms
Sarabanda & Marin-Neto,[96] 2011	Death caused by Chagas disease	LVEF <40%
Bestetti et al,[97] 2011	Death or cardiac transplantation	Lack of β-blocker use, need for inotropic support, LVSD
Nunes et al,[98] 2012	Death or cardiac transplantation	NYHA functional class, LVEF, right ventricular function, left atrial volume, E/e' ratio and interaction (LVEF and E/e' ratio)

Abbreviations: ECG, electrocardiogram; E/e' ratio, ratio of the early transmitral velocity to the tissue Doppler mitral annular early diastolic velocity; ICD, implantable cardioverter defibrillator; LVEF, left ventricular ejection fraction; LVSD, left ventricular systolic dimension; NYHA, New York Heart Association; VT, ventricular tachycardia.

Adapted from Ribeiro AL, Nunes MP, Teixeira MM, et al. Diagnosis and management of Chagas disease and cardiomyopathy. Nat Rev Cardiol 2012;9(10):582; with permission.

Proposed algorithm to guide mortality risk assessment and therapeutic decision-making in patients with Chagas disease

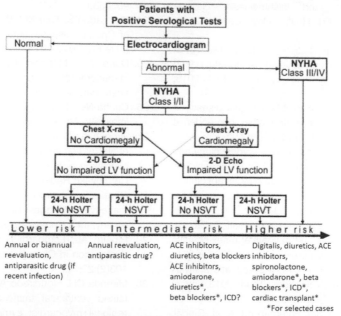

Fig. 7. Mortality risk assessment in Chagas disease. LV, left ventricle; NSVT, nonsustained VT; NYHA, New York heart association. (*Adapted from* Rassi A Jr, Rassi A, Rassi SG, et al. Predictors of mortality in chronic Chagas disease: a systematic review of observational studies. Circulation 2007;115:1107; with permission.)

Ten-year mortality in patients with 12 to 20 points was 84% to 85% (for the original and validation cohorts, respectively); for patients with 7 to 11 points, it was 37% to 44%, and for patients with 0 to 6 points, it was 9% to 10%. The combination of left ventricular systolic dysfunction and nonsustained VT was associated with particularly high risk (15.1-fold increased risk of death).[81] The presence of nonsustained VT alone was associated with a 2.15-fold increased risk of death.

SUMMARY

Chagas cardiomyopathy is a chronic condition and remains a significant cause of morbidity and mortality in Latin America. The diagnosis and treatment require specific knowledge about the acute and chronic forms of the disease. Chronic Chagas cardiomyopathy manifests as disorders of the heart's conduction system, heart failure, or pulmonary or cerebrovascular embolisms, leading to premature mortality and perpetuates the cycle of poverty in those affected. A strong surveillance system is required to monitor the foci of active transmission, diagnosed and estimated cases, health care coverage, and advances in vectoral control, as well as maintaining screening of blood donors and pregnant women.

REFERENCES

1. Chagas C. Nova trypanozomiaze humana. Mem Inst Oswaldo Cruz 1909;1(2):159–218.
2. Kirchhoff LV. American trypanosomiasis (Chagas' disease)—a tropical disease now in the United States. N Engl J Med 1993;329(9):639–14.
3. Schmunis GA. Epidemiology of Chagas disease in non-endemic countries: the role of international migration. Mem Inst Oswaldo Cruz 2007;102(Suppl 1):75–85.
4. Schmunis GA, Yadon ZE. Chagas disease: a Latin American health problem becoming a world health problem. Acta Trop 2010;115(1–2):14–21.
5. Hotez PJ, Dumonteil E, Woc-Colburn L, et al. Chagas disease: "the new HIV/AIDS of the Americas". PLoS Negl Trop Dis 2012;6(5):e1498.
6. Shikanai-Yasuda MA, Carvalho NB. Oral transmission of Chagas disease. Clin Infect Dis 2012;54(6): 845–52.
7. Dias JC. Evolution of Chagas disease screening programs and control programs: historical perspective. Glob Heart 2015;10(3):193–202.
8. WHO. Control of Chagas disease: second report of a WHO expert committee. Geneva: World Health Organization; 2002. p. 64.
9. WHO. Research priorities for Chagas disease, human African trypanosomiasis and leishmaniasis.

In: Technical Report of the Special Programme for Research and Training in Tropical Diseases Reference Group on Chagas Diseaes, human African trympanosomiasis and leishmaniasis. Geneva (Switzerland): World Health Organization; 2012. p. 11.

10. World Health Organization. Chagas disease in Latin America: an epidemiological update based on 2010 estimates. Wkly Epidemiol Rec 2015; 90(6):33–44.

11. Gascon J, Bern C, Pinazo MJ. Chagas disease in Spain, the United States and other non-endemic countries. Acta Trop 2010;115(1–2):22–7.

12. CDC. American trypanosomiasis: epidemiology and risk factors. Atlanta (Georgia): CDC; 2013. Available at: http://www.cdc.gov/parasites/chagas/epi.html.

13. Stanaway JD, Roth G. The burden of Chagas disease. Glob Heart 2015;10:139–44.

14. GBD 2013 Mortality and Causes of Death Collaborators. Global, regional, and national age-sex specific all-cause and cause-specific mortality for 240 causes of death, 1990-2013: a systematic analysis for the Global Burden of Disease Study 2013. Lancet 2015;385(9963):117–71.

15. Murray CJ, Barber RM, Foreman KJ, et al. Global, regional, and national disability-adjusted life years (DALYs) for 306 diseases and injuries and healthy life expectancy (HALE) for 188 countries, 1990-2013: quantifying the epidemiological transition. Lancet 2015;386(10009):2145–91.

16. Lee BY, Bacon KM, Bottazzi ME, et al. Global economic burden of Chagas disease: a computational simulation model. Lancet Infect Dis 2013;13(4):342–8.

17. Bonney KM, Engman DM. Chagas heart disease pathogenesis: one mechanism or many? Curr Mol Med 2008;8(6):510–8.

18. Tanowitz HB, Machado FS, Spray DC, et al. Developments in the management of Chagas cardiomyopathy. Expert Rev Cardiovasc Ther 2015;13(12): 1393–409.

19. Marin-Neto JA, Cunha-Neto E, Maciel BC, et al. Pathogenesis of chronic Chagas heart disease. Circulation 2007;115(9):1109–23.

20. Sabino EC, Ribeiro AL, Lee TH, et al. Detection of *Trypanosoma cruzi* DNA in blood by PCR is associated with Chagas cardiomyopathy and disease severity. Eur J Heart Fail 2015;17(4): 416–23.

21. Schijman AG, Vigliano CA, Viotti RJ, et al. *Trypanosoma cruzi* DNA in cardiac lesions of Argentinean patients with end-stage chronic Chagas heart disease. Am J Trop Med Hyg 2004;70(2): 210–20.

22. Zhang L, Tarleton RL. Parasite persistence correlates with disease severity and localization in chronic Chagas' disease. J Infect Dis 1999;180(2): 480–6.

23. Machado FS, Tanowitz HB, Ribeiro AL. Pathogenesis of Chagas cardiomyopathy: role of inflammation and oxidative stress. J Am Heart Assoc 2013;2(5): e000539.

24. Machado FS, Tyler KM, Brant F, et al. Pathogenesis of Chagas disease: time to move on. Front Biosci (Elite Ed) 2012;4:1743–58.

25. Dutra WO, Menezes CA, Magalhaes LM, et al. Immunoregulatory networks in human Chagas disease. Parasite Immunol 2014;36(8):377–87.

26. Cunha-Neto E, Teixeira PC, Nogueira LG, et al. Autoimmunity. Adv Parasitol 2011;76:129–52.

27. Junqueira Junior LF, Beraldo PS, Chapadeiro E, et al. Cardiac autonomic dysfunction and neuroganglionitis in a rat model of chronic Chagas' disease. Cardiovasc Radiol 1992;26(4):324–9.

28. Oliveira E, Ribeiro AL, Assis SF, et al. The Valsalva maneuver in Chagas disease patients without cardiopathy. Int J Control 2002;82(1):49–54.

29. Ribeiro AL, Lombardi F, Sousa MR, et al. Vagal dysfunction in Chagas disease. Int J Control 2005; 103(2):225–6.

30. Miranda CH, Figueiredo AB, Maciel BC, et al. Sustained ventricular tachycardia is associated with regional myocardial sympathetic denervation assessed with 123I-metaiodobenzylguanidine in chronic Chagas cardiomyopathy. J Nucl Med 2011;52(4):504–10.

31. Marin-Neto JA, Simoes MV, Rassi JA. Pathogenesis of chronic Chagas cardiomyopathy: the role of coronary microvascular derangements. Rev Soc Bras Med Trop 2013;46(5):536–41.

32. Ribeiro AL, Rocha MO. Indeterminate form of Chagas disease: considerations about diagnosis and prognosis. Rev Soc Bras Med Trop 1998;31(3): 301–14 [in Portuguese].

33. Andrade JP, Marin-Neto JA, Paola AA, et al. Latin American guidelines for the diagnosis and treatment of Chagas cardiomyopathy. Arq Bras Cardiol 2011; 96(6):434–42.

34. Laranja FS, Dias E, Miranda A, et al. Chagas' disease; a clinical, epidemiologic, and pathologic study. Circulation 1956;14(6):1035–60.

35. Laranja FS, Dias E, Nobrega G. Clínica e terapêutica da Doença de Chagas. Mem Inst Oswaldo Cruz 1948;46(2):57.

36. Reunião de Pesquisa Aplicada em Doença de Chagas. Validade do conceito de forma indeterminada da doença de Chagas. Rev Soc Bras Med Trop 1985;18(46):1.

37. Gallo L, Neto JA, Manço JC, et al. Abnormal heart rate responses during exercise in patients with Chagas' disease. Cardiology 1975;60(3): 147–62.

38. Pereira MH, Brito FS, Ambrose JA, et al. Exercise testing in the latent phase of Chagas' disease. Clin Cardiol 1984;7(5):261–5.

39. Arreaza N, Puigbó JJ, Acquatella H, et al. Radionuclide evaluation of left-ventricular function in chronic Chagas' cardiomyopathy. J Nucl Med 1983;24(7): 563–7.

40. Marin-Neto JA, Bromberg-Marin G, Pazin-Filho A, et al. Cardiac autonomic impairment and early myocardial damage involving the right ventricle are independent phenomena in Chagas' disease. Int J Cardiol 1998;65(3):261–9.

41. Sousa AC, Marin-Neto JA, Maciel BC. Systolic and diastolic dysfunction in the indeterminate, digestive and chronic cardiac forms of Chagas' disease. Arq Bras Cardiol 1988;50(5):293–9 [in Portuguese].

42. Ortiz J, Barretto AC, Matsumoto AY, et al. Segmental contractility changes in the indeterminate form of Chagas' disease. Echocardiographic study. Arq Bras Cardiol 1987;49(4):217–20 [in Portuguese].

43. Barros MV, Rocha MO, Ribeiro AL, et al. Doppler tissue imaging to evaluate early myocardium damage in patients with undetermined form of Chagas' disease and normal echocardiogram. Echocardiography 2001;18(2):131–6.

44. Ribeiro AL, Rocha MO, Barros MV, et al. A narrow QRS does not predict a normal left ventricular function in Chagas' disease. Pacing Clin Electrophysiol 2000;23(11 Pt 2):2014–7.

45. Acquatella H. Echocardiography in Chagas heart disease. Circulation 2007;115(9):1124–31.

46. Dias JC. The indeterminate form of human chronic Chagas' disease. A clinical epidemiological review. Rev Soc Bras Med Trop 1989;22(3):147–56.

47. Sabino EC, Ribeiro AL, Salemi VM, et al. Ten-year incidence of Chagas cardiomyopathy among asymptomatic Trypanosoma cruzi-seropositive former blood donors. Circulation 2013;127(10): 1105–15.

48. Nascimento BR, Araújo CG, Rocha MO, et al. The prognostic significance of electrocardiographic changes in Chagas disease. J Electrocardiol 2012; 45(1):43–8.

49. Nunes MC, Dones W, Morillo CA, et al. Chagas disease: an overview of clinical and epidemiological aspects. J Am Coll Cardiol 2013;62(9): 767–76.

50. Andrade JP, Marin Neto JA, Paola AA, et al. I Latin American Guidelines for the diagnosis and treatment of Chagas' heart disease: executive summary. Arq Bras Cardiol 2011;96(6):434–42.

51. Ribeiro AL, Sabino EC, Marcolino MS, et al. Electrocardiographic abnormalities in Trypanosoma cruzi seropositive and seronegative former blood donors. PLoS Negl Trop Dis 2013;7(2): e2078.

52. Ribeiro AL, Marcolino MS, Prineas RJ, et al. Electrocardiographic abnormalities in elderly Chagas disease patients: 10-year follow-up of the bambui cohort study of aging. J Am Heart Assoc 2014; 3(1):e000632.

53. Kaplinski M, Jois M, Galdos-Cardenas G, et al. Sustained domestic vector exposure is associated with increased Chagas cardiomyopathy risk but decreased parasitemia and congenital transmission risk among young women in Bolivia. Clin Infect Dis 2015;61(6):918–26.

54. Marcolino MS, Palhares DM, Ferreira LR, et al. Electrocardiogram and Chagas disease: a large population database of primary care patients. Glob Heart 2015;10(3):167–72.

55. Sarabanda AV, Sosa E, Simoes MV, et al. Ventricular tachycardia in Chagas' disease: a comparison of clinical, angiographic, electrophysiologic and myocardial perfusion disturbances between patients presenting with either sustained or nonsustained forms. Int J Control 2005;102(1):9–19.

56. Paixão LC, Ribeiro AL, Valacio RA, et al. Chagas disease: independent risk factor for stroke. Stroke 2009;40(12):3691–4.

57. Oliveira-Filho J, Viana LC, Vieira-de-Melo RM, et al. Chagas disease is an independent risk factor for stroke: baseline characteristics of a Chagas disease cohort. Stroke 2005;36(9):2015–7.

58. Nunes MC, Barbosa MM, Ribeiro AL, et al. Ischemic cerebrovascular events in patients with Chagas cardiomyopathy: a prospective follow-up study. J Neurol Sci 2009;278(1–2):96–101.

59. Strauss DG, Cardoso S, Lima JA, et al. ECG scar quantification correlates with cardiac magnetic resonance scar size and prognostic factors in Chagas' disease. Heart 2011;97(5):357–61.

60. Pierimarchi P, Cerni L, Alarcon de NB, et al. Rapid Chagas diagnosis in clinical settings using a multiparametric assay. Diagn Microbiol Infect Dis 2013; 75(4):381–9.

61. Dias JCP. Acute Chagas' disease. Mem Inst Oswaldo Cruz 1984;79:85–91.

62. Viotti R, Vigliano C, Lococo B, et al. Long-term cardiac outcomes of treating chronic Chagas disease with benznidazole versus no treatment: a nonrandomized trial. Ann Intern Med 2006;144(10):724–34.

63. Garcia S, Ramos CO, Senra JF, et al. Treatment with benznidazole during the chronic phase of experimental Chagas' disease decreases cardiac alterations. Antimicrob Agents Chemother 2005;49(4): 1521–8.

64. Viotti R, Vigliano C, Armenti H, et al. Treatment of chronic Chagas' disease with benznidazole: clinical and serologic evolution of patients with long-term follow-up. Am Heart J 1994;127(1): 151–62.

65. Morillo CA, Marin-Neto JA, Avezum A, et al. Randomized trial of benznidazole for chronic Chagas' cardiomyopathy. N Engl J Med 2015;373(14): 1295–306.

66. McMurray JJ, Adamopoulos S, Anker SD, et al. ESC guidelines for the diagnosis and treatment of acute and chronic heart failure 2012: The Task Force for the Diagnosis and Treatment of Acute and Chronic Heart Failure 2012 of the European Society of Cardiology. Developed in collaboration with the Heart Failure Association (HFA) of the ESC. Eur J Heart Fail 2012;14(8):803–69.

67. Yancy CW, Jessup M, Bozkurt B, et al. 2013 ACCF/AHA guideline for the management of heart failure: a report of the American College of Cardiology Foundation/American Heart Association Task Force on practice guidelines. Circulation 2013;128(16): e240–327.

68. Ribeiro AL, Nunes MP, Teixeira MM, et al. Diagnosis and management of Chagas disease and cardiomyopathy. Nat Rev Cardiol 2012;9(10):576–89.

69. Botoni FA, Poole-Wilson PA, Ribeiro AL, et al. A randomized trial of carvedilol after renin-angiotensin system inhibition in chronic Chagas cardiomyopathy. Am Heart J 2007;153(4):544.e1-8.

70. Taylor AL, Ziesche S, Yancy C, et al. Combination of isosorbide dinitrate and hydralazine in blacks with heart failure. N Engl J Med 2004;351(20):2049–57.

71. Pitt B, Zannad F, Remme WJ, et al. The effect of spironolactone on morbidity and mortality in patients with severe heart failure. Randomized Aldactone Evaluation Study Investigators. N Engl J Med 1999;341(10):709–17.

72. Zannad F, McMurray JJ, Krum H, et al. Eplerenone in patients with systolic heart failure and mild symptoms. N Engl J Med 2011;364(1):11–21.

73. Pitt B, Remme W, Zannad F, et al. Eplerenone, a selective aldosterone blocker, in patients with left ventricular dysfunction after myocardial infarction. N Engl J Med 2003;348(14):1309–21.

74. Bocchi EA, Fiorelli A. The paradox of survival results after heart transplantation for cardiomyopathy caused by *Trypanosoma cruzi*. First Guidelines Group for Heart Transplantation of the Brazilian Society of Cardiology. Ann Thorac Surg 2001;71(6): 1833–8.

75. Sousa AS, Xavier SS, Freitas GR, et al. Prevention strategies of cardioembolic ischemic stroke in Chagas' disease. Arq Bras Cardiol 2008;91(5):306–10.

76. Barbosa MP, Carmo AA, Rocha MO, et al. Ventricular arrhythmias in Chagas disease. Rev Soc Bras Med Trop 2015;48(1):4–10.

77. Barbosa MP, da Costa Rocha MO, de Oliveira AB, et al. Efficacy and safety of implantable cardioverter-defibrillators in patients with Chagas disease. Europace 2013;15(7):957–62.

78. Martinelli M. Implantable cardioverter-defibrillator efficacy in Chagas disease patients depends not only on the device performance: optimizing the adjunct therapy is essential. Europace 2014; 16(6):939.

79. Hotez PJ, Molyneux DH, Fenwick A, et al. Control of neglected tropical diseases. N Engl J Med 2007; 357(10):1018–27.

80. Yamagata Y, Nakagawa J. Control of Chagas disease. Adv Parasitol 2006;61:129–65.

81. Rassi A, Little WC, Xavier SS, et al. Development and validation of a risk score for predicting death in Chagas' heart disease. N Engl J Med 2006; 355(8):799–808.

82. Rocha MO, Ribeiro AL. A risk score for predicting death in Chagas' heart disease. N Engl J Med 2006;355(23):2488–9 [author reply: 2490–1].

83. Salles G, Xavier S, Sousa A, et al. Prognostic value of QT interval parameters for mortality risk stratification in Chagas' disease: results of a long-term follow-up study. Circulation 2003;108(3):305–12.

84. Basquiera AL, Sembaj A, Aguerri AM, et al. Risk progression to chronic Chagas cardiomyopathy: influence of male sex and of parasitaemia detected by polymerase chain reaction. Heart 2003;89(10): 1186–90.

85. Viotti RJ, Vigliano C, Laucella S, et al. Value of echocardiography for diagnosis and prognosis of chronic Chagas disease cardiomyopathy without heart failure. Heart 2004;90(6):655–60.

86. Viotti R, Vigliano C, Lococo B, et al. Clinical predictors of chronic chagasic myocarditis progression. Rev Esp Cardiol 2005;58(9):1037–44 [in Spanish].

87. Benchimol Barbosa PR. Noninvasive prognostic markers for cardiac death and ventricular arrhythmia in long-term follow-up of subjects with chronic Chagas' disease. Braz J Med Biol Res 2007;40(2):167–78.

88. Cardinalli-Neto A, Bestetti RB, Cordeiro JA, et al. Predictors of all-cause mortality for patients with chronic Chagas' heart disease receiving implantable cardioverter defibrillator therapy. J Cardiovasc Electrophysiol 2007;18(12):1236–40.

89. Ribeiro AL, Cavalvanti PS, Lombardi F, et al. Prognostic value of signal-averaged electrocardiogram in Chagas disease. J Cardiovasc Electrophysiol 2008;19(5):502–9.

90. Theodoropoulos TA, Bestetti RB, Otaviano AP, et al. Predictors of all-cause mortality in chronic Chagas' heart disease in the current era of heart failure therapy. Int J Cardiol 2008; 128(1):22–9.

91. Nunes MC, Barbosa MM, Ribeiro AL, et al. Left atrial volume provides independent prognostic value in patients with Chagas cardiomyopathy. J Am Soc Echocardiogr 2009;22(1):82–8.

92. Gonçalves JG, Dias Silva VJ, Calzada Borges MC, et al. Mortality indicators among chronic Chagas patients living in an endemic area. Int J Cardiol 2010; 143(3):235–42.

93. Lima-Costa MF, Matos DL, Ribeiro AL. Chagas disease predicts 10-year stroke mortality in

community-dwelling elderly: the Bambui cohort study of aging. Stroke 2010;41(11):2477–82.

94. Pedrosa RC, Salles JH, Magnanini MM, et al. Prognostic value of exercise-induced ventricular arrhythmia in Chagas' heart disease. Pacing Clin Electrophysiol 2011;34(11):1492–7.

95. Ribeiro AL, Rocha MO, Terranova P, et al. T-wave amplitude variability and the risk of death in Chagas disease. J Cardiovasc Electrophysiol 2011;22(7): 799–805.

96. Sarabanda AV, Marin-Neto JA. Predictors of mortality in patients with Chagas' cardiomyopathy and ventricular tachycardia not treated with implantable cardioverter-defibrillators. Pacing Clin Electrophysiol 2011;34(1):54–62.

97. Bestetti RB, Otaviano AP, Cardinalli-Neto A, et al. Effects of B-Blockers on outcome of patients with Chagas' cardiomyopathy with chronic heart failure. Int J Cardiol 2011;151(2):205–8.

98. Nunes MP, Colosimo EA, Reis RC, et al. Different prognostic impact of the tissue Doppler-derived E/e' ratio on mortality in Chagas cardiomyopathy patients with heart failure. J Heart Lung Transplant 2012;31(6):634–41.

Electrophysiology in the Developing World
Challenges and Opportunities

Michael Bestawros, MD, MPH

KEYWORDS

- Electrophysiology • Developing world • Developing countries • Atrial fibrillation • Anticoagulation
- Pacemaker • Stroke • Ventricular tachycardia

KEY POINTS

- Coincident with the epidemiologic transition in low-income and middle-income countries (LMICs), the burden of cardiac electrophysiologic disorders is significant and growing.
- The growth of handheld and wireless technologies allows a unique opportunity to provide arrhythmia diagnosis in remote areas of the world.
- With an estimated need for 1 million pacemakers worldwide per year, philanthropic donations of new pacemakers need to be supplemented by alternative sources of pacemakers, such as pacemaker reuse.
- Atrial fibrillation rates are expected to increase rapidly in LMICs, but its treatment, especially stroke-preventing anticoagulation, is poorly managed throughout much of the world.
- Supraventricular tachycardias can often be cured by an ablation, which is not only cost-effective, but cost saving.

INTRODUCTION

In the past 15 years, the United Nations General Assembly has only met once to tackle a global health crisis.[1] The meeting was in 2011, and the crisis was noncommunicable diseases (NCDs).[1] Thirty-eight million people die annually from noncommunicable diseases, and almost 75% of these deaths occur in low-income and middle-income countries (LMICs).[2] Eighty-two percent of premature deaths from NCDs (people aged <70 years) occur in LMICs, thereby disproportionately affecting their citizens during their most productive years. Cardiovascular disease accounts for 30% of all deaths worldwide and has twice the mortality of human immunodeficiency virus, malaria, and tuberculosis combined.[3,4] The burden of cardiovascular disease in LMICs is likely underrecognized.

The disparities in cardiovascular health between high-income countries and LMICs are evident, and there are few fields in which this is more evident than electrophysiology. Not only do arrhythmia treatment and recent advances in device therapy for heart failure treatment often require subspecialized expertise and high-tech equipment that are often not available in LMICs, but endemic diseases such as Chagas disease and rheumatic heart disease often manifest with sinus node dysfunction, atrial fibrillation (Afib), various degrees of atrioventricular block, bundle branch blocks, prolonged QT intervals, premature beats, ventricular tachycardia, and heart failure.[5–9] The diagnostic and treatment challenges of electrophysiology in the developing world deserve to be explored further.

Disclosure: The author has nothing to disclose.
New Mexico Heart Institute, 502 Elm Street North East, Albuquerque, NM 87102, USA
E-mail address: mbestaw@gmail.com

Cardiol Clin 35 (2017) 49–58
http://dx.doi.org/10.1016/j.ccl.2016.09.002
0733-8651/17/© 2016 Elsevier Inc. All rights reserved.

DIAGNOSTIC CHALLENGES

The accurate diagnosis of arrhythmias requires heart rhythm monitoring. In developing nations' rural communities, electrocardiogram (ECG) machines are often not available and generally cost $1000 or more.[10] Even when they are available, lack of ECG paper, limited numbers of electrodes, limited electricity, and limited expertise in interpretation restrict their use. Because of these limitations, patients with syncope, stroke, chest pain, or palpitations do not receive this basic indicated test.[11]

However, resources beyond philanthropic donation exist to address access to ECGs in LMICs. The wide availability of wireless technologies creates opportunities for both obtaining and interpreting basic ECGs. A 1-lead ECG, which is sufficient for most arrhythmia screening, can be obtained with dedicated handheld ECG monitors or smartphone cases with integrated electrodes, such as the AliveCor Kardia monitor (https://www.alivecor.com).[12,13] This Kardia monitor can perform HIPAA-compliant transmissions and is 98% specific and 97% sensitive in the diagnosis of Afib compared with 12-lead ECGs.[14] Majors and colleagues[15] presented an ECG chair concept that uses electrodes placed on a clinic chair's armrests to produce a single-lead ECG that could be interpreted locally or transmitted wirelessly. In India, mobile vans equipped with ECGs and satellite terminals can transmit ECGs for expert interpretation.[16] For diagnoses that require more long-term monitoring, devices such as the ZIO Patch by iRhythm Technologies or the Seeq MCT monitor by Medtronic offer more portable options than other Holter and event monitors, although their current pricing structures limit their use in LMICs.

BRADYARRHYTHMIAS AND PACEMAKER IMPLANTATION
Indications

Two diagnoses require pacemaker implantation: sinus node dysfunction and high-grade atrioventricular (AV) block. Manifestations of sinus node dysfunction vary from mild fatigue or dyspnea to frank syncope. High-grade AV block can be life threatening and, in the developed world, often leads to pacemaker implantation within 24 hours of diagnosis. In the absence of a reversible cause, these diagnoses are treated with a pacemaker.

Worldwide Inequalities Based on Income

The disparity of pacemaker implantation between high-income countries and LMICs is vast. The last world survey of cardiac pacing included 61

countries representing more than 80% of pacemaker and implantable cardioverter-defibrillator (ICD) implants worldwide.[17] Of note, 42 of the represented countries were high income, and more than 100 LMICs did not report any implants (**Fig. 1**).[17] Germany, France, and the United States all had more than 750 new implants per million population, whereas Bangladesh, Indonesia, Myanmar, Nepal, Pakistan, the Philippines, Vietnam, and Sudan had less than 10 new implants per million population.[17] Outside of Europe and North America, only Australia, Israel, and Uruguay had more than 300 new implants per million population.[17]

These differences affect both individual patients and their communities. The average life expectancy for patients with complete heart block without a pacemaker is 2.5 years.[18] Pacemakers can give back many productive years of life. In a South African study of pacemaker patients between 21 and 50 years old, those without structural heart disease lived as long as controls in the general population.[19] Among patients with and without structural heart disease who were alive 1 year after pacemaker implantation, 70% were alive at 20 years.[19]

Barriers to Pacemaker Use in Low-income and Middle-income Countries

Expertise
Although most countries have the necessary operating rooms and fluoroscopy, pacemaker implantation requires both expertise and long-term follow-up. Some countries do not have a single physician trained to implant pacemakers and follow pacemaker patients. In addition, physicians who go to high-income countries to receive such training often do not return.

Several methods of developing this expertise within LMICs exist. First, philanthropic provision of services through short-term trips are increasingly common. Project Pacer International has freely provided pacemaker implantation in Bolivia for more than 25 years and has expanded its services to India and other countries in South America and Africa.[20,21] Second, electrophysiologists have committed to regular training visits to some LMICs. Over the past 2 decades, French electrophysiologists have worked with the Cercle de Rythmologie Africain to increase pacemaker implantation rates in 12 French-speaking African nations from less than 0.5 per million to 3.3 per million.[22] Third, providing pacemaker training for physicians and technicians without comprehensive electrophysiology training may be effective. The Pan-African Society of Cardiology fellowships

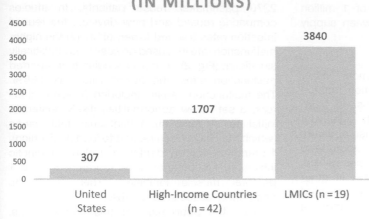

TOTAL POPULATION REPRESENTED (IN MILLIONS)

United States: 307
High-Income Countries (n = 42): 1707
LMICs (n = 19): 3840

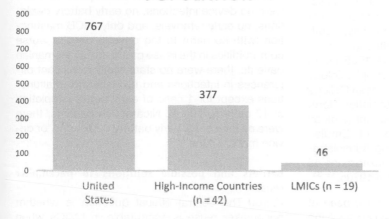

NEW IMPLANTS PER MILLION POPULATION

United States: 767
High-Income Countries (n = 42): 377
LMICs (n = 19): 46

Fig. 1. The 11th World Survey of Cardiac Pacing: population versus new implants per million population in LMICs, high-income countries, and the United States. (*Data from* Mond HG, Proclemer A. The 11th World Survey of Cardiac Pacing and Implantable Cardioverter-Defibrillators: calendar year 2009–a World Society of Arrhythmia's project. Pacing Clin Electrophysiol 2011;34(8):1013–27; and World Bank. Which are the World Bank Country and Lending Groups? 2016. Available at: https://datahelpdesk.worldbank.org/knowledgebase/articles/906519. Accessed June 26, 2016.)

in cardiac pacing provide 6 months of training at the University of Cape Town for selected African physicians and 3 months of training for nonphysician clinicians or nurses in cardiac pacing and follow-up.[23] The eventual goal of this program is to have at least 1 trained implanter in every African country.[23] The first graduate of this program is a physician based in Eldoret, Kenya.[24]

Cost

The most common objection to expanding pacemaker implantation programs is the assumption that it is not cost-effective. A 2007 cost-effectiveness model for single-chamber pacemaker implantation in patients with complete heart block made the conservative estimate of zero cost if no pacemaker is implanted and estimated that the cost of pacemaker implantation was $773 per life-year saved.[18] This model assumed a cost of $1750 for a single-chamber pacemaker, 50%

mortality at 2.5 years without a pacemaker, 68% mortality at 5 years without a pacemaker, a 4% complication rate, 7-year device longevity, 10-year follow-up, and mean age at implantation of 55 years. Varying the age at implantation between 50 and 70 years of age and the duration of follow-up between 10 and 30 years did not significantly affect the cost-effectiveness. By the World Health Organization's definition of cost-effectiveness, this $773 per life-year saved suggests that pacemaker implantation for complete heart block is cost-effective for every country in the world.[25] However, not all pacemaker implants are single-chamber pacemakers for complete heart block.

When pacemakers cannot be purchased, donations are required. For decades, STIMUBANK in France has collected pacemakers that are previously used or past their shelf lives and shipped these to LMICs.[26] Since 1984, Heartbeat International, which is present in 24 countries, has been responsible for more than 10,000 implantations of devices nearing the end of their shelf lives.[27,28] However, with an estimated need of 1 million pacemakers per year, the gap between supply and demand remains wide.[27]

Pacemaker reuse

Pacemaker reuse is probably the most widely researched and debated cost-reduction method of pacemaker implantation in LMICs. In high-income countries, pacemakers with significant battery life are often explanted because of death, infection, heart transplant, or need to upgrade to a different device. For $100 or less per device, these devices can be cleaned, sterilized in either the donor or recipient country, and then donated to patients who could otherwise not afford a pacemaker.[29]

History Pacemaker reuse has been performed in at least 15 countries, including India, Romania, Sweden, Hungary, Israel, Australia, Finland, Norway, Brazil, Canada, France, Holland, Italy, South Africa, and the Philippines.[29–31] Although pacemaker reuse was supported by the 1985 North American Society of Pacing and Electrophysiology Policy Conference and the 2002 American College of Cardiology/American Heart Association/North American Society of Pacing and Electrophysiology Guideline Update for Implantation of Cardiac Pacemakers, the US Food and Drug Administration has officially referred to pacemaker reuse as an "objectionable practice" since the 1970s.[32–34]

Safety Since the late 1960s, there have been at least 23 studies done in 15 countries and involving 3081 reused pacemakers and ICDs.[29–31,35] These studies have primarily focused on the safety and efficacy of pacemaker reuse. In 2011, Baman and colleagues[36] published a meta-analysis of 18 studies that reported infection rates in a total of 2270 pacemaker reuse patients. In studies comparing reused and new devices, the reused infection rates trended lower, although the higher malfunction rate in reused devices was statistically significant (**Fig. 2**). In the 17 studies that reported malfunction rates, the overall rate was 0.68%. The malfunction causes included 5 technical errors, 3 set screw abnormalities (likely related to initial device removal), 1 ventricular tachycardia (which may have been related to lead positioning), 1 premature battery depletion, 1 electromagnetic inhibition, 1 spontaneous reprogramming, and 1 pectoral muscle inhibition. There were no pacemaker-associated deaths.

Since the publication of this meta-analysis, several further studies have continued to present data on the safety of reuse. Jama and colleagues[30] reported that, in 126 South African patients, there were no device infections, no early battery depletions, no early removals, and only 1 ICD malfunction (with no harm to the patient) despite worse comorbidities in the reuse group. In 127 Romanian patients, there were no statistically significant differences in infections and no generator malfunctions except for 1 case of early battery depletion at 17 months.[35] In 17 Nicaraguan patients, there were no infections, early battery depletions, or device malfunctions.[31]

Barriers and possible solutions to pacemaker reuse

Ethical The central ethical question is whether pacemaker reuse is acceptable in LMICs when the practice is not performed in high-income countries. Egalitarianism may suggest that if a device is not acceptable in the donor country, then it should

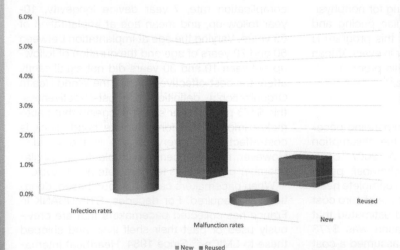

Fig. 2. New versus reused: infection and malfunction rates. (*Data from* Baman TS, Meier P, Romero J, et al. Safety of pacemaker reuse: a meta-analysis with implications for underserved nations Circ Arrhythm Electrophysiol 2011;4(3):318–23.)

not be acceptable elsewhere.[1] Ideally, everyone who needs a pacemaker would receive a new pacemaker. However, this ideal has led to great inequalities in LMICs, including poorer health outcomes and lost productivity.[1] From a utilitarian perspective, pacemaker reuse probably provides significantly more overall benefit than harm to individuals and society, assuming that quality care and distribution to the most in need are assured.[1] From a justice perspective, pacemaker reuse can allow recipients a wider range of life opportunities than no pacemaker or being pushed into poverty by the cost of a new pacemaker.[1] The World Health Organization estimates that health care expenses usher 100 million people into poverty every year.[1] In addition, informed consent to pacemaker reuse and its risks, benefits, uncertainties, and alternatives must be considered by providers, recipient nations, and patients.

Legal Liability issues remain unresolved. The device manufacturers initially sell these devices as single-use devices, so they are unlikely to be held responsible. In the European Union, the reprocessor assumes all the obligations of the initial manufacturer.[37]

Device ownership also remains unclear. In Sweden, pacemakers are the state's property, so device removal may occur without patient or family consent, whereas in Canada and India the patient owns the device on implantation.[38,39] However, possible device owners in many countries, such as the United States and the United Kingdom, include the patient, the patient's family, the device manufacturer, the payer, and the hospital.[34,39]

Legal obstacles exist in both high-income countries and LMICs. Project My Heart–Your Heart (MHYH) in Michigan is working with several recipient nations and the Food and Drug Administration to address some of these legal and regulatory issues. Recipient countries such as Vietnam and the Philippines have already deemed that importation and reuse of pacemakers is legal, and pilot programs for reuse have been established.[28,29] Zambia and Sierra Leone have granted acceptance letters to MHYH for importing refurbished pacemakers and pacemakers that are past their shelf lives (Constantine Akwanalo, personal communication, 2016).

Logistical Logistical barriers include stakeholders' impressions of device donation and reuse, obtaining devices, managing device recalls, and ensuring that the devices are distributed fairly.

Stakeholders include donors, recipients, and those who facilitate the intermediate steps. In a 2007 survey of device patients, 91% were willing to donate their devices to a medically underserved

nation.[40] According to the Cremation Association of North America, the 2025 cremation rate is predicted at 59%, and all pacemakers and ICDs must be explanted before cremation.[29] Eighty-four percent of funeral homes discard explanted devices or store them with no intended purpose.[41] In a survey of funeral directors, 89% were willing to donate devices to charity.[29]

If other barriers are addressed, obtaining used pacemakers is likely to be more straightforward. In a 2012 study of 3176 devices from crematories or funeral homes, 21% had at least 75% or 4 years of the battery life remaining.[42] Hughey and colleagues[34] have estimated that, if all devices were collected postmortem, nearly 40% of these devices would have approximately 7 years of battery life remaining.

Although much research has addressed the willingness of donors to donate devices, fewer studies have investigated the potential reused pacemaker recipients. In some cultures, cultural norms and religious beliefs may lead to unwillingness to receive devices from cadavers because of respect for the dead, beliefs about what happens to the deceased after death, beliefs about reincarnation, and the perception of receiving second-hand goods.[43] Although providing education about the refurbishing process may allay some of those concerns, there will still be some people who would refuse such a device. Given that the worldwide need for these potentially lifesaving devices far outstrips the supply, these concerns are unlikely to pose a barrier in most cases.

For the benefit of all stakeholders, a registry would need to be created for the purposes of follow-up and tracking for device recalls, and charitable device implantation requires proving financial need. Ensuring that pacemakers are fairly distributed requires clear criteria, a transparent selection process, and audits by either the donor agencies or independent agencies.[34] Acting as a coordinating center for pacemaker donation, Heartbeat International has shown for decades that these duties can be successfully performed.[27]

ATRIAL FIBRILLATION
Epidemiology

Approximately 33 million people live with Afib, and as the population ages, the prevalence of Afib will continue to increase along with its associated disability-adjusted life-years.[44,45] By 2050, India is projected to have more than 3 times as many people more than 60 years old, and in Africa this number will more than quadruple.[45] The increased Afib burden will probably disproportionately affect LMICs.

Afib prevalence is generally lower in people without European ancestry, but nonwhite ethnicities in LMICs present at younger ages.[46] In the RE-LY AF registry, patients with Afib in Africa, India, and the Middle East were 9 to 12 years younger on average than similar patients in other areas.[47] Compared with the overall study population, African patients with Afib had twice as much heart failure (64% vs 35%) and 11-fold more rheumatic heart disease (22% vs 2%).[47] In the Study of Genetics of Atrial Fibrillation in an African Population (SIGNAL), patients with valvular Afib were younger than patients with nonvalvular Afib by nearly 30 years (38 vs 68 years).[48] The epidemiologic transition in LMICs to longer life and unhealthy lifestyles is expected to lead to increased obesity, hypertension, diabetes, coronary artery disease, and heart failure, which are risk factors for Afib and its stroke risk.[45]

Prognosis and Stroke Risk

Afib carries an average risk of stroke of 4.4% per year, and these strokes are more severe and have higher 28-day mortalities than nonembolic strokes.[49,50] Patients with Afib admitted for stroke have longer hospitalizations, increased disability, and higher health care costs.[45] Among Medicare beneficiaries, patients with Afib with Hispanic or African ancestry carry a 2-fold increased stroke risk.[51] In medically underserved regions of the world, stroke-related mortality and disability rates are 10 times higher than in high-income countries.[52]

Afib also leads to increased risks of heart failure, myocardial infarction, dementia, chronic kidney disease, and mortality.[45] Patients with Afib with heart failure or myocardial infarction have increased mortality compared with those without Afib.[53,54] During an average of 318 days of follow-up of 172 patients with Afib in cardiology offices in Cameroon, 30% died, 16% had a nonlethal stroke, and 26% had severe heart failure symptoms.[55]

Rate Versus Rhythm Control

The AFFIRM (The Atrial Fibrillation Follow-up Investigation of Rhythm Management) trial, which only included patients with Afib for whom rate control was considered a reasonable alternative to rhythm control, showed no difference in mortality.[56] However, patients who maintain sinus rhythm with a rhythm control strategy have fewer symptoms and better quality-of-life indices.[57–59] In contrast with high-income countries, rate control strategies are used more than rhythm control strategies in LMICs. Compared with high-income countries, LMICs have more permanent Afib (likely because of delayed diagnoses), less access to antiarrhythmic medication or ablation, and less familiarity with antiarrhythmics. Digoxin, which is only indicated as adjunctive therapy and has significant potential toxicities, is used in a minority of patients with Afib in high-income countries and in most patients with Afib in LMICs.[60,61]

Anticoagulation

Oral anticoagulation in patients with Afib reduces stroke risk by 64% and mortality by 26%.[62] Worldwide adherence to anticoagulation guidelines to prevent stroke in patients with Afib is poor (**Fig. 3**). In the GARFIELD (The Global Anticoagulant Registry in the Field) registry of 10,607 adults with Afib in 19 countries, 62% of patients with indications for oral anticoagulation received it, and 49% of patients without indications for oral anticoagulation were on anticoagulation.[63] However, the numbers in many LMICs are even worse. Percentages as low as 1.5% in Brazil, 2.7% to 11.2% in China, 7.1% in Moldova, 16% in Malaysia, 21.5% in patients with Asian ancestry, 27% in Kosovo, and 34% in Cameroon have been published.[47,55,64–67] In the ROCKET-AF trial,

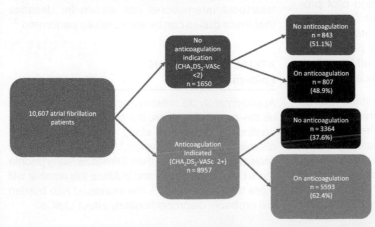

Fig. 3. Anticoagulation guideline adherence in worldwide GARFIELD registry. (*Data from* Kakkar AK, Mueller I, Bassand JP, et al. Risk profiles and antithrombotic treatment of patients newly diagnosed with atrial fibrillation at risk of stroke: perspectives from the international, observational, prospective GARFIELD registry. PLoS One 2013;8(5):e63479.)

subtherapeutic anticoagulation percentages were 44% in India, 37% in East Asia, 35% in Eastern Europe, and 27% in Latin America.[68] Newer anticoagulants that do not have the interaction restraints and monitoring requirements of warfarin could be better therapeutic options in LMICs. The INVICTUS (Investigation of Rheumatic AF Treatment Using Vitamin K Antagonists, Rivaroxaban, or Aspirin Studies) trial is a noninferiority trial that is currently recruiting 4500 patients with rheumatic heart disease and Afib to be randomized to rivaroxaban or warfarin.[69] However, newer anticoagulants still remain cost prohibitive in many settings. Left atrial appendage closure devices such as the WATCHMAN and Amplatzer Cardiac Plug allow stroke reduction through a 1-time procedure, although expertise in these currently costly procedures is still lacking even in more developed nations.[70,71]

TACHYARRHYTHMIAS
Supraventricular Tachycardia

Supraventricular tachycardias (SVTs) often cause significant morbidity associated with palpitations, lightheadedness, dyspnea, fatigue, chest pain, and/or syncope. Treatment options include medical therapy and often curative ablation. Because of lack of expertise and the initial expense of ablation, medical therapy is the mainstay of treatment in many LMICs. In contrast, for symptomatic SVT, ablation is often the preferred management strategy in most high-income nations.[72]

Although development of expertise requires many of the same training options as described for pacemakers earlier, the notion that cost is an insurmountable barrier deserves exploration. In high-income countries, ablation is more cost-effective than medical therapy.[73,74] Limited data in LMICs strongly suggest that not only is ablation cost-effective but it may also be cost saving. In a study of Guatemalan children and adolescents, the cost of ablation at 13 months ($1668) was 4.9 times higher than medical therapy, but after 5.1 years the cost of medical therapy began to exceed that of ablation.[75] In another study of Guatemalan adults, ablation cost $7993 less than medical therapy and led to 1.46 quality-adjusted life-years gained ($5480 per quality-adjusted life-year gained).[76] Sensitivity analyses adjusted treatment success rates, inflation, and complication rates and found a 78% chance of cost saving and a 92% chance of a cost-effectiveness ratio of less than $3500 per quality-adjusted life-year.[76] The investigators concluded that, "This demonstrates that radiofrequency ablation dominates medical therapy in the management of SVT."[76] Ablation generally costs less in developing nations because of the lower cost of staff as well as frequent catheter reuse. For example, closed-lumen catheters can be used at least 5 times without an increased risk of infection or decreased function.[77]

Ventricular Tachyarrhythmia

Ventricular tachyarrhythmias are likely the most difficult arrhythmias to manage worldwide. Medical therapy is available but often insufficient. Ablation can be effective, but, with the possible exception of idiopathic ventricular tachycardia, it is generally not stand-alone therapy. In addition, ICDs are lifesaving treatments with costs that are often several-fold higher than pacemaker treatment and with potentially more complex follow-up.

Given the complexity of these issues, the limited literature focuses on defining the scope of the problem. In 2003, Millar and Mayosi[78] reported that South Africa was the only sub-Saharan country implanting ICDs, and only 3 of the 35 ICDs implanted (0.8/million) were in state-funded public hospitals. In 2012, Vedanthan and colleagues[79] reviewed the literature available on sudden cardiac death in LMICs and reported that, because of limited data and data quality, no epidemiologic conclusions could be made without more comprehensive studies. One of the more impressive collaborations is the ongoing Pan-African Sudden Cardiac Death study, a prospective registry evaluating the incidence, prevalence, causes, characteristics, and outcomes of sudden cardiac arrest in participating countries.[80] Multiple such studies are needed to further define the disease burden, associated problems, and potential solutions.

SUMMARY

Along with the growing epidemic of cardiovascular morbidity and mortality in LMICs, the burden related to heart rhythm disorders is likely to increase significantly. Effective diagnostic and treatment modalities exist, but financial resources and expertise are limited. Cost-effective strategies exist to address most of these limitations, but many surmountable barriers need to be overcome to improve electrophysiologic care in LMICs.

REFERENCES

1. VanArtsdalen J, Goold SD, Kirkpatrick JN, et al. Pacemaker reuse for patients in resource poor countries: is something always better than nothing? Prog Cardiovasc Dis 2012;55(3):300–6.
2. WHO. Global status report on noncommunicable diseases 2014. World Health Organization; 2014.

3. Mendis S, Lindholm LH, Mancia G, et al. World Health Organization (WHO) and International Society of Hypertension (ISH) risk prediction charts: assessment of cardiovascular risk for prevention and control of cardiovascular disease in low and middle-income countries. J Hypertens 2007;25(8):1578–82.

4. Lopez AD, Mathers CD, Ezzati M, et al. Measuring the global burden of disease and risk factors, 1990-2001. In: Lopez AD, Mathers CD, Ezzati M, et al, editors. Global burden of disease and risk factors. Washington, DC: The International Bank for Reconstruction and Development/The World Bank Group; 2006. p. 8.

5. Ribeiro AL, Marcolino MS, Prineas RJ, et al. Electrocardiographic abnormalities in elderly Chagas disease patients: 10-year follow-up of the Bambui Cohort Study of Aging. J Am Heart Assoc 2014; 3(1):e000632.

6. Salles G, Xavier S, Sousa A, et al. Prognostic value of QT interval parameters for mortality risk stratification in Chagas' disease: results of a long-term follow-up study. Circulation 2003;108(3):305–12.

7. Healy C, Viles-Gonzalez JF, Saenz LC, et al. Arrhythmias in chagasic cardiomyopathy. Card Electrophysiol Clin 2015;7(2):251–68.

8. Zuhlke LJ, Steer AC. Estimates of the global burden of rheumatic heart disease. Glob Heart 2013;8(3): 189–95.

9. Sharma SK, Verma SH. A clinical evaluation of atrial fibrillation in rheumatic heart disease. J Assoc Physicians India 2015;63(6):22–5.

10. Day A, Oldroyd C, Godfrey S, et al. Availability of cardiac equipment in general practice premises in a cardiac network: a survey. Br J Cardiol 2008;15: 141–4.

11. Yameogo NV, Samadoulougou A, Millogo G, et al. Delays in the management of acute coronary syndromes with ST-ST segment elevation in Ouagadougou and factors associated with an extension of these delays: a cross-sectional study about 43 cases collected in the CHU-Yalgado Ouedraogo [in French]. Pan Afr Med J 2012;13:90.

12. Olgun Kucuk H, Kucuk U, Yalcin M, et al. Time to use mobile health devices to diagnose paroxysmal atrial fibrillation. Int J Cardiol 2016;222:1061.

13. Tarakji KG, Wazni OM, Callahan T, et al. Using a novel wireless system for monitoring patients after the atrial fibrillation ablation procedure: the iTransmit study. Heart Rhythm 2015;12(3):554–9.

14. Lau JK, Lowres N, Neubeck L, et al. iPhone ECG application for community screening to detect silent atrial fibrillation: a novel technology to prevent stroke. Int J Cardiol 2013;165(1):193–4.

15. Majors C, Pauly H, Hollabaugh S, et al. Low-Resource electrocardiogram chair. Presented at the Rice University global health technologies design competition. Houston, TX, April 2012.

16. Bagchi S. Telemedicine in rural India. PLoS Med 2006;3(3):e82.

17. Mond HG, Proclemer A. The 11th World Survey of Cardiac Pacing and Implantable Cardioverter-Defibrillators: calendar year 2009–a World Society of Arrhythmia's project. Pacing Clin Electrophysiol 2011;34(8):1013–27.

18. Mehra R, Koehler J. Incidence of complete heart block and cost-effectiveness of pacemaker therapy in India. 5th IET International Seminar on appropriate healthcare technologies for developing countries. London, May 21-22, 2008.

19. Mayosi BM, Little F, Millar RN. Long-term survival after permanent pacemaker implantation in young adults: 30 year experience. Pacing Clin Electrophysiol 1999;22(3):407–12.

20. Chute R, Otieno H, Turek F, et al. Project pacer international brings cardiac electrophysiology to East Africa. 2010;10(7).

21. Vivas Y, Ferrufino O, Zurita C, et al. Cardiac electrophysiology in Bolivia. Heart Rhythm 2009;6(7):1076.

22. Jouven X. Cardiac pacing program in Africa. 11th PASCAR Congress. Dakar(Senegal), May 15-19, 2013.

23. Sani M, Chin A, Mayosi B. The PASCAR programme for the recycling of pacemakers and ICDs. 11th PASCAR Congress. Dakar, Senegal.2013.

24. Binanay CA, Akwanalo CO, Aruasa W, et al. Building sustainable capacity for cardiovascular care at a public hospital in western Kenya. J Am Coll Cardiol 2015;66(22):2550–60.

25. Table: Threshold values for intervention cost-effectiveness by region. Available at: http://www.who.int/choice/costs/CER_levels/en/. Accessed June 25, 2016.

26. Anilkumar R, Balachander J. Refurbishing pacemakers: a viable approach. Indian Pacing Electrophysiol J 2004;4(1):1–2.

27. Mond HG, Mick W, Maniscalco BS. Heartbeat International: making "poor" hearts beat better. Heart Rhythm 2009;6(10):1538–40.

28. Kirkpatrick JN, Papini C, Baman TS, et al. Reuse of pacemakers and defibrillators in developing countries: logistical, legal, and ethical barriers and solutions. Heart Rhythm 2010;7(11):1623–7.

29. Baman TS, Kirkpatrick JN, Romero J, et al. Pacemaker reuse: an initiative to alleviate the burden of symptomatic bradyarrhythmia in impoverished nations around the world. Circulation 2010;122(16): 1649–56.

30. Jama ZV, Chin A, Badri M, et al. Performance of re-used pacemakers and implantable cardioverter defibrillators compared with new devices at Groote Schuur Hospital in Cape Town, South Africa. Cardiovasc J Afr 2015;26(4):181–7.

31. Hasan R, Ghanbari H, Feldman D, et al. Safety, efficacy, and performance of implanted recycled

cardiac rhythm management (CRM) devices in underprivileged patients. Pacing Clin Electrophysiol 2011;34(6):653–8.

32. Boal BH, Escher DJ, Furman S, et al. Report of the policy conference on pacemaker reuse sponsored by the North American Society of Pacing and Electrophysiology. J Am Coll Cardiol 1985; 5(3):808–10.

33. Gregoratos G, Abrams J, Epstein AE, et al. ACC/AHA/NASPE 2002 guideline update for implantation of cardiac pacemakers and antiarrhythmia devices–summary article: a report of the American College of Cardiology/American Heart Association Task Force on Practice Guidelines (ACC/AHA/NASPE Committee to Update the 1998 Pacemaker Guidelines). J Am Coll Cardiol 2002;40(9):1703–19.

34. Hughey AB, Baman TS, Eagle KA, et al. Pacemaker reuse: an initiative to help those in underserved nations in need of life-saving device therapy. Expert Rev Med Devices 2013;10(5):577–9.

35. Sosdean R, Mornos C, Enache B, et al. Safety and feasibility of biventricular devices reuse in general and elderly population–a single-center retrospective cohort study. Clin Interv Aging 2015;10:1311–8.

36. Baman TS, Meier P, Romero J, et al. Safety of pacemaker reuse: a meta-analysis with implications for underserved nations. Circ Arrhythm Electrophysiol 2011;4(3):318–23.

37. Ryden L. Re-use of devices in cardiology. Proceedings from a policy conference at the European Heart House, 1998. Eur Heart J 1998;19(11):1628–01.

38. Namboodiri KK, Sharma YP, Bali HK, et al. Re-use of explanted DDD pacemakers as VDD- clinical utility and cost effectiveness. Indian Pacing Electrophysiol J 2004;4(1):3–9.

39. Glister J, Glister T. Property in recyclable artificial implants. J Law Med 2013;21(2):357–63.

40. Kirkpatrick JN, Ghani SN, Burke MC, et al. Postmortem interrogation and retrieval of implantable pacemakers and defibrillators: a survey of morticians and patients. J Cardiovasc Electrophysiol 2007; 18(5):478–82.

41. Gakenheimer L, Lange DC, Romero J, et al. Societal views of pacemaker reutilization for those with untreated symptomatic bradycardia in underserved nations. J Interv Card Electrophysiol 2011;30(3): 261–6.

42. Baman TS, Crawford T, Sovitch P, et al. Feasibility of postmortem device acquisition for potential reuse in underserved nations. Heart Rhythm 2012;9(2):211–4.

43. Ochasi A, Clark P. Reuse of pacemakers in Ghana and Nigeria: medical, legal, cultural and ethical perspectives. Dev World Bioeth 2015;15(3):125–33.

44. Chugh SS, Havmoeller R, Narayanan K, et al. Worldwide epidemiology of atrial fibrillation: a global burden of disease 2010 study. Circulation 2014; 129(8):837–47.

45. Rahman F, Kwan GF, Benjamin EJ. Global epidemiology of atrial fibrillation. Nat Rev Cardiol 2014; 11(11):639–54.

46. Shen AY, Contreras R, Sobnosky S, et al. Racial/ethnic differences in the prevalence of atrial fibrillation among older adults–a cross-sectional study. J Natl Med Assoc 2010;102(10):906–13.

47. Oldgren J, Healey JS, Ezekowitz M, et al. Variations in cause and management of atrial fibrillation in a prospective registry of 15,400 emergency department patients in 46 countries: the RE-LY Atrial Fibrillation Registry. Circulation 2014;129(15):1568–76.

48. Bloomfield GS, Temu TM, Akwanalo CO, et al. Genetic mutations in African patients with atrial fibrillation: rationale and design of the study of genetics of atrial fibrillation in an African population (SIGNAL). Am Heart J 2015;170(3):455–64.e5.

49. Gage BF, Waterman AD, Shannon W, et al. Validation of clinical classification schemes for predicting stroke: results from the National Registry of Atrial Fibrillation. JAMA 2001;285(22):2864–70.

50. Kimura K, Minematsu K, Yamaguchi T, et al. Atrial fibrillation as a predictive factor for severe stroke and early death in 15,831 patients with acute ischaemic stroke. J Neurol Neurosurg Psychiatry 2005; 76(5):679–83.

51. Birman-Deych E, Radford MJ, Nilasena DS, et al. Use and effectiveness of warfarin in Medicare beneficiaries with atrial fibrillation. Stroke 2006;37(4): 1070–4.

52. Norrving B, Kissela B. The global burden of stroke and need for a continuum of care. Neurology 2013;80(3 Suppl 2):S5–12.

53. Chamberlain AM, Redfield MM, Alonso A, et al. Atrial fibrillation and mortality in heart failure: a community study. Circ Heart Fail 2011;4(6):740–6.

54. Ruff CT, Bhatt DL, Steg PG, et al. Long-term cardiovascular outcomes in patients with atrial fibrillation and atherothrombosis in the REACH Registry. Int J Cardiol 2014;170(3):413–8.

55. Ntep-Gweth M, Zimmermann M, Meiltz A, et al. Atrial fibrillation in Africa: clinical characteristics, prognosis, and adherence to guidelines in Cameroon. Europace 2010;12(4):482–7.

56. Wyse DG, Waldo AL, DiMarco JP, et al. A comparison of rate control and rhythm control in patients with atrial fibrillation. N Engl J Med 2002; 347(23):1825–33.

57. Thrall G, Lane D, Carroll D, et al. Quality of life in patients with atrial fibrillation: a systematic review. Am J Med 2006;119(5):448.e1-19.

58. Guglin M, Chen R, Curtis AB. Sinus rhythm is associated with fewer heart failure symptoms: insights from the AFFIRM trial. Heart Rhythm 2010;7(5):596–601.

59. Hsu LF, Jais P, Sanders P, et al. Catheter ablation for atrial fibrillation in congestive heart failure. N Engl J Med 2004;351(23):2373–83.

60. Dewhurst MJ, Adams PC, Gray WK, et al. Strikingly low prevalence of atrial fibrillation in elderly Tanzanians. J Am Geriatr Soc 2012;60(6):1135–40.

61. Shavadia J, Yonga G, Mwanzi S, et al. Clinical characteristics and outcomes of atrial fibrillation and flutter at the Aga Khan University Hospital, Nairobi. Cardiovasc J Afr 2013;24(2):6–9.

62. Hart RG, Pearce LA, Aguilar MI. Meta-analysis: antithrombotic therapy to prevent stroke in patients who have nonvalvular atrial fibrillation. Ann Intern Med 2007;146(12):857–67.

63. Kakkar AK, Mueller I, Bassand JP, et al. Risk profiles and antithrombotic treatment of patients newly diagnosed with atrial fibrillation at risk of stroke: perspectives from the international, observational, prospective GARFIELD registry. PLoS One 2013; 8(5):e63479.

64. Wen-Hang QI, Society of Cardiology CMA. Retrospective investigation of hospitalised patients with atrial fibrillation in mainland China. Int J Cardiol 2005;105(3):283–7.

65. Gamra H, Murin J, Chiang CE, et al. Use of antithrombotics in atrial fibrillation in Africa, Europe, Asia and South America: insights from the International RealiseAF Survey. Arch Cardiovasc Dis 2014; 107(2):77–87.

66. Nguyen TN, Hilmer SN, Cumming RG. Review of epidemiology and management of atrial fibrillation in developing countries. Int J Cardiol 2013;167(6): 2412–20.

67. Marcolino MS, Palhares DM, Benjamin EJ, et al. Atrial fibrillation: prevalence in a large database of primary care patients in Brazil. Europace 2015; 17(12):1787–90.

68. Singer DE, Hellkamp AS, Piccini JP, et al. Impact of global geographic region on time in therapeutic range on warfarin anticoagulant therapy: data from the ROCKET AF clinical trial. J Am Heart Assoc 2013;2(1):e000067.

69. Investigation of Rheumatic AF Treatment Using Vitamin K Antagonists, Rivaroxaban or Aspirin Studies, Non-Inferiority (INVICTUS-VKA). 2016. Available at: https://clinicaltrials.gov/ct2/show/NCT02832544? term=invictus&rank=2. Accessed August 15, 2016.

70. Holmes DR, Reddy VY, Turi ZG, et al. Percutaneous closure of the left atrial appendage versus warfarin therapy for prevention of stroke in patients with atrial fibrillation: a randomised non-inferiority trial. Lancet 2009;374(9689):534–42.

71. Urena M, Rodes-Cabau J, Freixa X, et al. Percutaneous left atrial appendage closure with the AMPLATZER cardiac plug device in patients with nonvalvular atrial fibrillation and contraindications to anticoagulation therapy. J Am Coll Cardiol 2013; 62(2):96–102.

72. Page RL, Joglar JA, Caldwell MA, et al. 2015 ACC/AHA/HRS guideline for the management of adult patients with supraventricular tachycardia: a report of the American College of Cardiology/American Heart Association Task Force on Clinical Practice Guidelines and the Heart Rhythm Society. J Am Coll Cardiol 2016;67(13):e27–115.

73. Hogenhuis W, Stevens SK, Wang P, et al. Cost-effectiveness of radiofrequency ablation compared with other strategies in Wolff-Parkinson-White syndrome. Circulation 1993;88(5 Pt 2):II437–446.

74. Cheng CH, Sanders GD, Hlatky MA, et al. Cost-effectiveness of radiofrequency ablation for supraventricular tachycardia. Ann Intern Med 2000; 133(11):864–76.

75. Vida VL, Calvimontes GS, Macs MO, et al. Radiofrequency catheter ablation of supraventricular tachycardia in children and adolescents: feasibility and cost-effectiveness in a low-income country. Pediatr Cardiol 2006;27(4):434–9.

76. Rodriguez BC, Leal S, Calvimontes G, et al. Cost-effectiveness of radiofrequency ablation for supraventricular tachycardia in Guatemala: patient outcomes and economic analysis from a low-middle-income country. Value Health Reg Issues 2015;8:92–8.

77. Pantos I, Efstathopoulos EP, Katritsis DG. Reuse of devices in cardiology: time for a reappraisal. Hellenic J Cardiol 2013;54(5):376–81.

78. Millar RN, Mayosi BM. Utilization of implantable defibrillators in Africa. Card Electrophysiol Rev 2003; 7(1):14–6.

79. Vedanthan R, Fuster V, Fischer A. Sudden cardiac death in low- and middle-income countries. Glob Heart 2012;7(4):353–60.

80. Bonny A, Ngantcha M, Amougou SN, et al. Rationale and design of the Pan-African Sudden Cardiac Death survey: the Pan-African SCD study. Cardiovasc J Afr 2014;25(4):176–84.

Cardiac Disease Associated with Human Immunodeficiency Virus Infection

Gerald S. Bloomfield, MD[a],*, Claudia Leung, BS[b]

KEYWORDS

- Human immunodeficiency virus • Cardiovascular diseases/epidemiology
- Cardiovascular diseases/management • HIV infections/Complications

KEY POINTS

- Typical causes and presentations of cardiac disease in patients infected with human immunodeficiency virus (HIV) differ in high-income countries (HIC) and low-income and middle-income countries (LMIC).
- In LMIC, cardiac disease is often related to end-stage manifestations of HIV/acquired immunodeficiency syndrome, including HIV-associated cardiomyopathy, pericarditis, pulmonary arterial hypertension, and complications of opportunistic infections.
- In HIC, disease causes related to aging and inflammation, particularly atherosclerosis, are more common.
- Both the HIV virus and prolonged antiretroviral therapy use are associated with dyslipidemia and are associated with increased risk of subclinical vascular disease and atherothrombotic cardiovascular events.
- Cardiovascular screening and risk factor management are important considerations in HIV care.

INTRODUCTION

Cardiac disease among patients infected with human immunodeficiency virus (HIV) has drastically changed with the advent and availability of antiretroviral therapy (ART). Early in the HIV epidemic, the predominant presentations of HIV-associated cardiac disease were dilated cardiomyopathy, pericardial disease, pulmonary hypertension, HIV-associated malignancies, and opportunistic infections (OIs). Appropriate ART has rendered HIV a chronic disease, and, with proper disease management, the life expectancy of individuals infected with HIV in high-income countries (HICs) approaches that of the uninfected population.[1] However, prolonged ART use predisposes to dyslipidemia, hyperglycemia, and lipodystrophy, among other side effects. In HICs, these effects, compounded with the cardiac effects of aging and inflammation, contribute to an increased risk of numerous cardiovascular diseases (CVDs).

In low resource settings, the burden of HIV-associated CVD differs because of variances in resources, infrastructure, and comorbid disease

Disclosure: The authors have nothing to disclose.
[a] Division of Cardiology, Duke Global Health Institute, Duke Clinical Research Institute, Duke University, 2400 Pratt Street, Durham, NC 27705, USA; [b] Feinberg School of Medicine, Northwestern University, 420 East Superior Street, Chicago, IL 60611, USA
* Corresponding author.
E-mail address: gerald.bloomfield@duke.edu

0733-8651/17/© 2016 Elsevier Inc. All rights reserved.

cardiology.theclinics.com

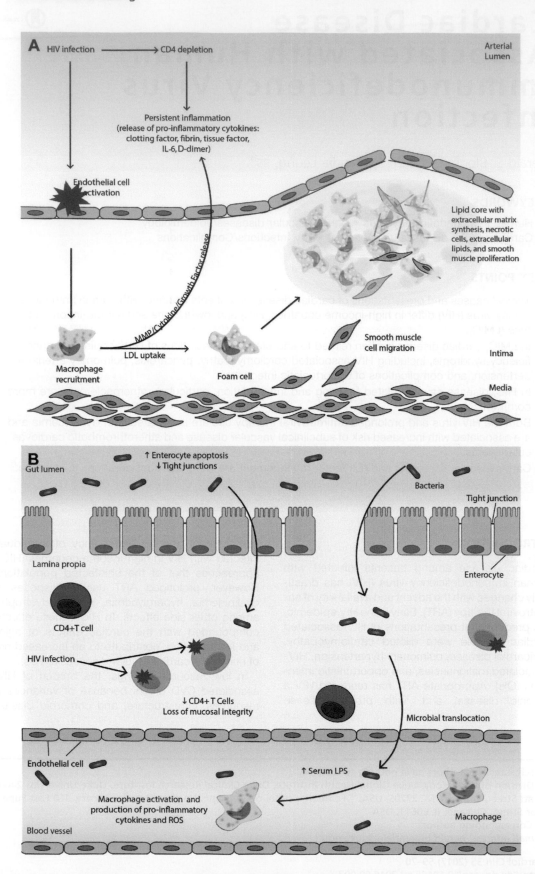

A

HIV infection ─────────→ CD4 depletion

Arterial Lumen

Persistent inflammation
(release of pro-inflammatory cytokines:
clotting factor, fibrin, tissue factor,
IL-6, D-dimer)

Endothelial cell activation

Lipid core with
extracellular matrix
synthesis, necrotic
cells, extracellular
lipids, and smooth
muscle proliferation

MMP/Cytokine/Growth Factor release

LDL uptake

Smooth muscle
cell migration

Intima

Macrophage
recruitment

Foam cell

Media

B

↑ Enterocyte apoptosis
↓ Tight junctions

Gut lumen

Bacteria

Tight junction

Lamina propia

Enterocyte

CD4+T cell

HIV infection

↓ CD4+ T Cells
Loss of mucosal integrity

Microbial translocation

Endothelial cell

↑ Serum LPS

Macrophage activation and
production of pro-inflammatory
cytokines and ROS

Macrophage

Blood vessel

burden. In regions where ART initiation is often delayed and access is limited, the predominant manifestations are still related to opportunistic, infection-related myopericardial disease.[2] However, CVD risk factors are increasingly common, especially in urban areas,[3] driven by increasing socioeconomic status and lifestyle changes. These changes characterize an epidemiologic transition in which forms of cardiac disease that were previously restricted to the aging HIV population of HICs are becoming more common in low-income and middle-income countries (LMICs). This article focuses on the most common presentations of cardiac disease among patients with HIV in both HICs and LMICs, focusing on epidemiologic trends, pathophysiology, clinical presentation, disease management, and future directions.

PATHOPHYSIOLOGY

The pathophysiology of HIV-associated CVD includes an intricate interplay of inflammation, direct effects of HIV proteins, immune dysfunction, drug effects, malnutrition, and other factors. Inflammation and dyslipidemias drive the pathophysiology of coronary artery disease (CAD) in patients infected with HIV. In particular, persistent HIV viral replication,[4] microbial translocation,[5] and coinfections (eg, cytomegalovirus)[6] contribute to a proinflammatory milieu that accelerates atherosclerosis (**Fig. 1**). Higher rates of acute myocardial infarction in individuals infected with HIV[7] are associated with higher levels of inflammatory biomarkers interleukin (IL)-6 and D-dimer, which are in turn associated with increased rates of all-cause mortality in individuals infected with HIV.[8] Protease inhibitors (PIs), particularly older generation PIs (ie, indinavir, nelfinavir, and ritonavir), are commonly implicated in ART-associated dyslipidemia (**Table 1**), and are associated with greater risk of acute myocardial infarction (AMI).[9,10] They are postulated to increase CVD risk by inducing dyslipidemia and reactive oxygen species (ROS) production, with resultant mitochondrial dysfunction,

fatty infiltration in liver and muscle, and insulin resistance.[11]

Inflammation is also a key driver of HIV-associated cardiomyopathy, as well as cardiac autoimmunity, drug effects, and nutritional deficiencies (eg, selenium and vitamin D deficiencies).[12–15] HIV-induced derangements in cell-mediated immunity also result in an increased risk of developing tuberculosis (TB) pericarditis.[16,17] In addition, HIV proteins tat, gp120, and nef promote endothelial dysfunction, resulting in the intimal and medial hyperplasia of pulmonary arteries (endarteritis obliterans) in patients with HIV-associated pulmonary arterial hypertension (PAH).[18] Depletion of T-regulatory cells, which normally function to limit vascular injury, results in increased pulmonary vasculature injury and loss of self-tolerance.[19]

CORONARY ARTERY DISEASE
Epidemiology

CAD is a major cause of death and disability among patients with HIV.[20] In the Veterans Aging Cohort Study–Virtual Cohort (VACS-VC), the rate of AMI was almost twice as high in patients infected with HIV compared with uninfected patients, even after adjustment for traditional CVD risk factors, comorbidities, and substance use.[7] The Data Collection on Adverse Events of Anti-HIV Drugs (D:A:D) study among patients infected with HIV in 21 HICs reported an incidence rate of first cardiovascular or cerebrovascular events in patients infected with HIV to be 5.7 per 1000 person-years.[9] Epidemiologic studies suggest an increasing prevalence of CAD and related risk factors, particularly in developing urban centers in LMICs.[21–23] Although data from LMICs on CAD in patients infected with HIV are scarce, the INTERHEART study reported a high global prevalence of common CVD risk factors in 52 countries, including smoking, diabetes mellitus, hypertension, abdominal obesity, and increased apolipoprotein B/apolipoprotein A-1 ratio.[24] INTERHEART was not a study of HIV-associated CVD, but these results highlight the growing burden of CVD risk factors worldwide.

Fig. 1. (A) HIV-induced endothelial cell activation results in monocyte recruitment and macrophage transformation in the subendothelial lining. Proinflammatory mediators and HIV-induced cluster of differentiation 4 (CD4) depletion contribute to persistent inflammation. HIV nef protein facilitates macrophage uptake of low-density lipoprotein (LDL), forming foam cells. Eventual foam cell apoptosis forms a cholesterol-rich necrotic core, and matrix metalloproteinases (MMPs) released by macrophages create an unstable plaque that is prone to rupture. (B) HIV infection results in early and irreversible CD4 T-cell depletion in the mucosal gastrointestinal tract, enterocyte apoptosis, and tight junction disruption. As a result, HIV damages the structural integrity of the intestinal epithelium, allowing translocation of microbial products to the lamina propria. Global dysfunction of the mucosal immune system, particularly CD4 cell depletion, fails to prevent systemic microbial translocation once microbial products enter the lamina propria. Bacterial lipopolysaccharide in the bloodstream stimulates an innate immune response, contributing to ongoing immune activation. LPS, lipopolysaccharide; ROS, reactive oxygen species.

Table 1
Antiretroviral therapy effects on selected serum lipids

Drug	HDL-c	LDL-c	TG	TC
PIs				
Ritonavir-boosted PIs	↓	↑	↑↑	↑↑
Lopinavir/ritonavir	↓	↑	↑↑↑	↑↑↑
Fosamprenavir/ritonavir	↓	↑	↑↑↑	↑↑↑
Darunavir/ritonavir	↓	↑	↑↑	↑↑
Atazanavir/ritonavir	↓	↑	↑↑	↑↑
Nelfinavir	a/↓		↑	↑
Saquinavir	↑/a		↑	↑
NNRTIs				
Efavirenz			↑↑	↑↑
Nevirapine			↑	↑
NRTIs				
Stavudine		↑↑↑	↑↑↑	
Zidovudine		↑↑	↑↑	
Abacavir		↑	↑	

Abbreviations: HDL-c, high-density lipoprotein cholesterol; LDL-c, low-density lipoprotein cholesterol; NNRTIs, nonnucleoside reverse transcriptase inhibitors; NRTIs, nucleoside reverse transcriptase inhibitors; TC, total cholesterol; TG, triglycerides.
[a] Refers to no change in lipid levels.

Small studies in sub-Saharan Africa and southeast Asia show overlap between HIV and CVD risk factors.[23,25]

Clinical Presentation

The spectrum of CAD in patients with HIV is similar to that of the general population, including silent ischemia, stable angina, and acute coronary syndrome (ACS). However, the profile of a typical patient with HIV and ACS is a young (<50 years) man with long known duration of HIV, and presence of other comorbidities such as dyslipidemia, hypertension, and diabetes mellitus.[26] In LMICs, thrombosis is more common than atherosclerosis, and patients infected with HIV with ACS have a greater degree of thrombophilia compared with uninfected persons.[27] Noncalcified, soft plaques are more prevalent and extensive in patients infected with HIV, and represent an early stage of atherosclerosis that is more prone to rupture and thrombus formation.[28,29] Certain behavioral risk factors, including illicit drug use (eg, cocaine) and tobacco smoking, are more common in the HIV population, and compound the risk of CAD. Because patients infected with HIV with ACS are often chest pain free on presentation and have fewer typical symptoms,[26] recognition of the increased risk of CAD in patients with HIV is important to mitigate the risk of delayed diagnosis and treatment.

Management and Prognosis

In the acute setting, procedural success of percutaneous coronary intervention (PCI) is similar to that of the general population[30]; however, patients infected with HIV with ACS have a higher risk for recurrent coronary revascularization and AMI than the general population.[31] Post-PCI, there is a high incidence of rehospitalization for recurrent coronary event (45%),[32] restenosis (9%–43%),[33] and percutaneous revascularization (20%).[31] Several reports show successful thrombolysis in patients with HIV presenting with AMI.[34] In the Prognosis of Acute Coronary Syndrome (PACS) study, recurrent ACS was 6.5 times more frequent at 1-year follow-up,[30] and 3.4 times more frequent at 3-year follow-up,[35] in patients infected with HIV compared with uninfected persons. HIV status and lipid parameters were the only independent predictors of recurrence.[30] Despite this, the most commonly used CVD risk estimating techniques for patients with ACS do not take into account HIV infection.

There are few specific guidelines for the management of stable CAD in patients with HIV, and current practice follows the same approach as for the general population. Blood pressure control, lipid management, lifestyle changes, and smoking cessation are cornerstones of management.[36] Recent lipid management guidelines from the National Lipid Association (NLA) recommend first-line statin therapy (atorvastatin, rosuvastatin, or pitavastatin) for patients infected with HIV with increased low-density lipoprotein cholesterol and non–high-density lipoprotein cholesterol, and fibrate or omega-3 fatty acids for increased triglyceride levels.[37] Given the significant contribution of inflammation to the pathophysiology of HIV-associated cardiac disease, statins may also be beneficial for their antiinflammatory effects. Statins are metabolized by hepatic cytochrome P450 (CYP3A4) and should be used with caution in patients on PIs, which are CYP3A4 inhibitors (**Table 2**), because of potential liver and muscle toxicity.[38] A systematic review of 18 clinical trials found pravastatin, rosuvastatin, and pitavastatin to be safe and efficacious in treating hyperlipidemia when coadministered with ART without dose adjustment.[39] Concerns remain regarding the risk of diabetes with statin use.[40,41] A large trial powered for clinical end points is underway to better elucidate the risks and benefits of statin use in the HIV-infected population.[42,43]

HUMAN IMMUNODEFICIENCY VIRUS–ASSOCIATED CARDIOMYOPATHY
Epidemiology

With the advent of ARTs, HIV-associated cardiomyopathy (HIVAC) has become less common[44]

but HIV remains a significant risk factor for heart failure.[45] A meta-analysis of 11 studies of left ventricular function in patients infected with HIV and on ART reported 8.3% prevalence of systolic dysfunction and 43.4% for diastolic dysfunction.[46] Systolic dysfunction was significantly associated with chronic inflammation, tobacco smoking, and history of myocardial infarction. Diastolic dysfunction was significantly associated with hypertension and age.[46]

Clinical Presentation

In the Heart of Soweto study of HIV-associated cardiac diseases in sub-Saharan Africa, HIVAC was the most common cardiac presentation among individuals infected with HIV (38%).[47] HIVAC is most often associated with low socioeconomic status, longer duration of HIV infection, low total lymphocyte count, low CD4 count (<100/mm^3), high HIV-1 viral load, and low plasma levels of selenium.[12] In contrast with the pre-ART era,[48] the current presentation of HIVAC in HIC is most commonly minimally symptomatic with mildly reduced left ventricular (LV) systolic function or impaired diastolic function. In regions with delayed ART initiation and high prevalence of OIs, symptomatic systolic dysfunction and dilated cardiomyopathies are still common.[49]

Table 2
Metabolism and dosing precautions of select lipid level–lowering therapies

Drug	Hepatic Metabolism	Note	
		Use with PIs	Use with NNRTIs
Statins			
Atorvastatin	CYP3A4	Start with low dose	Consider higher dose
Fluvastatin	CYP2C9; CYP3A4 (minor)	Consider higher dose	Consider higher dose
Lovastatin	CYP3A4	Contraindicated	Consider higher dose
Pitavastatin	CYP2C9	Start at usual dose	Start at usual dose
Pravastatin	No P450 interactions	First line, consider higher dose	Consider higher dose
Rosuvastatin	CYP2C9<10%	Consider higher dose	Consider higher dose
Simvastatin	CYP3A4	Contraindicated	Consider higher dose
Fibrates			
Bezafibrate[a] Fenofibrate Gemfibrozil	No P450 interactions; glucuronidation with renal elimination	No known interactions with PIs or NRTIs; gemfibrozil interacts with statins	
Cholesterol Absorption Inhibitor			
Ezetimibe	No P450 interactions	Use with statins, or alone if statin not tolerated	
PCSK9 Inhibitors			
Alirocumab Evolocumab	No P450 interactions	No known interactions with PIs or NRTIs	

Abbreviations: CYP, cytochrome P450; PCSK9, proprotein convertase subtilisin/kexin type 9.
[a] Available in the United States as an investigational drug.

Management and Prognosis

Management of patients infected with HIV presenting with cardiomyopathy should prioritize identification of other concomitant causes of cardiomyopathy that may require specific therapies, including OIs, cardiotoxic drugs, and CAD.[50,51] In the absence of guidelines or controlled trials addressing the most effective strategies for treating for HIVAC, treatment should follow current society consensus recommendations. LV function is an independent predictor of death in children[52] and adults infected with HIV,[53] and the likelihood of developing HIVAC increases with progressive immunosuppression, particularly CD4 count less than 100 cells/μL. In retrospective studies, both ART and prevention of OIs are associated with lower incidence of cardiomyopathy.[54] Thus, treatment should include appropriate ART initiation with the goals of restoring immune status, suppressing viral load, and preventing OIs. Avoidance of cardiotoxic drugs; preventing adverse drug-drug interactions; and prolonging survival with β-blockers, angiotensin-converting enzyme inhibitors, and spironolactone are also critical.[49] There are limited data regarding the efficacy of antiinflammatory therapies (eg, anti–tumor necrosis factor [TNF] therapy) in HIVAC, and further investigation should be directed toward patients with cardiomyopathies of inflammatory causes. The current experience with cytokine inhibition in heart failure is limited to patients who are not infected with HIV,[55] but small studies on anti-TNF therapy that have included individuals infected with HIV show no adverse infectious events with etanercept or infliximab.[56]

PERICARDIAL DISEASE IN HUMAN IMMUNODEFICIENCY VIRUS
Epidemiology

Worldwide, pericarditis (usually as a result of TB infection) is the most common cardiac disorder associated with HIV.[57] Since the early 1980s, HIV has emerged as the most important predisposing factor to TB, increasing the risk by 20 times overall, and by 120 times in patients with AIDS.[58] In some regions of Africa, up to 80% of patients with TB are also infected with HIV.[59]

Clinical Presentation

Clinically, pericarditis can present as pericardial effusion, constrictive pericarditis, and effusive-constrictive pericarditis. Pericardial effusion is most common (80%), followed by effusive-constrictive pericarditis (15%).[60] Patients infected with HIV are more likely to present with disseminated

TB and pericardial tamponade,[2] but less likely to have constrictive pericarditis at 6 months.[61] Patients with advanced immunosuppression are also more likely to have diminished granuloma formation (systemically and within the pericardium),[62] myopericarditis, dyspnea, and hemodynamic instability.[60] Atrial fibrillation is also common in patients with TB pericardial effusion, particularly in those with evidence of LV dysfunction.[63]

Management and Prognosis

In patients with TB pericarditis, the cornerstones of management are adequate diagnosis, timely pericardiocentesis for relief of tamponade and sampling of pericardial fluid, antituberculosis chemotherapy, appropriate follow-up for management of HIV, and recognizing the onset of constrictive pericarditis. HIV status and immunocompetence are important determinants of mortality.[57] Early initiation of ART among patients infected with HIV with tuberculosis significantly increases survival despite an increased risk of TB-related immune reconstitution inflammatory syndrome.[64] In the Investigation of the Management of Pericarditis in Africa (IMPI Africa) registry of TB pericarditis, immunocompromised patients (those with clinical signs of HIV infection) had a 6-month mortality of 40% versus 17% for immunocompetent patients.[61] The IMPI Africa trial compared adjunctive prednisolone therapy and *Mycobacterium indicus pranii* immunotherapy with placebo in 1400 patients infected and uninfected with HIV with suspected or probable TB pericarditis. Neither therapy had a significant effect on the composite end point of death, cardiac tamponade requiring pericardiocentesis, and constrictive pericarditis. Prednisolone, compared with placebo, significantly reduced the incidence of constrictive pericarditis and the incidence of hospitalization. Both prednisolone and *M indicus pranii*, compared with placebo, were significantly associated with an increased risk of HIV-associated malignancy, possibly caused by a synergistic effect between the two therapies among immunocompromised patients.[65]

HUMAN IMMUNODEFICIENCY VIRUS–ASSOCIATED PULMONARY ARTERIAL HYPERTENSION
Epidemiology

The few reports on HIV-associated pulmonary arterial hypertension (HIVPAH) suggest a higher prevalence in LMICs (0.6%–13% in sub-Saharan Africa)[47,66] than in HICs (0.5%),[67] possibly caused by a high burden of comorbid pulmonary diseases. There are no known specific risk factors; however,

HIVPAH seems to be more prevalent among intravenous drug users.[68]

Clinical Presentation

Patients with HIVPAH can present at any stage of HIV infection; there is no association with serum CD4 count or viral load.[69] Patients are more often male and tend to present at a younger age (average, 35 years) than those with other forms of PAH.[68] The most common presenting symptom is dyspnea (93%). Other signs are pedal edema, syncope, fatigue, nonproductive cough, and chest pain. Diagnostic work-up often reveals cardiomegaly and pulmonary artery enlargement on chest radiograph; right ventricular hypertrophy and right atrial dilatation on electrocardiogram; and right ventricular dilatation, right atrial dilatation, and tricuspid regurgitation on echocardiogram.[70] The gold standard diagnosis is right heart catheterization measuring mean pulmonary artery pressure greater than 25 mm Hg and pulmonary artery wedge pressure less than 15 mm Hg.

Management and Prognosis

There is no cure for HIVPAH, and currently there are no specific guidelines for management. Similar to other forms of PAH, treatment includes supportive treatment (oxygen therapy, diuretics, oral anticoagulants) and PAH-specific therapies (prostaglandins, endothelin receptor antagonists, calcium channel blockers, and phosphodiesterase inhibitors). Calcium channel blockers and phosphodiesterase inhibitors should be titrated carefully because coadministration with antiretrovirals, including ritonavir and indinavir, may increase plasma concentrations of calcium channel blockers.[71,72] In general, HIVPAH is unresponsive to treatment of comorbid infection, oxygen therapy, or vasodilators.[18] A higher CD4 count at diagnosis is associated with better survival,[68] and although ART does not seem to prevent the development of HIVPAH, it may delay its onset and reduce risk of secondary pulmonary infection, which can exacerbate PAH and lead to early mortality.[73] Thus, ART initiation is recommended in all patients with HIVPAH irrespective of CD4 count.[74] However, most die within 1 year of diagnosis because of complications of PAH.[70]

CARDIOVASCULAR SCREENING AND RISK STRATIFICATION

Conventional cardiovascular risk calculators do not take into account novel risk factors associated with HIV, such as inflammation and immune activation, coagulation disorders, kidney disease, and ART exposure (**Table 3**). Accordingly, both the Framingham Risk Score (FRS) and the American College of Cardiology (ACC)/American Heart Association (AHA) Risk Calculator underestimate 5-year and 10-year CVD event rates by 20% to 25% in patients infected with HIV.[75,76] The D:A:D study group developed an HIV-specific risk assessment tool that predicts 5-year AMI and CAD risk better than the FRS, and incorporates traditional risk factors, cumulative exposure to ART drugs, current use of abacavir, and CD4 count.[77] Biomarkers associated with CVD in patients with HIV include high-sensitivity C-reactive protein, IL-6, D-dimer,[78] and LpPLA2 (lipoprotein-associated phospholipase A2),[79] and have been proposed to improve risk stratification, but have not been incorporated in any of the developed models. More research is needed to evaluate and validate their use for CVD risk stratification.

TREATMENT THRESHOLDS

Guidelines for lipid management in patients infected with HIV have been developed by the Infectious Disease Society of America[80] and the European AIDS Clinical Society,[81] which recommend estimation of 10-year AMI risk using the FRS. The NLA guidelines consider HIV a major risk factor for CVD, and recommend estimation of risk using either the FRS or the ACC/AHA Risk Calculator.[37] However, both the FRS and the ACC/AHA guidelines have not been formally validated in patients infected with HIV and multiple studies report imprecise risk prediction in this group.[75,76] NLA guidelines recommend the same treatment goals for patients infected with HIV as for the general population.[37] Treatment of diabetes mellitus also warrants attention. The US Department of Health and Human Services recommends fasting plasma glucose testing 1 to 3 months after ART initiation and every 6 to 12 months thereafter.[82] Treatment with oral medications and insulin therapy follows standard guidelines with special considerations to potential drug interactions, particularly PIs. Hemoglobin A1c (HbA1c) underestimates glycemia in patients infected with HIV, especially those with higher mean corpuscular volume, abacavir use, and lower CD4 count.[83] Thus, clinicians may consider a more stringent HbA1c goal or recommended testing alternatives (fasting plasma glucose or oral glucose tolerance testing).[84]

Management of hypertension in patients with HIV should generally follow the recent Joint National Committee guidelines,[85] with attention to potential drug-drug interactions between antihypertensives and ART, particularly certain

Table 3
Characteristics of cardiovascular risk scores

Characteristic	ACC/AHA	Framingham MI	Framingham Total CVD	Score	QRISK2	D:A:D Risk Calculator
Age	●	●	●	●	●	●
Sex	●	●	●	●	●	●
Smoking tobacco	●	●	●	●	●	●
Diabetes	●	●	●	○	●	●
Race/ethnicity	●	○	○	○	●	○
Social deprivation	○	○	○	○	●	○
Lipids	●	●	●	●	●	●
Hypertension therapy	●	●	●	○	●	○
Blood pressure	●	●	●	●	●	●
Body mass index	○	○	○	○	●	○
Family history of premature CVD/CHD	○	○	○	○	●	●
Chronic kidney disease	○	○	○	○	●	○
Atrial fibrillation	○	○	○	○	●	○
Rheumatoid arthritis	○	○	○	○	●	○
Cummulative exposure to PIs and NRTIs	○	○	○	○	○	●
Current use of ABC	○	○	○	○	○	●
Output						
Five-year prediction						
Stroke, fatal or nonfatal CHD					✓	✓
Ten-year prediction						
Fatal or nonfatal ASCVD	✓					
CHD, TIA or stroke, or CVD death			✓			
Fatal or nonfatal MI		✓				
Fatal CVD				✓		
Lifetime prediction						
Fatal or nonfatal ASCVD	✓					

Green boxes, characteristics included in risk calculation; red boxes, characteristics not included in risk calculation.

Abbreviations: ABC, abacavir; ACC, American College of Cardiology; AHA, American Heart Association; ASCVD, atherosclerotic cardiovascular disease; CHD, coronary heart disease; MI, myocardial infarction; TIA, transient ischemic attack.

Table 4
Elimination pathways of select antihypertensive drugs

Drug	Elimination (%)	
	Hepatic	Renal
β-Blockers		
Atenolol	—	85–100
Carvedilol	CYP2D6, <10	—
Labetalol	CYP2D6/biliary	<5
Metoprolol	CYP2D6, 3–10	—
Propranolol	CYP2D6, 3A4, 2C19, <1	—
Calcium Channel Blockers		
Dihydropyridines (eg, nifedipine)	CYP3A metabolism, 90 Biliary excretion, 15	80–90, 10 unchanged
Phenylalkylamines (eg, verapamil)	CYP3A metabolism, 90 Biliary excretion, 20–25	70, 3–4 unchanged
Benzothiazepines (eg, diltiazem)	CYP3A metabolism, 90 Biliary excretion, 65	35, 2–4 unchanged
Angiotensin II Receptor Blockers		
Candesartan	CYP2C9 metabolism (minor) Unchanged/biliary excretion, 40	60
Irbesartan	CYP2C9 metabolism with biliary excretion, 80	20
Losartan	CYP2C9 active metabolite, 90 CYP3A4 (minor)	10
Olmesartan	Biliary excretion, 65	35
Telmisartan	Unchanged/biliary excretion, 99	1
Valsartan	Unchanged/biliary excretion, 70	30

non-nucleoside reverse transcriptase inhibitors and PIs based on route of elimination (**Table 4**).[86] Target blood pressure for patients with HIV and comorbidities should be less than 140/90 mm Hg, until evidence indicates otherwise.

SUMMARY

The typical cause and clinical presentation of cardiac disease in patients with HIV differ in HICs and LMICs. In HICs where ART access is more pervasive, CVD is characterized by complications related to aging, immune activation, and ART use. In LMICs and resource-limited regions of HICs with limited ART access, CVD is commonly related to OIs and end-stage manifestations of HIV/AIDS, including HIVAC, pericarditis, and HIV-PAH. Increasing ART access has drastically improved the life expectancy of patients infected with HIV. As a result, more attention needs to be devoted to cardiovascular screening, prevention, and risk factor management in the care of patients infected with HIV.

REFERENCES

1. Samji H, Cescon A, Hogg RS, et al. Closing the gap: increases in life expectancy among treated HIV-positive individuals in the United States and Canada. PLoS One 2013;8(12):e81355.
2. Ntsekhe M, Mayosi BM. Cardiac manifestations of HIV infection: an African perspective. Nat Clin Pract Cardiovasc Med 2009;6(2):120–7.
3. Bovet P, Ross AG, Gervasoni J-P, et al. Distribution of blood pressure, body mass index and smoking habits in the urban population of Dar es Salaam, Tanzania, and associations with socioeconomic status. Int J Epidemiol 2002;31(1):240–7.
4. Yukl SA, Shergill AK, McQuaid K, et al. Effect of raltegravir-containing intensification on HIV burden and T-cell activation in multiple gut sites of HIV-positive adults on suppressive antiretroviral therapy. AIDS 2010;24(16):2451–60.
5. Brenchley JM, Price DA, Schacker TW, et al. Microbial translocation is a cause of systemic immune activation in chronic HIV infection. Nat Med 2006; 12(12):1365–71.

6. Hsue PY, Hunt PW, Sinclair E, et al. Increased carotid intima-media thickness in HIV patients is associated with increased cytomegalovirus-specific T-cell responses. AIDS 2006;20(18):2275–83.

7. Freiberg MS, Chang C-CH, Kuller LH, et al. HIV infection and the risk of acute myocardial infarction. JAMA Intern Med 2013;173(8):614–22.

8. Kuller LH, Tracy R, Belloso W, et al. Inflammatory and coagulation biomarkers and mortality in patients with HIV infection. PLoS Med 2008;5(10):e203.

9. Sabin CA, Worm SW, Weber R, et al, D:A:D Study Group. Use of nucleoside reverse transcriptase inhibitors and risk of myocardial infarction in HIV-infected patients enrolled in the D:A:D study: a multi-cohort collaboration. Lancet 2008;371(9622):1417–26.

10. Friis-Møller N, Reiss P, Sabin CA, et al. Class of antiretroviral drugs and the risk of myocardial infarction. N Engl J Med 2007;356(17):1723–35.

11. Anuurad E, Bremer A, Berglund L. HIV protease inhibitors and obesity. Curr Opin Endocrinol Diabetes Obes 2010;17(5):478–85.

12. Twagirumukiza M, Nkeramihigo E, Seminega B, et al. Prevalence of dilated cardiomyopathy in HIV-infected African patients not receiving HAART: a multicenter, observational, prospective, cohort study in Rwanda. Curr HIV Res 2007;5(1):129–37.

13. Ross AC, Judd S, Kumari M, et al. Vitamin D is linked to carotid intima-media thickness and immune reconstitution in HIV-positive individuals. Antivir Ther 2011;16(4):555–63.

14. Wang TJ, Pencina MJ, Booth SL, et al. Vitamin D deficiency and risk of cardiovascular disease. Circulation 2008;117(4):503–11.

15. Lai H, Gerstenblith G, Fishman EK, et al. Vitamin D deficiency is associated with silent coronary artery disease in cardiovascularly asymptomatic African Americans with HIV infection. Clin Infect Dis 2012;54(12):1747–55.

16. Matthews K, Ntsekhe M, Syed F, et al. HIV-1 infection alters CD4+ memory T-cell phenotype at the site of disease in extrapulmonary tuberculosis. Eur J Immunol 2012;42(1):147–57.

17. Mayosi BM, Burgess LJ, Doubell AF. Tuberculous pericarditis. Circulation 2005;112(23):3608–16.

18. Butrous G. Human immunodeficiency virus-associated pulmonary arterial hypertension: considerations for pulmonary vascular diseases in the developing world. Circulation 2015;131(15):1361–70.

19. Nicolls MR, Taraseviciene-Stewart L, Rai PR, et al. Autoimmunity and pulmonary hypertension: a perspective. Eur Respir J 2005;26(6):1110–8.

20. Palella FJ Jr, Baker RK, Moorman AC, et al. Mortality in the highly active antiretroviral therapy era: changing causes of death and disease in the HIV outpatient study. J Acquir Immune Defic Syndr 2006;43(1):27–34.

21. Lawoyin TO, Asuzu MC, Kaufman J, et al. Prevalence of cardiovascular risk factors in an African, urban inner city community. West Afr J Med 2002;21(3):208–11.

22. Njelekela M, Negishi H, Nara Y, et al. Cardiovascular risk factors in Tanzania: a revisit. Acta trop 2001;79(3):231–9.

23. Jantarapakde J, Phanuphak N, Chaturawit C, et al. Prevalence of metabolic syndrome among antiretroviral-naive and antiretroviral-experienced HIV-1 infected Thai adults. AIDS Patient Care STDS 2014;28(7):331–40.

24. Yusuf S, Hawken S, Ounpuu S, et al. Effect of potentially modifiable risk factors associated with myocardial infarction in 52 countries (the INTERHEART study): case-control study. Lancet 2004;364(9438):937–52.

25. Muyanja D, Muzoora C, Muyingo A, et al. High prevalence of metabolic syndrome and cardiovascular disease risk among people with HIV on stable ART in southwestern Uganda. AIDS Patient Care STDS 2016;30(1):4–10.

26. Perello R, Calvo M, Miro O, et al. Clinical presentation of acute coronary syndrome in HIV infected adults: a retrospective analysis of a prospectively collected cohort. Eur J Intern Med 2011;22(5):485–8.

27. Becker AC, Jacobson B, Singh S, et al. The thrombotic profile of treatment-naive HIV-positive black South Africans with acute coronary syndromes. Clin Appl Thromb Hemost 2011;17(3):264–72.

28. Post WS, Budoff M, Kingsley L, et al. Associations between HIV infection and subclinical coronary atherosclerosis. Ann Intern Med 2014;160(7):458–67.

29. D'Ascenzo F, Cerrato E, Calcagno A, et al. High prevalence at computed coronary tomography of non-calcified plaques in asymptomatic HIV patients treated with HAART: a meta-analysis. Atherosclerosis 2015;240(1):197–204.

30. Boccara F, Mary-Krause M, Teiger E, et al. Acute coronary syndrome in human immunodeficiency virus-infected patients: characteristics and 1 year prognosis. Eur Heart J 2011;32(1):41–50.

31. D'Ascenzo F, Cerrato E, Biondi-Zoccai G, et al. Acute coronary syndromes in human immunodeficiency virus patients: a meta-analysis investigating adverse event rates and the role of antiretroviral therapy. Eur Heart J 2012;33(7):875–80.

32. Matetzky S, Domingo M, Kar S, et al. Acute myocardial infarction in human immunodeficiency virus-infected patients. Arch Intern Med 2003;163(4):457–60.

33. Boccara F, Lang S, Meuleman C, et al. HIV and coronary heart disease: time for a better understanding. J Am Coll Cardiol 2013;61(5):511–23.

34. Boccara F, Cohen A. Coronary artery disease and stroke in HIV-infected patients: prevention and

pharmacological therapy. Adv Cardiol 2003;40: 163–84.

35. Boccara F, Mary-Krause M, Teiger E. HIV-infected status is associated with increased recurrence of acute coronary syndrome. Results of long term follow up of the PACS-HIV study. Archives of Cardiovascular Disease Supplements 2012. http://dx.doi.org/10.1016/S1878-6480(12)70419-6.

36. Escarcega RO, Franco JJ, Mani BC, et al. Cardiovascular disease in patients with chronic human immunodeficiency virus infection. Int J Cardiol 2014; 175(1):1–7.

37. Jacobson TA, Maki KC, Orringer CE, et al. National lipid association recommendations for patient-centered management of dyslipidemia: part 2. J Clin Lipidol 2015;9(6 Suppl):S1–122.e1.

38. Chauvin B, Drouot S, Barrail-Tran A, et al. Drug-drug interactions between HMG-CoA reductase inhibitors (statins) and antiviral protease inhibitors. Clin Pharmacokinet 2013;52(10):815–31.

39. Feinstein MJ, Achenbach CJ, Stone NJ, et al. A systematic review of the usefulness of statin therapy in HIV-infected patients. Am J Cardiol 2015; 115(12):1760–6.

40. Culver AL, Ockene IS, Balasubramanian R, et al. Statin use and risk of diabetes mellitus in postmenopausal women in the women's health initiative. Arch Intern Med 2012;172(2):144–52.

41. Erlandson KM, Jiang Y, Debanne SM, et al. Rosuvastatin worsens insulin resistance in HIV-infected adults on antiretroviral therapy. Clin Infect Dis 2015;61(10):1566–72.

42. National Institute of Allergy and Infectious Diseases (NIAID), National Heart Lung and Blood Institute NHLBI. Evaluating the Use of Pitavastatin to Reduce the Risk of Cardiovascular Disease in HIV-Infected Adults (REPRIEVE). Bethesda (MD) Available at: https://clinicaltrials.gov/ct2/show/NCT02344290. Accessed September 29, 2016.

43. Longenecker CT, Triant VA. Initiation of antiretroviral therapy at high CD4 cell counts: does it reduce the risk of cardiovascular disease? Curr Opin HIV AIDS 2014;9(1):54–62.

44. Lumsden RH, Bloomfield GS. The causes of HIV-associated cardiomyopathy: a tale of two worlds. Biomed Res Int 2016;2016(4):1–9.

45. Butt AA, Chang C-C, Kuller L, et al. Risk of heart failure with human immunodeficiency virus in the absence of prior diagnosis of coronary heart disease. Arch Intern Med 2011;171(8):737–43.

46. Cerrato E, D'Ascenzo F, Biondi-Zoccai G, et al. Cardiac dysfunction in pauci symptomatic human immunodeficiency virus patients: a meta-analysis in the highly active antiretroviral therapy era. Eur Heart J 2013;34(19):1432–6.

47. Sliwa K, Carrington MJ, Becker A, et al. Contribution of the human immunodeficiency virus/acquired immunodeficiency syndrome epidemic to de novo presentations of heart disease in the Heart of Soweto Study cohort. Eur Heart J 2012;33(7):866–74.

48. Magula NP, Mayosi BM. Cardiac involvement in HIV-infected people living in Africa: a review. Cardiovasc J S Afr 2003;14(5):231–7.

49. Bloomfield GS, Alenezi F, Barasa FA, et al. Human immunodeficiency virus and heart failure in low- and middle-income countries. JACC Heart Fail 2015;3(8):579–90.

50. Monsuez J-J, Escaut L, Teicher E, et al. Cytokines in HIV-associated cardiomyopathy. Int J Cardiol 2007; 120(2):150–7.

51. Barbaro G. Cardiovascular manifestations of HIV infection. Circulation 2002;106(11):1420–5.

52. Lipshultz SE, Easley KA, Orav EJ, et al. Cardiac dysfunction and mortality in HIV-infected children: the prospective P2C2 HIV multicenter study. Pediatric Pulmonary and Cardiac Complications of Vertically Transmitted HIV Infection (P2C2 HIV) study group. Circulation 2000;102(13):1542–8.

53. Moyers BS, Secemsky EA, Vittinghoff E, et al. Effect of left ventricular dysfunction and viral load on risk of sudden cardiac death in patients with human immunodeficiency virus. Am J Cardiol 2014;113(7):1260–5.

54. Pugliese A, Isnardi D, Saini A, et al. Impact of highly active antiretroviral therapy in HIV-positive patients with cardiac involvement. J Infect 2000;40(3):282–4.

55. Mann DL, McMurray JJV, Packer M, et al. Targeted anticytokine therapy in patients with chronic heart failure: results of the Randomized Etanercept Worldwide Evaluation (RENEWAL). Circulation 2004; 109(13):1594–602.

56. Calabrese LH, Zein N, Vassilopoulos D. Safety of antitumour necrosis factor (anti-TNF) therapy in patients with chronic viral infections: hepatitis C, hepatitis B, and HIV infection. Ann Rheum Dis 2004; 63(suppl_2):ii18–24.

57. Ntsekhe M, Mayosi BM. Tuberculous pericarditis with and without HIV. Heart Fail Rev 2013;18(3): 367–73.

58. Zumla A, Malon P, Henderson J, et al. Impact of HIV infection on tuberculosis. Postgrad Med J 2000; 76(895):259–68.

59. Syed FF, Sani MU. Recent advances in HIV-associated cardiovascular diseases in Africa. Heart 2013;99(16):1146–53.

60. Mayosi BM, Wiysonge CS, Ntsekhe M, et al. Clinical characteristics and initial management of patients with tuberculous pericarditis in the HIV era: the Investigation of the Management of Pericarditis in Africa (IMPI Africa) registry. BMC Infect Dis 2006;6(1):1.

61. Mayosi BM, Wiysonge CS, Ntsekhe M, et al. Mortality in patients treated for tuberculous pericarditis in sub-Saharan Africa. S Afr Med J 2008;98(1):36–40.

62. Reuter H, Burgess LJ, Schneider J, et al. The role of histopathology in establishing the diagnosis of

tuberculous pericardial effusions in the presence of HIV. Histopathology 2006;48(3):295–302.

63. Syed FF, Mayosi BM. A modern approach to tuberculous pericarditis. Prog Cardiovasc Dis 2007; 50(3):218–36.

64. Blanc F-X, Sok T, Laureillard D, et al. Earlier versus later start of antiretroviral therapy in HIV-infected adults with tuberculosis. N Engl J Med 2011; 365(16):1471–81.

65. Mayosi BM, Ntsekhe M, Bosch J, et al. Prednisolone and *Mycobacterium indicus pranii* in tuberculous pericarditis. N Engl J Med 2014;371(12): 1121–30.

66. Chillo P, Bakari M, Lwakatare J. Echocardiographic diagnoses in HIV-infected patients presenting with cardiac symptoms at Muhimbili National Hospital in Dar es Salaam, Tanzania. Cardiovasc J Afr 2012; 23(2):90–7.

67. Sitbon O, Lascoux-Combe C, Delfraissy J-F, et al. Prevalence of HIV-related pulmonary arterial hypertension in the current antiretroviral therapy era. Am J Respir Crit Care Med 2012;177(1):108–13.

68. Nunes H, Humbert M, Sitbon O, et al. Prognostic factors for survival in human immunodeficiency virus-associated pulmonary arterial hypertension. Am J Respir Crit Care Med 2003;167(10):1433–9.

69. Thienemann F, Sliwa K, Rockstroh JK. HIV and the heart: the impact of antiretroviral therapy: a global perspective. Eur Heart J 2013;34(46):3538–46.

70. Janda S, Quon BS, Swiston J. HIV and pulmonary arterial hypertension: a systematic review. HIV Med 2010;11(10):620–34.

71. Glesby MJ, Aberg JA, Kendall MA, et al. Pharmacokinetic interactions between indinavir plus ritonavir and calcium channel blockers. Clin Pharmacol Ther 2005;78(2):143–53.

72. Barnett CF, Hsue PY. Human immunodeficiency virus-associated pulmonary arterial hypertension. Clin Chest Med 2013;34(2):283–92.

73. Degano B, Guillaume M, Savale L, et al. HIV-associated pulmonary arterial hypertension: survival and prognostic factors in the modern therapeutic era. AIDS 2010;24(1):67–75.

74. Zuber J-P, Calmy A, Evison JM, et al. Pulmonary arterial hypertension related to HIV infection: improved hemodynamics and survival associated with antiretroviral therapy. Clin Infect Dis 2004; 38(8):1178–85.

75. Regan S, Meigs JB, Massaro J, et al. Evaluation of the ACC/AHA CVD risk prediction algorithm among HIV-infected patients. CROI 2015;6:390–9.

76. Thompson-Paul A, Lichtenstein K, Armon C, et al. Cardiovascular disease risk prediction in the HIV Outpatient Study (HOPS). Clin Infect Dis 2016. [Epub ahead of print].

77. Friis-Møller N, Thiebaut R, Reiss P, et al. Predicting the risk of cardiovascular disease in HIV-infected patients: the data collection on adverse effects of anti-HIV drugs study. Eur J Cardiovasc Prev Rehabil 2010;17(5):491–501.

78. Worm SW, Hsue P. Role of biomarkers in predicting CVD risk in the setting of HIV infection? Curr Opin HIV AIDS 2010;5(6):467–72.

79. Mangili A, Ahmad R, Wolfert RL, et al. Lipoprotein-associated phospholipase A2, a novel cardiovascular inflammatory marker, in HIV-infected patients. Clin Infect Dis 2014;58(6):893–900.

80. Dube MP, Stein JH, Aberg JA, et al. Guidelines for the evaluation and management of dyslipidemia in human immunodeficiency virus (HIV)-infected adults receiving antiretroviral therapy: recommendations of the HIV Medicine Association of the infectious Disease Society of AMERICA and the Adult AIDS Clinical Trials Group. Clin Infect Dis 2003;37(5):613–27.

81. Lundgren JD, Battegay M, Behrens G, et al. European AIDS Clinical Society (EACS) guidelines on the prevention and management of metabolic diseases in HIV. HIV Med 2008;9(2):72–81.

82. Panel on Antiretroviral Guidelines for Adults and Adolescents. Guidelines for the use of antiretroviral agents in HIV-1-infected adults and adolescents. Department of Health and Human Services. Available at: http://www.aidsinfo.nih.gov/ContentFiles/AdultandAdolescentGL.pdf. Accessed September 29, 2016.

83. Kim PS, Woods C, Georgoff P, et al. A1C underestimates glycemia in HIV infection. Diabetes care 2009;32(9):1591–3.

84. Monroe AK, Glesby MJ, Brown TT. Diagnosing and managing diabetes in HIV-infected patients: current concepts. Clin Infect Dis 2015;60(3):453–62.

85. Abrass CK, Applebaum JS, Boyd CM, et al. The HIV and aging consensus project. Report from the HIV & Aging Consensus Project: recommended treatment strategies for clinicians managing older patients with HIV infection. Washington, DC: American Academy of HIV Medicine; 2011. p. 1–76. Available at: http://hiv-age.org/.

86. Peyriere H, Eiden C, Macia JC, et al. Antihypertensive drugs in patients treated with antiretrovirals. Ann Pharmacother 2012;46(5):703–9.

Environmental Exposures and Cardiovascular Disease

A Challenge for Health and Development in Low- and Middle-Income Countries

Melissa S. Burroughs Peña, MD, MS[a],*, Allman Rollins, MD[b]

KEYWORDS

- Environmental health • Air pollution • Household air pollution • Heavy metals • Lead • Arsenic
- Cadmium • Cardiovascular disease

KEY POINTS

- Environmental exposures, including air pollution and heavy metal and metalloid contamination, are more prevalent in low- and middle-income countries.
- Exposure to air pollution in the form of ambient air pollution and household air pollution from biomass fuel use is associated with hypertension, acute myocardial infarction, heart failure, arrhythmia, sudden cardiac death, and cardiovascular mortality.
- Lead, arsenic, and cadmium exposures are associated with hypertension, coronary heart disease, and cardiovascular mortality.
- There is increasing epidemiologic evidence of an association of environmental exposures with cardiovascular risk factors and cardiovascular disease, yet most of the research has been conducted in high-income countries.

INTRODUCTION

In the wake of large-scale economic development in low- and middle-income countries (LMIC), environmental pollution has been a challenge that has spurred tension within countries and across regions.[1] The use of fossil fuel combustion to increase access to electricity and transportation for millions of people has simultaneously modernized a multitude of rural and urban communities while locally polluting the air and globally increasing air temperatures.[2–4] Extractive industries, such as mining, have fueled the economies of many middle-income countries, lifting large swaths of the population out of poverty while contaminating water with heavy metals.[5] The conflict over environmental pollution is so intense in some regions that large-scale demonstrations and even violence have erupted, thus threatening national and regional security.[5] Although many have argued that poverty reduction and economic growth justify the subsequent damage to the environment, the health consequences of environmental pollution, particularly for the populations residing in LMIC, must also be taken into account.[6,7]

The authors report no conflicts of interest.

[a] Division of Cardiology, Department of Medicine, University of California, San Francisco, 505 Parnassus Avenue, 11th Floor, Room 1180D, San Francisco, CA 94143, USA; [b] Department of Medicine, University of California, 505 Parnassus Avenue, San Francisco, CA 94143, USA

* Corresponding author.

E-mail address: Melissa.Burroughspena@ucsf.edu

Exposure to environmental pollution is associated with multiple adverse health outcomes in children and adults. Although environmental pollution often evokes concerns for neurologic development, cancer, and pulmonary disease, cardiovascular disease must be considered as well.[8] Cardiovascular disease is the top cause of mortality worldwide and has been identified as a target for large-scale, multisectoral intervention at the population level.[9,10] Taking into account the necessary integration of public and private sector activities to reduce the population burden of cardiovascular disease, the substantial impact of environmental exposures on the burden of cardiovascular disease at the population level must be acknowledged and addressed.[11–13] Understanding the impact of environmental exposures on cardiovascular disease has the potential to yield greater insight into the full human cost of economic development.[14]

This review discusses the extent of the exposure, mechanisms of disease pathogenesis, and the impact on cardiovascular disease for the following 5 environmental exposures: air pollution, household air pollution, lead, arsenic, and cadmium (**Fig. 1**). Although the selected environmental exposures described in this review do not represent an exhaustive list of every exposure with an observed

association with cardiovascular disease, these pollutants represent the most widely studied exposures. While the focus of this review is to discuss the impact of these exposures on cardiovascular disease in LMIC, data from studies of high-income countries are incorporated as needed to better illustrate the full impact of these exposures on cardiovascular disease risk factors and outcomes (**Table 1**).

AMBIENT AIR POLLUTION

Fossil fuels power economic development in LMIC, fueling the expansion of industry, housing, and transportation. However, fossil fuel combustion releases a heterogeneous mixture of gases and particles, all of which are components of ambient air pollution. Particulate matter is defined as particles suspended in the air of varying chemical composition and can be separated by particle size: coarse particulate matter less than 10 μm in diameter (PM_{10}), fine particulate matter less than 2.5 μm in diameter ($PM_{2.5}$), and ultrafine particulate matter less than 0.1 μm in diameter ($PM_{<0.1}$). The gaseous products of fossil fuel combustion include carbon monoxide (CO), nitrogen dioxide, sulfur dioxide, nitrogen oxides, and ozone. PM are heterogeneous in chemical composition and

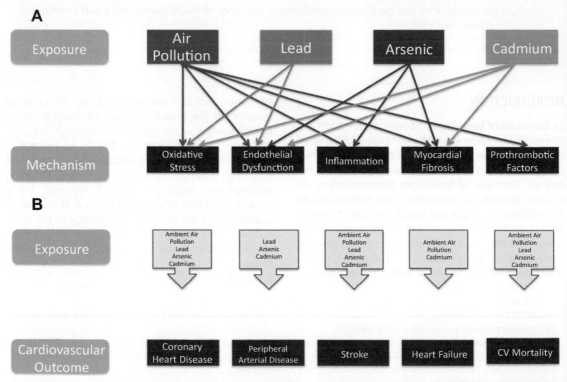

Fig. 1. Summary of the association between environmental exposures, pathophysiologic mechanisms, and cardiovascular disease. (*A*) Multiple mechanisms by which selected environmental exposures cause cardiovascular injury. (*B*) Multiple cardiovascular (CV) outcomes that are associated with environmental exposures.

Table 1
The origin of the peer-reviewed literature on the association between selected environmental exposures and cardiovascular disease by World Bank Country income level

	Hypertension	Subclinical Atherosclerosis	Cardiac Structure and Function	Coronary Heart Disease	Heart Failure	Cardiovascular Hospitalization	Arrhythmia	Stroke	Cardiovascular Mortality
Ambient air pollution	Both	High-income	Both	Both	Both	Both	High-income	High-income	Both
Biomass fuel air pollution	LMIC	LMIC	LMIC	LMIC					
Lead	Both	Both	Both	High-income				High-income	High-income
Arsenic	Both	Both	LMIC	Both	High-income			Both	Both
Cadmium	Both	High-income		High-income	Both			High-income	High-income

Legend: ■, data derived from LMIC; ■, data derived from high-income countries; ■, data derived from both LMIC and high-income countries.

can contain different metallic and nonmetallic compounds from different sources and may exert differential health effects. Ambient air pollution is the most robustly studied environmental exposure that has been linked to cardiovascular disease.

Extent of the Exposure

Exposure to ambient air pollution in urban and periurban communities in LMIC is often much higher than what is observed in the large metropolitan areas of high-income countries. According to the 2016 Urban Air Quality Database, 98% of urban centers with more than 100,000 inhabitants in LMIC are annually exposed to $PM_{2.5}$ levels greater than 10 $\mu g/m^3$ and PM_{10} greater than 20 $\mu g/m^3$; these levels are guidelines set forth by the World Health Organization (WHO).[15,16] Lack of robust regulation of the sources of air pollution likely contributes to disproportionate air pollution exposure in LMIC.[17] Although this database did not identify the sources of PM, common sources include diesel exhaust, industrial smokestack emissions, and biomass combustion.

For example, all of the Latin American major metropolitan areas with 2013 air quality data exceed the WHO standards for $PM_{2.5}$ and PM_{10}, with Bogotá, Colombia and Lima, Peru leading the cities with highest annual mean $PM_{2.5}$ concentration at 35.1 $\mu g/m^3$ and 31.5 $\mu g/m^3$, respectively.[2,3] However, air pollution in China's capital Beijing largely exceeds cities in Latin America with an annual mean $PM_{2.5}$ concentration greater than 80 $\mu g/m^3$ in 2015.[18] In addition, although much of the air pollution exposure in sub-Saharan Africa results from household air pollution from biomass fuel combustion and data on ambient air pollution exposure in the region are few, it is estimated that 32% of all West Africans are exposed to $PM_{2.5}$ levels that exceed the WHO limit.[18] Considerable heterogeneity of air pollution exposure can exist within large metropolitan areas as well, often disproportionately affecting low-income communities.[19] Looking to the future, the effect of temperature on $PM_{2.5}$ concentration raises concern that the impact of air pollution exposure on health might continue to increase in the wake of climate change, differentially affecting LMIC with warm climates.[4,20]

Mechanisms of Disease

Ambient air pollution affects cardiovascular health largely because of systemic inflammation from the incorporation of fine particulate matter into the pulmonary interstitium.[21–23] In addition, ultrafine particulate matter and the gaseous components of air pollution have the potential to directly enter the bloodstream.[24,25] In the presence of air pollutants, multiple biochemical effects have been observed, including increased oxidative stress through increased production of reactive oxygen species; increased inflammatory biomarkers, including interleukin-6 (IL-6) and C-reactive protein (CRP); increased prothrombotic factors, including D-dimer, platelet activation, increased fibrinogen, thrombin generation, and impaired fibrinolysis; increased expression of adhesive molecules on monocytes and leukocytes; and impaired endothelial function, including nitric oxide (NO)-mediated vasodilation.[22,26–35] The acute physiologic response to exposure to ambient air pollution includes increased plasma viscosity, reduced heart rate variability, impaired vasoreactivity, vasoconstriction, increased blood pressure, and increased insulin resistance.[28,32,33,36–48]

Impact on Cardiovascular Disease

Chronic exposure to ambient air pollution has been associated with risk factors for cardiovascular disease in multiple cohorts. The association between chronic air pollution exposure and elevated blood pressure has been extensively studied, including data from multiethnic cohorts in several countries.[39,49–51] In addition, some evidence has emerged supporting an association between air pollution exposure with elevated fasting glucose and type 2 diabetes mellitus.[49,52,53] Nevertheless, the data have not been entirely consistent, and additional studies on the factors that increase vulnerability to the blood pressure effects of air pollution exposure are needed, including a greater understanding of the specific air pollutants that account for the observed cardiometabolic effects.[54,55] Most of the studies of ambient air pollution and cardiovascular risk factors were conducted in high-income countries, with very few studies conducted in LMIC.[43]

Exposure to ambient air pollution is associated with multiple measures of subclinical cardiovascular disease. Ambient air pollution has been associated with measures of subclinical atherosclerosis, including carotid-intimal thickness and aortic atherosclerotic plaques.[56–60] There is evidence that air pollution exposure is also associated with the progression of coronary calcium.[61] In addition, air pollution exposure has also been associated with adverse cardiac remodeling, including right and left ventricular hypertrophy.[57,62,63] Although most of these studies were conducted in high-income countries, several small studies in LMIC have recently emerged, including a study of occupational air pollution exposure and cardiac structure and function in Iran.[64]

Beyond subclinical cardiovascular disease, large studies have demonstrated a strong association between ambient air pollution exposure and adverse cardiovascular outcomes. Acute ambient air pollution exposure has been associated with angina, stroke, acute myocardial infarction, heart failure hospitalization, arrhythmias, cardiac arrest, heart failure hospitalization, and cardiovascular mortality.[50,65–83] Data that are specific to LMIC are largely conducted in upper middle-income countries, including China and in Latin America.[50,84–91] Of note, almost no studies of air pollution and cardiovascular disease in sub-Saharan Africa have been published. The discrepancy between the relatively high exposure to ambient air pollution in LMIC and the lack of data specific to LIMC suggest that the public health impact is potentially underestimated.

HOUSEHOLD AIR POLLUTION FROM BIOMASS FUEL USE

Although economic development in LMIC has improved access to electricity, natural gas, and liquefied petroleum gas, many communities depend on biomass fuels for daily needs.[92] Biomass fuels include wood, charcoal, dung, and crop residue, which are burned in indoor and outdoor stoves for cooking and heating. Similar to fossil fuel combustion, biomass fuels produce gases and particulate matter that are suspended in air, including CO and fine particulate matter ($PM_{2.5}$). Exposure to the components of biomass fuel combustion has been studied in several contexts in relation to cardiovascular disease risk factors and outcomes.

The Extent of the Exposure

Household air pollution from biomass fuel use affects 3 billion people worldwide, including 6.5 million Americans.[92,93] Although biomass fuel use can be found on every continent, it is more prevalent in resource-poor settings, disproportionately affecting low-income individuals in high-income countries and LMIC.[93] In many cultures, women are more likely to perform household cooking, and thus, are more highly exposed to smoke from biomass fuel use, along with small children in the home. The geographic distribution of biomass fuel use can vary by region due to social, cultural, economic, and climate differences. For example, in the Andean region of South America, daily biomass fuel use is primarily confined to rural communities.[94] In contrast, a large study in periurban Malawi found that 70.9% of the 6445 households surveyed use wood and/or charcoal for cooking.[95] Furthermore, older age and low education were associated with the use of wood for

cooking. Understanding and addressing the social and cultural factors that contribute to biomass fuel use is critical and has implications for the implementation of improved cook-stove interventions.

Mechanisms of Disease

The biochemical and physiologic response to the air pollutants released from biomass fuel combustion has not been as extensively studied as air pollution from fossil fuel combustion. Although both forms of combustion release fine particulate matter, the chemical composition of the particulate matter varies according to fuel source, and some studies suggest that the chemical composition and diameter of particulate matter have a differential impact on cardiovascular disease outcomes.[71,96–98] Coarse particulate matter is often found in ocean spray, dust, and construction byproducts. Acute exposure to wood smoke has been shown to cause arterial stiffness and decreased heart rate variability.[99] In addition, observational studies conducted in women in villages in eastern India observed increased proinflammatory cytokines, higher serum CRP, and higher reactive oxygen species generation in the women exposed to biomass fuel smoke.[100] Another study of women in rural India observed an increase in systolic blood pressure during cooking times during which there was also an increase in exposure to the air pollutant black carbon, a major component of soot.[101] Additional research on the acute biochemical and physiologic response to household air pollution from biomass fuel combustion is needed to better understand how this exposure differs from ambient air pollution.

Impact on Cardiovascular Disease

Exposure to biomass fuel smoke has been associated with cardiovascular risk factors in multiple observational studies. The most common cardiovascular risk factor associated with biomass fuel use is elevated blood pressure. Multiple cohort studies in China, Peru, Guatemala, and Nicaragua have identified an association between exposure to biomass fuel smoke and elevated blood pressure.[102–107] Replacement of traditional cook-stoves with cleaner burning cook-stoves was associated with lower blood pressure.[104] In addition to observing differences in blood pressure, 2 large studies in China and Peru also observed an increased prevalence of hypertension in daily biomass fuel users.[103,106]

Exposure to biomass fuel smoke has also been associated with subclinical cardiovascular disease in several small studies. In Guatemala, biomass fuel use was associated with changes in the ST segment of the electrocardiogram in women before participating in an improved cook-stove trial.[108] These changes improved after the cook-stove intervention, suggesting an improvement in myocardial ischemia. In addition, a cross-sectional study of 266 individuals in Puno, Peru found that chronic exposure to biomass fuel smoke was associated with increased carotid intima media thickness and a higher prevalence of carotid atherosclerotic plaques.[109] However, contrary to what was previously hypothesized, in a sample from the same Peruvian cohort, there was no association between biomass fuel use with elevated NT pro-BNP or right ventricular systolic pressure by echocardiography.[110] A small echocardiography study in a single hospital in Turkey observed that biomass fuel users had increased right ventricular systolic pressure and decreased left and right ventricular myocardial indices, indicating decreased biventricular systolic function.[111] However, the relationship between biomass fuel smoke exposure and cardiac structure and function is currently undergoing further examination in population-based cohorts.

There have been conflicting results in studies of the association of household air pollution from biomass fuel use with outcomes, such as coronary heart disease and cardiovascular mortality. Although the Global Burden of Disease Study estimated the global impact of household air pollution due to biomass fuel use based on the observed relationship between ambient air pollution exposure and cardiovascular events, very few studies have examined cardiovascular outcomes in biomass fuel users. Emerging data suggest an association between biomass fuel use and coronary heart disease.[112] In a study of participants living in the Brazilian Amazon, elderly individuals with increased exposure to biomass fuel smoke had increased cardiovascular mortality when compared with age-matched controls.[113] However, large cohorts in Iran and Bangladesh have failed to demonstrate an association between chronic biomass fuel use and cardiovascular mortality.[114,115] Additional studies that prospectively study cardiovascular outcomes in biomass fuel users compared with nonusers are needed to better quantify the impact of household air pollution on cardiovascular disease.

LEAD

The acute and chronic neurologic effects of lead exposure have been widely described in both high-income countries and LMIC.[116] However, less public attention has been paid to the cardiovascular impact of chronic lead exposure and the contribution of heavy metal exposure on

the burden of cardiovascular disease in LMIC. Globally, it is estimated that lead exposure ranks number 26 as a risk factor for disability-adjusted life-years lost, yet in subregions of Latin America and Southern Africa, this ranking increases to number 20.[92] Lead exposure in LMIC deserves close examination as a modifiable risk factor for cardiovascular disease and a potential target for intervention at the population level.

Extent of the Exposure

Globally, an estimated 26 million people are at risk for lead toxicity, resulting in a loss of 9 million disability-adjusted life-years.[117] Although lead exposure exists in high-income countries and LMIC alike from lead pipes and paint, in general, the prevalence of lead exposure has not decreased in LMIC to the degree that has been observed in many high-income countries.[118,119] Tobacco use is a common mode of lead exposure in high-income countries and LMIC; however, there are multiple sources of lead exposure that are specific to the industries and cultures of LMIC.[120] Although leaded petroleum was banned from high-income countries many decades ago, its use in LMIC continues in Yemen, Algeria, and Iraq, polluting the air and soil.[117,121,122] In addition, occupational exposures in battery manufacturing and recycling factories have been well described, particularly in Kenya and several South Asian countries.[123–125] Mining operations in Peru, Tanzania, Nigeria, and Zambia have been associated with lead exposure not only for the workers at the mine but also for the local communities located near the mines.[126–128] Toxic waste from other industrial sources is also known to contaminate water and soil with lead.[116] Fishing and hunting with lead tools fashioned from industrial sources are associated with chronic lead exposure in Peruvian Amazon River Basin communities.[129] Moreover, the artisanal use of lead in pottery has also been a source of lead exposure in Latin America and Africa,[117,118,130,131] and leaded paints are still being sold and used in some LMIC, as noted in a recent study in Cambodia.[132] Independent of the source of the lead contamination, children are often the most vulnerable population exposed to lead, with often unmeasured detriment to the present and future neurologic and cardiovascular health.[116,127,131,133–135]

Mechanisms of Disease

By promoting the generation of reactive oxygen species, lead increases oxidative stress in cardiovascular tissues and endothelial cells.[136] The increase in oxidative stress in the setting of lead exposure is also associated with decreased NO availability. Decreased NO availability in turn has been shown to cause sodium retention, vasoconstriction, and increased adrenergic tone.[136] In addition, NF-κB activation due to increased oxidative stress in the setting of lead exposure leads to the oxidation of low-density lipoprotein, increases the expression of adhesive molecules on monocytes, and increases foam cell formation.[136] These processes in addition to platelet activation and vascular remodeling are the basis by which lead-associated cardiovascular disease occurs.[136]

Impact of Cardiovascular Disease

Hypertension is the cardiovascular risk factor most greatly associated with lead exposure. Multiple studies in the United States in addition to several studies in LMIC have demonstrated a convincing association between even low levels of lead exposure and increased blood pressure, gestational hypertension incidence, and hypertension prevalence.[123,137–139] Moreover, some evidence suggests the lead exposure is also associated with decreased heart rate variability.[137] However, emerging evidence suggests that lead exposure is also associated with other cardiometabolic derangements, including increased fasting glucose, decreased high-density lipoprotein, increased total cholesterol, and increased prevalence of the metabolic syndrome.[130,140,141] Several of these studies of cardiometabolic impairment in the setting of lead exposure were conducted in LMIC settings, including multiple settings in West Africa and the Americas, thus highlighting the potential role of environmental exposures on noncommunicable disease risk in LMIC.

Lead exposure is associated with subclinical cardiovascular disease and cardiovascular outcomes. Increased carotid intimal medial thickness has been observed in association with increased serum lead levels in a Turkish population with concomitant renal disease.[142] Lead exposure has also been associated with reduced heart rate variability and abnormalities of cardiac structure and function, including increased left ventricular hypertrophy and decreased ejection fraction.[137] Clinical atherosclerotic disease has been observed in association with lead exposure, including stroke, peripheral arterial disease, and coronary heart disease.[137,143] Increased exposure to lead has also been associated with increased cardiovascular mortality in several studies of the US population.[137,144,145] Despite the considerable exposure to lead in LMIC, there are limited published data on lead exposure and cardiovascular disease outcomes in LMIC populations.

ARSENIC

Arsenic is a naturally occurring metalloid and a contaminant of drinking water, soil, and food. In contrast to acute arsenic poisoning, chronic arsenic exposure can be more difficult to identify, but ultimately is associated with multiple adverse health outcomes, including cardiovascular disease.[117]

Extent of the Exposure

Chronic arsenic exposure has been described in countries of all income levels and most commonly occurs from drinking wells contaminated with arsenic naturally present in the soil.[117] Although arsenic contamination of wells within the United States has been well documented, particularly in Native American reservations, arsenic contamination in LMIC countries, including Bangladesh, India, Taiwan, and Turkey, has also been well documented.[146–150] Safe drinking water is more readily available within high-income countries, therefore arsenic contamination from well water disproportionately affects low-income communities, such as in Bangladesh, where an estimated 20 million inhabitants consume arsenic-contaminated water.[148,150,151] Arsenic contamination of food such as rice represents a particularly important exposure risk factor for inhabitants of LMIC and constituents of global trade partners.[151–153]

Mechanisms of Disease

Arsenic typically enters the body through the gastrointestinal tract and is metabolized in the liver, where it undergoes methylation, yielding toxic intermediates.[154] Arsenic exposure is associated with increased inflammatory markers, including IL-6 and IL-8, and matrix metalloproteinase-2 and -9.[155,156] In animal models, arsenic exposure leads to myocardial fibrosis, which is proposed to be the mechanism by which QT prolongation in electrocardiogram occurs in response to arsenic toxicity.[157] In addition, endothelial dysfunction associated with arsenic exposure has also been observed. In Bangladesh, gene by environment interaction in relation to increases in blood pressure from arsenic exposure has been well described, demonstrating variable cardiotoxicity due to variable methylation of arsenic.[158–160] In a separate Bangladesh study, folate supplementation promoted urinary excretion of arsenic and may attenuate arsenic toxicity.[161]

Impact on Cardiovascular Disease

Chronic arsenic exposure has been associated with cardiovascular risk factors. Although elevated blood pressure and hypertension in response to arsenic exposure have been observed in multiple

LIMC settings, including India, Bangladesh, Mexico, and China, this observation has not been consistent.[162–168] In addition, type 2 diabetes mellitus, elevated triglycerides, and elevated total cholesterol have also been observed in association with arsenic exposure.[148,166,169]

Chronic arsenic exposure is associated with subclinical cardiovascular disease, including increased carotid intimal medial thickness, which has been observed in several studies in LMIC, including Mexico and Bangladesh.[166,170,171] Moreover, left ventricular ejection fraction is reduced in children chronically exposed to arsenic in Mexico.[167] In terms of clinical cardiovascular disease, arsenic exposure is associated with peripheral arterial disease, cardiomyopathy, coronary heart disease, acute myocardial infarction, stroke, stroke mortality, and cardiovascular mortality.[172–181] Not only does arsenic exposure increase the risk of acquired heart disease, but also is associated with increased risk of congenital heart disease.[182] As more evidence is generated regarding the full spectrum of cardiovascular disease associated with chronic arsenic exposure, the potential cost of arsenic contamination in LMIC is being appreciated.

CADMIUM

Cadmium does not receive the same degree of attention from the lay public as lead or arsenic; however, the public health burden in relation to exposure to cadmium remains significant.[117] An estimated 5 million people are exposed chronically to cadmium, which has implications for cardiovascular disease risk at the population level in many LMIC.[117]

Extent of the Exposure

Similar to lead, cadmium exposure commonly occurs from tobacco smoking, an exposure that has been well described in high-income countries and LMIC.[138,183] In addition, cadmium from mining, smelting, refining, and industrial waste can also pollute air, water, and soil, leading to the contamination of foods, including leafy vegetables, fish, and shellfish.[117,183] Cadmium is also used in the production of plastics, fertilizers, and batteries.[117,184] Communities in LMIC, particularly low-income communities, may be chronically exposed to cadmium, an exposure that is only recently made apparent as heavy metal monitoring is implemented in communities, as illustrated by studies from Ghana and Uganda.[185,186] In fact, cadmium exposure is likely to increase in the coming decades in part due to electronic waste disposal, as seen in Nigeria.[187] Beyond contamination of the environment, serum levels of cadmium from individuals living in LMIC can be several orders of magnitude greater than what is observed in high-income countries.[188]

Mechanisms of Disease

Cadmium increases oxidative stress through the increased production and decreased metabolism of reactive oxygen species.[189] Moreover, cadmium has been shown to impair endothelial function.[190] Cadmium also has been associated with increased serum levels of galetin-3, a biomarker for myocardial fibrosis, in a population in Turkey.[191] Through these multiple mechanisms, cadmium exposure is thought to cause cardiovascular disease.

Impact on Cardiovascular Disease

Similar to other environmental exposures, cadmium exposure is associated with elevated blood pressure and hypertension.[192–195] Although much of the evidence was generated in high-income countries, several studies have been conducted in LMIC, including Thailand, China, and Pakistan.[196–198] Of note, there are several studies that did not find an association between measured cadmium exposure and hypertension, suggesting that additional data on the genetic and environmental risk factors for cadmium-related hypertension is needed.[199,200] Cadmium has also been associated with cardiometabolic derangement, including type 2 diabetes, as noted in a study from China.[198] In addition, increased carotid intimal medial thickness and carotid plaques also have been associated with cadmium exposure.[142]

The evidence regarding the association between cadmium exposure and cardiovascular disease outcomes overwhelmingly comes from high-income countries. Cadmium exposure is associated with diseases of atherosclerosis, including peripheral arterial disease, stroke, ischemic heart disease, and acute coronary syndromes.[193,201–204] Cadmium exposure has also been associated with incident heart failure, although it is unclear what percentage of heart failure cases are ischemic versus nonischemic in cause.[193,203,205] The largest studies of cadmium and cardiovascular disease are from US National Health and Nutrition Examination Survey data and the Strong Heart Study of US Native Americans. In these cohorts, cadmium exposure was associated with cardiovascular mortality, thus highlighting the likely unmeasured mortality burden that cadmium exposure potentially has in LMIC.[206–208]

SUMMARY

Environmental exposures in LMIC lie at the intersection of increased economic development and the rising public health burden of cardiovascular disease. Increasing evidence suggests an association of exposure to ambient air pollution, household air pollution from biomass fuel, lead, arsenic, and cadmium with multiple cardiovascular disease outcomes, including hypertension, coronary heart disease, stroke, and cardiovascular mortality. Although populations in LMIC are disproportionately exposed to environmental pollution, the bulk of evidence that links these exposures to cardiovascular disease is derived from populations in high-income countries. Low-income regions of high-income countries are at high risk of exposure. In order to better understand the extent to which environmental exposures contribute to the rising epidemic of cardiovascular disease in LMIC and develop interventions to reduce cardiovascular disease risk at the population level, additional research is needed.

REFERENCES

1. Landrigan PJ, Fuller R, Horton R. Environmental pollution, health, and development: a Lancet-Global Alliance on Health and Pollution-Icahn School of Medicine at Mount Sinai Commission. Lancet 2015;386(10002):1429–31.
2. Bell ML, Cifuentes LA, Davis DL, et al. Environmental health indicators and a case study of air pollution in Latin American cities. Environ Res 2011;111(1):57–66.
3. Green J, Sanchez S. Air quality in Latin America: an overview. Washington, DC: Clear Air Institute; 2013.
4. Patz JA, Frumkin H, Holloway T, et al. Climate change: challenges and opportunities for global health. JAMA 2014;312(15):1565–80.
5. Mining in Latin America: from conflict to cooperation. The Economist 2016.
6. Briggs D. Environmental pollution and the global burden of disease. Br Med Bull 2003;68:1–24.
7. Landrigan PJ, Fuller R. Global health and environmental pollution. Int J Public Health 2015;60(7): 761–2.
8. Bhatnagar A. Environmental cardiology: studying mechanistic links between pollution and heart disease. Circ Res 2006;99(7):692–705.
9. Beaglehole R, Bonita R, Alleyne G, et al. UN high-level meeting on non-communicable diseases: addressing four questions. Lancet 2011;378(9789): 449–55.
10. Lozano R, Naghavi M, Foreman K, et al. Global and regional mortality from 235 causes of death for 20 age groups in 1990 and 2010: a systematic analysis for the Global Burden of Disease Study 2010. Lancet 2012;380(9859): 2095–128.
11. Ordunez P. Cardiovascular health in the Americas: facts, priorities and the UN high-level meeting on non-communicable diseases. MEDICC Rev 2011; 13(4):6–10.
12. Ebrahim S, Pearce N, Smeeth L, et al. Tackling non-communicable diseases in low- and middle-income countries: is the evidence from high-income countries all we need? PLoS Med 2013; 10(1):e1001377.
13. Pearce N, Ebrahim S, McKee M, et al. Global prevention and control of NCDs: limitations of the standard approach. J Public Health Policy 2015;36(4): 408–25.
14. Burroughs Pena MS, Bloomfield GS. Cardiovascular disease research and the development agenda in low- and middle-income countries. Glob Heart 2015;10(1):71–3.
15. Osserian N, Chriscaden K. Air pollution levels rising in many of the world's poorest cities. 2016. Available at: http://www.who.int/mediacentre/news/releases/2016/air-pollution-rising/en. Accessed July 6, 2016.
16. Ambient (Outdoor) Air Quality and Health WHO website. Available at: http://www.who.int/mediacentre/factsheets/fs313/en. Accessed August 7, 2016.
17. Actions on air quality: regional reports, United Nations Environment Programme website. Available at: http://www.unep.org/transport/airquality/regionalreports.asp. Accessed August 10, 2016.
18. Energy and air pollution. Paris: International Energy Agency/OECD; 2016.
19. Bravo MA, Bell ML. Spatial heterogeneity of PM10 and O3 in Sao Paulo, Brazil, and implications for human health studies. J Air Waste Manag Assoc 2011;61(1):69–77.
20. Kioumourtzoglou MA, Schwartz J, James P, et al. PM2.5 and mortality in 207 US cities: modification by temperature and city characteristics. Epidemiology 2016;27(2):221–7.
21. Seaton A, MacNee W, Donaldson K, et al. Particulate air pollution and acute health effects. Lancet 1995;345(8943):176–8.
22. Mills NL, Donaldson K, Hadoke PW, et al. Adverse cardiovascular effects of air pollution. Nat Clin Pract Cardiovasc Med 2009;6(1):36–44.
23. Brook RD, Rajagopalan S, Pope CA 3rd, et al. Particulate matter air pollution and cardiovascular disease: an update to the scientific statement from the American Heart Association. Circulation 2010; 121(21):2331–78.
24. Nemmar A, Hoet PH, Vanquickenborne B, et al. Passage of inhaled particles into the blood circulation in humans. Circulation 2002;105(4): 411–4.
25. Mills NL, Amin N, Robinson SD, et al. Do inhaled carbon nanoparticles translocate directly into the

circulation in humans? Am J Respir Crit Care Med 2006;173(4):426–31.

26. Pekkanen J, Brunner EJ, Anderson HR, et al. Daily concentrations of air pollution and plasma fibrinogen in London. Occup Environ Med 2000; 57(12):818–22.

27. Peters A, Frohlich M, Doring A, et al. Particulate air pollution is associated with an acute phase response in men; results from the MONICA-Augsburg Study. Eur Heart J 2001;22(14):1198–204.

28. Mills NL, Tornqvist H, Robinson SD, et al. Diesel exhaust inhalation causes vascular dysfunction and impaired endogenous fibrinolysis. Circulation 2005;112(25):3930–6.

29. Frampton MW, Stewart JC, Oberdorster G, et al. Inhalation of ultrafine particles alters blood leukocyte expression of adhesion molecules in humans. Environ Health Perspect 2006;114(1):51–8.

30. Tornqvist H, Mills NL, Gonzalez M, et al. Persistent endothelial dysfunction in humans after diesel exhaust inhalation. Am J Respir Crit Care Med 2007;176(4):395–400.

31. Lucking AJ, Lundback M, Mills NL, et al. Diesel exhaust inhalation increases thrombus formation in man. Eur Heart J 2008;29(24):3043–51.

32. Strak M, Hoek G, Steenhof M, et al. Components of ambient air pollution affect thrombin generation in healthy humans: the RAPTES project. Occup Environ Med 2013;70(5):332–40.

33. Hajat A, Allison M, Diez-Roux AV, et al. Long-term exposure to air pollution and markers of inflammation, coagulation, and endothelial activation: a repeat-measures analysis in the Multi-Ethnic Study of Atherosclerosis (MESA). Epidemiology 2015; 26(3):310–20.

34. Adar SD, D'Souza J, Mendelsohn-Victor K, et al. Markers of inflammation and coagulation after long-term exposure to coarse particulate matter: a cross-sectional analysis from the multi-ethnic study of atherosclerosis. Environ Health Perspect 2015;123(6):541–8.

35. Li W, Wilker EH, Dorans KS, et al. Short-term exposure to air pollution and biomarkers of oxidative stress: the Framingham Heart Study. J Am Heart Assoc 2016;5(5).

36. Peters A, Doring A, Wichmann HE, et al. Increased plasma viscosity during an air pollution episode: a link to mortality? Lancet 1997; 349(9065):1582–7.

37. Brook RD, Brook JR, Urch B, et al. Inhalation of fine particulate air pollution and ozone causes acute arterial vasoconstriction in healthy adults. Circulation 2002;105(13):1534–6.

38. Urch B, Silverman F, Corey P, et al. Acute blood pressure responses in healthy adults during controlled air pollution exposures. Environ Health Perspect 2005;113(8):1052–5.

39. Auchincloss AH, Diez Roux AV, Dvonch JT, et al. Associations between recent exposure to ambient fine particulate matter and blood pressure in the Multi-Ethnic Study of Atherosclerosis (MESA). Environ Health Perspect 2008;116(4):486–91.

40. Brook RD, Rajagopalan S. Particulate matter, air pollution, and blood pressure. J Am Soc Hypertens 2009;3(5):332–50.

41. Brook RD, Urch B, Dvonch JT, et al. Insights into the mechanisms and mediators of the effects of air pollution exposure on blood pressure and vascular function in healthy humans. Hypertension 2009;54(3):659–67.

42. Park SK, Auchincloss AH, O'Neill MS, et al. Particulate air pollution, metabolic syndrome, and heart rate variability: the multi-ethnic study of atherosclerosis (MESA). Environ Health Perspect 2010; 118(10):1406–11.

43. Baccarelli A, Barretta F, Dou C, et al. Effects of particulate air pollution on blood pressure in a highly exposed population in Beijing, China: a repeated-measure study. Environ Health 2011;10:108.

44. Shields KN, Cavallari JM, Hunt MJ, et al. Traffic-related air pollution exposures and changes in heart rate variability in Mexico City: a panel study. Environ Health 2013;12:7.

45. Brook RD, Sun Z, Brook JR, et al. Extreme air pollution conditions adversely affect blood pressure and insulin resistance: the air pollution and cardiometabolic disease study. Hypertension 2016;67(1):77–85.

46. Green R, Broadwin R, Malig B, et al. Long- and short-term exposure to air pollution and inflammatory/hemostatic markers in midlife women. Epidemiology 2016;27(2):211–20.

47. Haberzettl P, O'Toole TE, Bhatnagar A, et al. Exposure to fine particulate air pollution causes vascular insulin resistance by inducing pulmonary oxidative stress. Environ Health Perspect 2016. [Epub ahead of print].

48. Ljungman PL, Wilker EH, Rice MB, et al. The impact of multipollutant clusters on the association between fine particulate air pollution and microvascular function. Epidemiology 2016;27(2):194–201.

49. Coogan PF, White LF, Jerrett M, et al. Air pollution and incidence of hypertension and diabetes mellitus in black women living in Los Angeles. Circulation 2012;125(6):767–72.

50. Langrish JP, Li X, Wang S, et al. Reducing personal exposure to particulate air pollution improves cardiovascular health in patients with coronary heart disease. Environ Health Perspect 2012;120(3): 367–72.

51. Kirwa K, Eliot MN, Wang Y, et al. Residential proximity to major roadways and prevalent hypertension among postmenopausal women: results from the Women's Health Initiative San Diego Cohort. J Am Heart Assoc 2014;3(5).

52. Peng C, Bind MC, Colicino E, et al. Particulate air pollution and fasting blood glucose in non-diabetic individuals: associations and epigenetic mediation in the normative aging study, 2000-2011. Environ Health Perspect 2016. [Epub ahead of print].

53. Yitshak Sade M, Kloog I, Liberty IF, et al. The association between air pollution exposure and glucose and lipids levels. J Clin Endocrinol Metab 2016; 101(6):2460–7.

54. Park SK, Adar SD, O'Neill MS, et al. Long-term exposure to air pollution and type 2 diabetes mellitus in a multiethnic cohort. Am J Epidemiol 2015; 181(5):327–36.

55. Coogan PF, White LF, Yu J, et al. PM2.5 and diabetes and hypertension incidence in the Black Women's Health Study. Epidemiology 2016;27(2):202–10.

56. Breton CV, Wang X, Mack WJ, et al. Carotid artery intima-media thickness in college students: race/ethnicity matters. Atherosclerosis 2011;217(2): 441–6.

57. Gill EA, Curl CL, Adar SD, et al. Air pollution and cardiovascular disease in the Multi-Ethnic Study of Atherosclerosis. Prog Cardiovasc Dis 2011; 53(5):353–60.

58. Breton CV, Wang X, Mack WJ, et al. Childhood air pollutant exposure and carotid artery intima-media thickness in young adults. Circulation 2012;126(13):1614–20.

59. Rivera M, Basagana X, Aguilera I, et al. Association between long-term exposure to traffic-related air pollution and subclinical atherosclerosis: the REGI-COR study. Environ Health Perspect 2013;121(2): 223–30.

60. Wilker EH, Mittleman MA, Coull BA, et al. Long-term exposure to black carbon and carotid intima-media thickness: the normative aging study. Environ Health Perspect 2013;121(9):1061–7.

61. Kaufman JD, Adar SD, Barr RG, et al. Association between air pollution and coronary artery calcification within six metropolitan areas in the USA (the Multi-Ethnic Study of Atherosclerosis and Air Pollution): a longitudinal cohort study. Lancet 2016; 388(10045):696–704.

62. Leary PJ, Kaufman JD, Barr RG, et al. Traffic-related air pollution and the right ventricle. The multi-ethnic study of atherosclerosis. Am J Respir Crit Care Med 2014;189(9):1093–100.

63. Liu Y, Goodson JM, Zhang B, et al. Air pollution and adverse cardiac remodeling: clinical effects and basic mechanisms. Front Physiol 2015;6:162.

64. Golshahi J, Sadeghi M, Saqira M, et al. Exposure to occupational air pollution and cardiac function in workers of the Esfahan Steel Industry, Iran. Environ Sci Pollut Res Int 2016;23(12):11759–65.

65. Dockery DW, Pope CA 3rd, Xu X, et al. An association between air pollution and mortality in six U.S. cities. N Engl J Med 1993;329(24):1753–9.

66. Hoffmann B, Moebus S, Stang A, et al. Residence close to high traffic and prevalence of coronary heart disease. Eur Heart J 2006;27(22):2696–702.

67. Miller KA, Siscovick DS, Sheppard L, et al. Long-term exposure to air pollution and incidence of cardiovascular events in women. N Engl J Med 2007; 356(5):447–58.

68. Peng RD, Chang HH, Bell ML, et al. Coarse particulate matter air pollution and hospital admissions for cardiovascular and respiratory diseases among Medicare patients. JAMA 2008; 299(18):2172–9.

69. Puett RC, Schwartz J, Hart JE, et al. Chronic particulate exposure, mortality, and coronary heart disease in the nurses' health study. Am J Epidemiol 2008;168(10):1161–8.

70. Bell ML, Peng RD, Dominici F, et al. Emergency hospital admissions for cardiovascular diseases and ambient levels of carbon monoxide: results for 126 United States urban counties, 1999-2005. Circulation 2009;120(11):949–55.

71. Peng RD, Bell ML, Geyh AS, et al. Emergency admissions for cardiovascular and respiratory diseases and the chemical composition of fine particle air pollution. Environ Health Perspect 2009;117(6):957–63.

72. Mustafic H, Jabre P, Caussin C, et al. Main air pollutants and myocardial infarction: a systematic review and meta-analysis. JAMA 2012;307(7):713–21.

73. Cesaroni G, Badaloni C, Gariazzo C, et al. Long-term exposure to urban air pollution and mortality in a cohort of more than a million adults in Rome. Environ Health Perspect 2013;121(3):324–31.

74. Chen H, Goldberg MS, Burnett RT, et al. Long-term exposure to traffic-related air pollution and cardiovascular mortality. Epidemiology 2013; 24(1):35–43.

75. Ensor KB, Raun LH, Persse D. A case-crossover analysis of out-of-hospital cardiac arrest and air pollution. Circulation 2013;127(11):1192–9.

76. Hart JE, Rimm EB, Rexrode KM, et al. Changes in traffic exposure and the risk of incident myocardial infarction and all-cause mortality. Epidemiology 2013;24(5):734–42.

77. Hoek G, Krishnan RM, Beelen R, et al. Long-term air pollution exposure and cardio- respiratory mortality: a review. Environ Health 2013;12(1):43.

78. Madrigano J, Kloog I, Goldberg R, et al. Long-term exposure to PM2.5 and incidence of acute myocardial infarction. Environ Health Perspect 2013; 121(2):192–6.

79. Shah AS, Langrish JP, Nair H, et al. Global association of air pollution and heart failure: a systematic review and meta-analysis. Lancet 2013;382(9897): 1039–48.

80. Wichmann J, Folke F, Torp-Pedersen C, et al. Out-of-hospital cardiac arrests and outdoor air pollution

exposure in Copenhagen, Denmark. PLoS One 2013;8(1):e53684.

81. Cesaroni G, Forastiere F, Stafoggia M, et al. Long term exposure to ambient air pollution and incidence of acute coronary events: prospective cohort study and meta-analysis in 11 European cohorts from the ESCAPE Project. BMJ 2014;348: f7412.

82. Milojevic A, Wilkinson P, Armstrong B, et al. Short-term effects of air pollution on a range of cardiovascular events in England and Wales: case-crossover analysis of the MINAP database, hospital admissions and mortality. Heart 2014; 100(14):1093–8.

83. Stockfelt L, Andersson EM, Molnar P, et al. Long term effects of residential NOx exposure on total and cause-specific mortality and incidence of myocardial infarction in a Swedish cohort. Environ Res 2015;142:197–206.

84. Martins LC, Pereira LA, Lin CA, et al. The effects of air pollution on cardiovascular diseases: lag structures. Rev Saude Publica 2006; 40(4):677–83.

85. O'Neill MS, Bell ML, Ranjit N, et al. Air pollution and mortality in Latin America: the role of education. Epidemiology 2008;19(6):810–9.

86. Liu L, Breitner S, Schneider A, et al. Size-fractioned particulate air pollution and cardiovascular emergency room visits in Beijing, China. Environ Res 2013;121:52–63.

87. Freitas CU, Leon AP, Juger W, et al. Air pollution and its impacts on health in Vitoria, Espirito Santo, Brazil. Rev Saude Publica 2016;50:4.

88. Huang F, Chen R, Shen Y, et al. The impact of the 2013 Eastern China smog on outpatient visits for coronary heart disease in Shanghai, China. Int J Environ Res Public Health 2016;13(7).

89. Phung D, Hien TT, Linh HN, et al. Air pollution and risk of respiratory and cardiovascular hospitalizations in the most populous city in Vietnam. Sci Total Environ 2016;557–558:322–30.

90. Ye X, Peng L, Kan H, et al. Acute effects of particulate air pollution on the incidence of coronary heart disease in Shanghai, China. PLoS One 2016;11(3):e0151119.

91. Zuniga J, Tarajia M, Herrera V, et al. Assessment of the possible association of air pollutants PM10, O3, NO2 with an increase in cardiovascular, respiratory, and diabetes mortality in Panama City: a 2003 to 2013 data analysis. Medicine 2016;95(2): e2464.

92. Lim SS, Vos T, Flaxman AD, et al. A comparative risk assessment of burden of disease and injury attributable to 67 risk factors and risk factor clusters in 21 regions, 1990-2010: a systematic analysis for the Global Burden of Disease Study 2010. Lancet 2012;380(9859):2224–60.

93. Rogalsky D, Mendola P, Metts T, et al. Estimating the number of low-income Americans exposed to household air pollution from burning solid fuels. Environ Health Perspect 2014;122(8):1–5.

94. Pollard SL, Williams DL, Breysse PN, et al. A cross-sectional study of determinants of indoor environmental exposures in households with and without chronic exposure to biomass fuel smoke. Environ Health 2014;13(1):21.

95. Piddock KC, Gordon SB, Ngwira A, et al. A cross-sectional study of household biomass fuel use among a periurban population in Malawi. Ann Am Thorac Soc 2014;11(6):915–24.

96. Meng Q, Richmond-Bryant J, Lu SE, et al. Cardiovascular outcomes and the physical and chemical properties of metal ions found in particulate matter air pollution: a QICAR study. Environ Health Perspect 2013;121(5):558–64.

97. Sun M, Kaufman JD, Kim SY, et al. Particulate matter components and subclinical atherosclerosis: common approaches to estimating exposure in a Multi-Ethnic Study of Atherosclerosis cross-sectional study. Environ Health 2013;12:39.

98. Kim SY, Sheppard L, Kaufman JD, et al. Individual-level concentrations of fine particulate matter chemical components and subclinical atherosclerosis: a cross-sectional analysis based on 2 advanced exposure prediction models in the multi-ethnic study of atherosclerosis. Am J Epidemiol 2014;180(7):718–28.

99. Unosson J, Blomberg A, Sandstrom T, et al. Exposure to wood smoke increases arterial stiffness and decreases heart rate variability in humans. Part Fibre Toxicol 2013;10:20.

100. Dutta A, Ray MR, Banerjee A. Systemic inflammatory changes and increased oxidative stress in rural Indian women cooking with biomass fuels. Toxicol Appl Pharmacol 2012;261(3):255–62.

101. Norris C, Goldberg MS, Marshall JD, et al. A panel study of the acute effects of personal exposure to household air pollution on ambulatory blood pressure in rural Indian women. Environ Res 2016; 147:331–42.

102. Baumgartner J, Schauer JJ, Ezzati M, et al. Indoor air pollution and blood pressure in adult women living in rural China. Environ Health Perspect 2011;119(10):1390–5.

103. Lee MS, Hang JQ, Zhang FY, et al. In-home solid fuel use and cardiovascular disease: a cross-sectional analysis of the Shanghai Putuo study. Environ Health 2012;11:18.

104. Clark ML, Bachand AM, Heiderscheidt JM, et al. Impact of a cleaner-burning cookstove intervention on blood pressure in Nicaraguan women. Indoor Air 2013;23(2):105–14.

105. Baumgartner J, Zhang Y, Schauer JJ, et al. Highway proximity and black carbon from cookstoves

as a risk factor for higher blood pressure in rural China. Proc Natl Acad Sci U S A 2014;111(36): 13229–34.

106. Burroughs Pena M, Romero KM, Velazquez EJ, et al. Relationship between daily exposure to biomass fuel smoke and blood pressure in high-altitude Peru. Hypertension 2015;65(5):1134–40.

107. Dutta A, Roychoudhury S, Chowdhury S, et al. Changes in sputum cytology, airway inflammation and oxidative stress due to chronic inhalation of biomass smoke during cooking in premenopausal rural Indian women. Int J Hyg Environ Health 2013;216(3):301–8.

108. McCracken J, Smith KR, Stone P, et al. Intervention to lower household wood smoke exposure in Guatemala reduces ST-segment depression on electrocardiograms. Environ Health Perspect 2011;119(11):1562–8.

109. Painschab MS, Davila-Roman VG, Gilman RH, et al. Chronic exposure to biomass fuel is associated with increased carotid artery intima-media thickness and a higher prevalence of atherosclerotic plaque. Heart 2013;99(14):984–91.

110. Caravedo MA, Painschab MS, Davila-Roman VG, et al. Lack of association between chronic exposure to biomass fuel smoke and markers of right ventricular pressure overload at high altitude. Am Heart J 2014;168(5):731–8.

111. Kargin R, Kargin F, Mutlu H, et al. Long-term exposure to biomass fuel and its relation to systolic and diastolic biventricular performance in addition to obstructive and restrictive lung diseases. Echocardiography 2011;28(1):52–61.

112. Fatmi Z, Coggon D. Coronary heart disease and household air pollution from use of solid fuel: a systematic review. Br Med Bull 2016;118(1):91–109.

113. Nunes KV, Ignotti E, Hacon Sde S. Circulatory disease mortality rates in the elderly and exposure to PM(2.5) generated by biomass burning in the Brazilian Amazon in 2005. Cad Saude Publica 2013; 29(3):589–98.

114. Alam D, Chowdhury M, Siddiquee A, et al. Adult cardiopulmonary mortality and indoor air pollution: a 10-year retrospective cohort study in a low-income rural setting. Glob Heart 2012;7(3): 215–21.

115. Mitter S, Vedanthan R, Islami F, et al. Household fuel use and cardiovascular disease mortality: Golestan Cohort Study. Circulation 2016;133:2360–9.

116. Chatham-Stephens K, Caravanos J, Ericson B, et al. The pediatric burden of disease from lead exposure at toxic waste sites in low and middle income countries. Environ Res 2014; 132:379–83.

117. World's Worst Pollution Problems. New York Pure Earth and Green Cross Switzerland;2015. Available at: www.worstpolluted.org.

118. Tong S, von Schirnding YE, Prapamontol T. Environmental lead exposure: a public health problem of global dimensions. Bull World Health Organ 2000;78(9):1068–77.

119. Muntner P, Menke A, DeSalvo KB, et al. Continued decline in blood lead levels among adults in the United States: the National Health and Nutrition Examination Surveys. Arch Intern Med 2005;165(18): 2155–61.

120. Richter PA, Bishop EE, Wang J, et al. Trends in tobacco smoke exposure and blood lead levels among youths and adults in the United States: the National Health and Nutrition Examination Survey, 1999-2008. Prev Chronic Dis 2013;10: E213.

121. Jones D, Diop A, Block M, et al. Assessment and remediation of lead contamination in Senegal. J Health Pollution 2011;2:37–47.

122. Leaded Petrol Phase-out: Global status as at June 2016, United Nations Environment Programme website. Available at: http://www.unep.org/Transport/new/PCFV/pdf/Maps_Matrices/world/lead/MapWorld Lead June2016.pdf. Accessed August 8, 2016.

123. Ahmad SA, Khan MH, Khandker S, et al. Blood lead levels and health problems of lead acid battery workers in Bangladesh. ScientificWorldJournal 2014;2014:974104.

124. Basit S, Karim N, Munshi AB. Occupational lead toxicity in battery workers. Pak J Med Sci 2015; 31(4):775–80.

125. Were FH, Moturi MC, Gottesfeld P, et al. Lead exposure and blood pressure among workers in diverse industrial plants in Kenya. J Occup Environ Hyg 2014;11(11):706–15.

126. van Geen A, Bravo C, Gil V, et al. Lead exposure from soil in Peruvian mining towns: a national assessment supported by two contrasting examples. Bull World Health Organ 2012;90(12):878–86.

127. Yabe J, Nakayama SM, Ikenaka Y, et al. Lead poisoning in children from townships in the vicinity of a lead-zinc mine in Kabwe, Zambia. Chemosphere 2015;119:941–7.

128. Getso K, Hadejia I, Sabitu K, et al. Prevalence and determinants of childhood lead poisoning in Zamfar State, Nigeria. J Health Pollution 2014;6:1–9.

129. Anticona C, Bergdahl IA, San Sebastian M. Lead exposure among children from native communities of the Peruvian Amazon basin. Rev Panam Salud Publica 2012;31(4):296–302.

130. Ademuyiwa O, Ugbaja RN, Idumebor F, et al. Plasma lipid profiles and risk of cardiovascular disease in occupational lead exposure in Abeokuta, Nigeria. Lipids Health Dis 2005;4:19.

131. Caravanos J, Dowling R, Tellez-Rojo MM, et al. Blood lead levels in Mexico and pediatric burden of disease implications. Ann Glob Health 2014; 80(4):269–77.

132. Lim S, Murphy T, Wilson K, et al. Leaded paint in Cambodia—Pilot-scale assessment. J Health Pollution 2015;9:18–24.

133. Caravanos J, Fuller R, Robinson S, Centers for Disease Control and Prevention (CDC). Notes from the field: severe environmental contamination and elevated blood lead levels among children—Zambia, 2014. MMWR Morb Mortal Wkly Rep 2014;63(44):1013.

134. Laborde A, Tomasina F, Bianchi F, et al. Children's health in Latin America: the influence of environmental exposures. Environ Health Perspect 2015; 123(3):201–9.

135. Suk WA, Ahanchian H, Asante KA, et al. Environmental pollution: an under-recognized threat to children's health, especially in low- and middle-income countries. Environ Health Perspect 2016; 124(3):A41–5.

136. Vaziri ND. Mechanisms of lead-induced hypertension and cardiovascular disease. Am J Physiol Heart Circ Physiol 2008;295(2):H454–65.

137. Navas-Acien A, Guallar E, Silbergeld EK, et al. Lead exposure and cardiovascular disease–a systematic review. Environ Health Perspect 2007; 115(3):472–82.

138. Afridi HI, Kazi TG, Kazi NG, et al. Evaluation of cadmium, lead, nickel and zinc status in biological samples of smokers and nonsmokers hypertensive patients. J Hum Hypertens 2010;24(1):34–43.

139. Shiue I. Higher urinary heavy metal, arsenic, and phthalate concentrations in people with high blood pressure: US NHANES, 2009-2010. Blood Press 2014;23(6):363–9.

140. Rhee SY, Hwang YC, Woo JT, et al. Blood lead is significantly associated with metabolic syndrome in Korean adults: an analysis based on the Korea National Health and Nutrition Examination Survey (KNHANES), 2008. Cardiovasc Diabetol 2013;12:9.

141. Ettinger AS, Bovet P, Plange-Rhule J, et al. Distribution of metals exposure and associations with cardiometabolic risk factors in the "Modeling the Epidemiologic Transition Study". Environ Health 2014;13:90.

142. Ari E, Kaya Y, Demir H, et al. The correlation of serum trace elements and heavy metals with carotid artery atherosclerosis in maintenance hemodialysis patients. Biol Trace Elem Res 2011; 144(1–3):351–9.

143. Arslan C, Altan H, Akgun OO, et al. Trace elements and toxic heavy metals play a role in Buerger disease and atherosclerotic peripheral arterial occlusive disease. Int Angiol 2010;29(6):489–95.

144. Schober SE, Mirel LB, Graubard BI, et al. Blood lead levels and death from all causes, cardiovascular disease, and cancer: results from the NHANES III mortality study. Environ Health Perspect 2006;114(10):1538–41.

145. Aoki Y, Brody DJ, Flegal KM, et al. Blood lead and other metal biomarkers as risk factors for cardiovascular disease mortality. Medicine 2016;95(1): e2223.

146. Flanagan SV, Johnston RB, Zheng Y. Arsenic in tube well water in Bangladesh: health and economic impacts and implications for arsenic mitigation. Bull World Health Organ 2012;90(11): 839–46.

147. Chen Y, Wu F, Liu M, et al. A prospective study of arsenic exposure, arsenic methylation capacity, and risk of cardiovascular disease in Bangladesh. Environ Health Perspect 2013;121(7):832–8.

148. Chen CJ. Health hazards and mitigation of chronic poisoning from arsenic in drinking water: Taiwan experiences. Rev Environ Health 2014;29(1–2): 13–9.

149. Gunduz O, Bakar C, Simsek C, et al. Statistical analysis of causes of death (2005-2010) in villages of Simav Plain, Turkey, with high arsenic levels in drinking water supplies. Arch Environ Occup Health 2015;70(1):35–46.

150. Joca L, Sacks JD, Moore D, et al. Systematic review of differential inorganic arsenic exposure in minority, low-income, and indigenous populations in the United States. Environ Int 2016;92-93:707–15.

151. Smith AH, Lingas EO, Rahman M. Contamination of drinking-water by arsenic in Bangladesh: a public health emergency. Bull World Health Organ 2000; 78(9):1093–103.

152. Gilbert-Diamond D, Cottingham KL, Gruber JF, et al. Rice consumption contributes to arsenic exposure in US women. Proc Natl Acad Sci U S A 2011;108(51):20656–60.

153. Davis MA, Mackenzie TA, Cottingham KL, et al. Rice consumption and urinary arsenic concentrations in U.S. children. Environ Health Perspect 2012;120(10):1418–24.

154. Sidhu MS, Desai KP, Lynch HN, et al. Mechanisms of action for arsenic in cardiovascular toxicity and implications for risk assessment. Toxicology 2015; 331:78–99.

155. Das N, Paul S, Chatterjee D, et al. Arsenic exposure through drinking water increases the risk of liver and cardiovascular diseases in the population of West Bengal, India. BMC Public Health 2012;12:639.

156. Islam MS, Mohanto NC, Karim MR, et al. Elevated concentrations of serum matrix metalloproteinase-2 and -9 and their associations with circulating markers of cardiovascular diseases in chronic arsenic-exposed individuals. Environ Health 2015; 14:92.

157. Chu W, Li C, Qu X, et al. Arsenic-induced interstitial myocardial fibrosis reveals a new insight into drug-induced long QT syndrome. Cardiovasc Res 2012; 96(1):90–8.

158. Wu F, Jasmine F, Kibriya MG, et al. Interaction between arsenic exposure from drinking water and genetic susceptibility in carotid intima-media thickness in Bangladesh. Toxicol Appl Pharmacol 2014; 276(3):195–203.

159. Farzan SF, Karagas MR, Jiang J, et al. Gene-arsenic interaction in longitudinal changes of blood pressure: findings from the Health Effects of Arsenic Longitudinal Study (HEALS) in Bangladesh. Toxicol Appl Pharmacol 2015;288(1): 95–105.

160. Wu F, Jasmine F, Kibriya MG, et al. Interaction between arsenic exposure from drinking water and genetic polymorphisms on cardiovascular disease in Bangladesh: a prospective case-cohort study. Environ Health Perspect 2015;123(5):451–7.

161. Gamble MV, Liu X, Ahsan H, et al. Folate and arsenic metabolism: a double-blind, placebo-controlled folic acid–supplementation trial in Bangladesh. Am J Clin Nutr 2006;84(5):1093–101.

162. Abhyankar LN, Jones MR, Guallar E, et al. Arsenic exposure and hypertension: a systematic review. Environ Health Perspect 2012;120(4):494–500.

163. Guha Mazumder D, Purkayastha I, Ghose A, et al. Hypertension in chronic arsenic exposure: a case control study in West Bengal. J Environ Sci Health A Tox Hazard Subst Environ Eng 2012;47(11): 1514–20.

164. Islam MR, Khan I, Attia J, et al. Association between hypertension and chronic arsenic exposure in drinking water: a cross-sectional study in Bangladesh. Int J Environ Res Public Health 2012;9(12):4522–36.

165. Li X, Li B, Xi S, et al. Prolonged environmental exposure of arsenic through drinking water on the risk of hypertension and type 2 diabetes. Environ Sci Pollut Res Int 2013;20(11):8151–61.

166. Stea F, Bianchi F, Cori L, et al. Cardiovascular effects of arsenic: clinical and epidemiological findings. Environ Sci Pollut Res Int 2014;21(1):244–51.

167. Osorio-Yanez C, Ayllon-Vergara JC, Arreola-Mendoza L, et al. Blood pressure, left ventricular geometry, and systolic function in children exposed to inorganic arsenic. Environ Health Perspect 2015;123(6):629–35.

168. Ameer SS, Engstrom K, Harari F, et al. The effects of arsenic exposure on blood pressure and early risk markers of cardiovascular disease: evidence for population differences. Environ Res 2015;140:32–6.

169. Mendez MA, Gonzalez-Horta C, Sanchez-Ramirez B, et al. Chronic exposure to arsenic and markers of cardiometabolic risk: a cross-sectional study in Chihuahua, Mexico. Environ Health Perspect 2016;124(1):104–11.

170. Osorio-Yanez C, Ayllon-Vergara JC, Aguilar-Madrid G, et al. Carotid intima-media thickness and plasma asymmetric dimethylarginine in Mexican children exposed to inorganic arsenic. Environ Health Perspect 2013;121(9):1090–6.

171. Wu F, Molinaro P, Chen Y. Arsenic exposure and subclinical endpoints of cardiovascular diseases. Curr Environ Health Rep 2014;1(2):148–62.

172. Cheng TJ, Ke DS, Guo HR. The association between arsenic exposure from drinking water and cerebrovascular disease mortality in Taiwan. Water Res 2010;44(19):5770–6.

173. Jovanovic DD, Paunovic K, Manojlovic DD, et al. Arsenic in drinking water and acute coronary syndrome in Zrenjanin municipality, Serbia. Environ Res 2012;117:75–82.

174. Moon K, Guallar E, Navas-Acien A. Arsenic exposure and cardiovascular disease: an updated systematic review. Curr Atheroscler Rep 2012;14(6): 542–55.

175. Chen Y, Karagas MR. Arsenic and cardiovascular disease: new evidence from the United States. Ann Intern Med 2013;159(10):713–4.

176. Moon KA, Guallar E, Umans JG, et al. Association between exposure to low to moderate arsenic levels and incident cardiovascular disease. A prospective cohort study. Ann Intern Med 2013; 159(10):649–59.

177. Rahman M, Sohel N, Yunus M, et al. A prospective cohort study of stroke mortality and arsenic in drinking water in Bangladeshi adults. BMC Public Health 2014;14:174.

178. D'Ippoliti D, Santelli E, De Sario M, et al. Arsenic in drinking water and mortality for cancer and chronic diseases in central Italy, 1990-2010. PLoS One 2015;10(9):e0138182.

179. Farzan SF, Chen Y, Rees JR, et al. Risk of death from cardiovascular disease associated with low-level arsenic exposure among long-term smokers in a US population-based study. Toxicol Appl Pharmacol 2015;287(2):93–7.

180. James KA, Byers T, Hokanson JE, et al. Association between lifetime exposure to inorganic arsenic in drinking water and coronary heart disease in Colorado residents. Environ Health Perspect 2015; 123(2):128–34.

181. Wade TJ, Xia Y, Mumford J, et al. Cardiovascular disease and arsenic exposure in Inner Mongolia, China: a case control study. Environ Health 2015; 14:35.

182. Rudnai T, Sandor J, Kadar M, et al. Arsenic in drinking water and congenital heart anomalies in Hungary. Int J Hyg Environ Health 2014;217(8): 813–8.

183. Riederer AM, Belova A, George BJ, et al. Urinary cadmium in the 1999-2008 U.S. National Health and Nutrition Examination Survey (NHANES). Environ Sci Technol 2013;47(2):1137–47.

184. Tellez-Plaza M, Jones MR, Dominguez-Lucas A, et al. Cadmium exposure and clinical

cardiovascular disease: a systematic review. Curr Atheroscler Rep 2013;15(10):356.

185. Vowotor M, Hood C, Sackey S, et al. An assessment of heavy metal pollution in sediments of a tropical lagoon: a case study of the Benya Lagoon, Komenda Edina Eguafo Abrem Municipality KEEA)- Ghana. J Health Pollution 2014;6:26–39.

186. Namuhani N, Kimumwe C. Soil contamination with heavy metals around Jinia Steel Rolling Mills in Jinja Municipality, Uganda. J Health Pollution 2015;9:61–7.

187. Schmidt CW. Unfair trade e-Waste in Africa. Environ Health Perspect 2006;114(4):A232–5.

188. Orisakwe O, Blum J, Zelikoff J. Metal pollution in Nigeria: a biomonitoring update. J Health Pollution 2014;6:40–52.

189. Valko M, Morris H, Cronin MT. Metals, toxicity and oxidative stress. Curr Med Chem 2005;12(10):1161–208.

190. Kaya Y, Ari E, Demir H, et al. Serum cadmium levels are independently associated with endothelial function in hemodialysis patients. Int Urol Nephrol 2012;44(5):1487–92.

191. Yazihan N, Kocak MK, Akcil E, et al. Involvement of galectin-3 in cadmium-induced cardiac toxicity. Anadolu Kardiyol Derg 2011;11(6):479–84.

192. Al-Saleh I, Shinwari N, Mashhour A, et al. Cadmium and mercury levels in Saudi women and its possible relationship with hypertension. Biol Trace Elem Res 2006;112(1):13–29.

193. Peters JL, Perlstein TS, Perry MJ, et al. Cadmium exposure in association with history of stroke and heart failure. Environ Res 2010;110(2):199–206.

194. Lee BK, Kim Y. Association of blood cadmium with hypertension in the Korean general population: analysis of the 2008-2010 Korean National Health and Nutrition Examination Survey data. Am J Ind Med 2012;55(11):1060–7.

195. Caciari T, Sancini A, Fioravanti M, et al. Cadmium and hypertension in exposed workers: a meta-analysis. Int J Occup Med Environ Health 2013;26(3):440–56.

196. Swaddiwudhipong W, Nguntra P, Kaewnate Y, et al. Human health effects from cadmium exposure: comparison between persons living in cadmium-contaminated and non-contaminated areas in northwestern Thailand. Southeast Asian J Trop Med Public Health 2015;46(1):133–42.

197. Afridi HI, Kazi TG, Talpur FN, et al. Distribution of arsenic, cadmium, lead, and nickel levels in biological samples of Pakistani hypertensive patients and control subjects. Clin Lab 2014;60(8):1309–18.

198. Liu B, Feng W, Wang J, et al. Association of urinary metals levels with type 2 diabetes risk in coke oven workers. Environ Pollut 2015;210:1–8.

199. Gallagher CM, Meliker JR. Blood and urine cadmium, blood pressure, and hypertension: a systematic review and meta-analysis. Environ Health Perspect 2010;118(12):1676–84.

200. Kurihara I, Kobayashi E, Suwazono Y, et al. Association between exposure to cadmium and blood pressure in Japanese peoples. Arch Environ Health 2004;59(12):711–6.

201. Lee MS, Park SK, Hu H, et al. Cadmium exposure and cardiovascular disease in the 2005 Korea National Health and Nutrition Examination Survey. Environ Res 2011;111(1):171–6.

202. Tellez-Plaza M, Navas-Acien A, Crainiceanu CM, et al. Cadmium and peripheral arterial disease: gender differences in the 1999-2004 US National Health and Nutrition Examination Survey. Am J Epidemiol 2010;172(6):671–81.

203. Tellez-Plaza M, Guallar E, Howard BV, et al. Cadmium exposure and incident cardiovascular disease. Epidemiology 2013;24(3):421–9.

204. Barregard L, Sallsten G, Fagerberg B, et al. Blood cadmium levels and incident cardiovascular events during follow-up in a population-based cohort of Swedish adults: the Malmo Diet and Cancer Study. Environ Health Perspect 2016;124(5):594–600.

205. Borne Y, Barregard L, Persson M, et al. Cadmium exposure and incidence of heart failure and atrial fibrillation: a population-based prospective cohort study. BMJ Open 2015;5(6):e007366.

206. Menke A, Muntner P, Silbergeld EK, et al. Cadmium levels in urine and mortality among U.S. adults. Environ Health Perspect 2009;117(2):190–6.

207. Tellez-Plaza M, Navas-Acien A, Menke A, et al. Cadmium exposure and all-cause and cardiovascular mortality in the U.S. general population. Environ Health Perspect 2012;120(7):1017–22.

208. Larsson SC, Wolk A. Urinary cadmium and mortality from all causes, cancer and cardiovascular disease in the general population: systematic review and meta-analysis of cohort studies. Int J Epidemiol 2016;45(3):782–91.

Diagnosis and Management of Endomyocardial Fibrosis

Andrea Beaton, MD[a],*, Ana Olga Mocumbi, MD, PhD[b]

KEYWORDS

- Endomyocarial fibrosis • Restrictive cardiomyopathy • Heart failure • Neglected diseases

KEY POINTS

- Endomyocardial fibrosis is an important cause of restrictive cardiomyopathy worldwide.
- The etiology of endomyocardial fibrosis remains elusive, and the disease is most often diagnosed in the late stages of disease.
- Medical management is of little benefit, and although surgical intervention offers some survival advantage, access is limited in low-resource settings.
- International collaboration, modern research techniques, and increased funding are needed to improve understanding of this neglected tropical disease.

INTRODUCTION

Endomyocardial fibrosis (EMF), one of the world's most neglected cardiovascular diseases, remains an important cause of restrictive cardiomyopathy. Worldwide prevalence is estimated at 10 to 12 million,[1] although systematic global epidemiology is extremely limited. Most cases occur in tropical, low-resource settings, and poverty is a multifactorial driver of disease development, contributes to late diagnosis, and limits access to appropriate medical and surgical care. Knowledge advancement around EMF has been slow, and significant questions remain on the etiology, natural history, and best therapeutic strategies. Increased awareness, advocacy, and research are needed to further understand this neglected tropical cardiomyopathy and to improve survival of those affected.

EPIDEMIOLOGY

EMF remains primarily a tropical cardiomyopathy with most cases coming from Africa, Asia, and South America. African cases have clustered in Uganda, Nigeria, the Ivory Coast, and the coastal areas of Mozambique, but 16 countries distributed across the continent have reported cases.[2] Outside of Africa, hotspots include Kerala State in India,[3–5] Guangzi providence in China,[6] and Brazil.[7]

Geographic restriction and regional variation within high prevalence countries has been noted. In Mozambique, almost two-thirds of patients presenting at a tertiary center with EMF resided in a single costal province.[8] Ethnic predisposition is reported, with EMF being more common among Rwandan and Burundian immigrants living in Uganda compared with native Ugandans,[9,10] although Rwanda and Burundi report few primary cases.

Conflicts of Interest: The authors have nothing to disclose.
[a] Division of Cardiology, Children's National Health System, 111 Michigan Avenue, Northwest, Washington, DC 20010, USA; [b] Chronic and Non-Communicable Disease Division, National Health Institutes and Eduardo Mondlane University, Avenida do Zimbábew, Maputo, Mozambique
* Corresponding author.
E-mail address: abeaton@childrensnational.org

Cardiol Clin 35 (2017) 87–98
http://dx.doi.org/10.1016/j.ccl.2016.08.005
0733-8651/17/© 2016 Elsevier Inc. All rights reserved.

Accurate estimates of the incidence and prevalence of EMF remain challenging. A single population screening, conducted in an endemic area of Mozambique, suggests EMF may have a much broader disease spectrum and much higher prevalence than previously thought. Echocardiographic screening of 948 residents of the Inharrime district found 19.8% with evidence of EMF, 77.3% of whom had mild disease.[11] Case detection was higher among family members, and risk increased with each additional positive case within a family, a finding previously reported in Uganda[12] and Zambia.[13]

EMF patients most typically come from the lowest socioeconomic groups, even within broadly low-income countries.[9,14] Classically, EMF presents in childhood and adolescence, although some sites report a bimodal distribution with second peak among women in childbearing years.[9,15] Extreme presentations in infancy[16,17] and the elderly[11] have also been reported. Several studies found no sex specific preponderance, whereas others show conflicting higher rates among women (Uganda[15]) and among men (Mozambique,[11] Nigeria[18]).

Evidence shows that incidence and prevalence of EMF may be decreasing in some regions, potentially because of improving socioeconomic conditions.[19] In the last half-century, parts of Nigeria have seen a decrease from 10% to less than 1% prevalence.[20] Similarly, high-incidence regions of India have reported dramatic declines.[19] In contrast, cases of EMF are being reported from countries that historically have not been affected (Malawi[21]), likely secondary to increasing availability of echocardiography.[2] Other regions, such as Uganda,[22] report no change, and in most affected countries, no trend data have been collected.

ETIOLOGY

There is no clear consensus on the etiology of EMF. Authentication and replication of individual hypotheses has been difficult. Poor recognition and characterization of the early disease state and the relative scarcity of contemporary investigations using modern techniques have further compounded this challenge. Poverty and geographic specificity have emerged as the most consistent risk factors and are intimately related to most proposed etiologies, which are grouped into the 3 main categories of eosinophilia and parasitic disease, diet and toxicity, and genetic susceptibility.[23]

EMF is most prevalent in tropical regions, which are also plagued by infectious and parasitic disease. Specific trigger pathogens have been proposed including malaria,[24,25] streptococcus,[26,27] fillariasis,[28–30] and schistosomiasis,[27,31] among others. However, imperfect matching of pathogens with EMF distribution[32,33] and inconsistent parasitic loads in affected patients[34] argue against direct infection as a single infectious trigger. A common immune overreaction, resulting from a variety of different pathogens, is more plausible. Associations with increased circulating IgE[28,35] and eosinophilia[31,36] have been reported, and specific hyperimmune conditions, such as malarial hypersplenomegaly syndrome have been linked to EMF development.[12] Here again, however, there are inconsistencies, suggesting that at most, the immune response is one of several components of EMF development.

Dietary deficiencies (magnesium[37]) and excesses (vitamin D[38]), ingested toxins (cerium, cyanogenic glycosides,[39] serotonin[40,41]), and herbal preparations[39] have also been proposed as causative. The right-sided predilection for EMF supports the potential role of a toxin, filtered from the blood in the pulmonary circulation.[19] Cassava, a root vegetable nearly ubiquitous to the diet of certain low-income countries, has been studied most extensively, with some evidence of endocardial thickening and fibrosis in mice fed a cassava-rich diet.[42] However, as happens with parasitic load,[43] cassava consumption is typically proportionate to poverty level.[19]

It is most likely that EMF results from the complex interplay of a susceptible host being exposed to environmental challenges through the conditions of extreme poverty (including infectious and dietary challenges). Familial clustering of EMF cases has been reported from Uganda,[12] Nigeria,[44] Zambia,[13] and Mozambique.[11] A single formal genetic analysis conducted in 2 populations found polymorphisms in the human leukocyte antigen system to be associated with a predisposition to EMF.[45] Further formal genetic studies, ideally unbiased genomewide investigations, are of critical importance and may find new insights into the pathogenesis of EMF.

NATURAL HISTORY

EMF patients typically present late, when serious cardiovascular symptoms and complications develop. Thus, although the late stages of EMF have been extensively reported, it has been more challenging to characterize the patterns and presentations of early disease. The current understanding of EMF involves progression through 3 disease stages: an active inflammatory stage, a transitional stage, and a chronic fibrotic stage,[23] but no prospective study has documented this progression in patients. Alternate presentations, similar to those described for rheumatic heart disease, are also likely, including an indolent course with only late disease detection, an aggressive presentation with early heart failure and death, and a transition to a subacute phase without cardiac sequale.[46]

CLINICAL PRESENTATION AND PATHOPHYSIOLOGY
Acute Phase

Knowledge of the acute inflammatory phase of EMF comes from a limited number of historical studies, with no corroborating contemporary data. High levels of eosinophilia have been reported, suggesting that the early disease phase may be an allergic or immune system overreaction, but laboratory findings are inconsistent.[34,43,47] A prospective study of Nigerian patients with eosinophilia greater than the 97th percentile found 29.5% (13 of 44) with new diagnosis of EMF.[48] These patients reported symptoms supportive of allergic/immune involvement with fever, itching, periorbital swelling, and hives. EMF should be considered in patients residing in endemic areas who present with those symptoms, but in reality, the acute phase of EMF is rarely detected, and most patients present in a chronic or an acute-on-chronic state.

Chronic or Advanced Phase

Patients with chronic or advanced EMF typically show a related group of symptoms including malnutrition, cachexia, stunted growth, and hypoalbuminemia. Signs of poor cardiac output including digital clubbing and male feminization can occur.[49] Severe ascites without peripheral edema is pathognomonic and hypothesized to result from concurrent peritoneal inflammation and fibrosis (**Fig. 1**).[34,50,51] Repeated paracentesis, often necessary for symptomatic relief, contributes to hypoalbuminemia. Skeletal muscle fibrosis has been documented and suggests EMF may be merely the cardiac portion of a more general inflammatory and fibrotic state.[34] Several other notable findings, including proptosis, hyperpigmentation of the lips and gums, parotid swelling, and central cyanosis are often seen, but their cause is not fully understood.[32,34,52]

Cardiac involvement is typically a pancarditis[53] progressing to patchy endocardial fibrosis, and then more diffuse fibrotic involvement (**Fig. 2**) and restrictive physiology.[43] Endocardial fibrosis is pronounced in the atrioventricular valves,

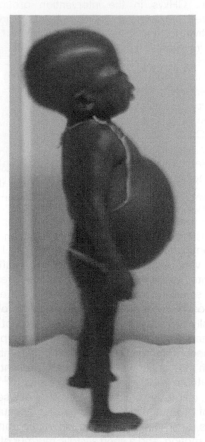

Fig. 1. A 2-year-old boy (one of the youngest patients reported) with RV EMF and the classic features of massive abdominal ascites without peripheral edema.

leading to mitral and tricuspid regurgitation, and in the ventricular apices, where thrombus can develop. The atria can also be affected by patchy fibrosis.[53–55] The combination of atrioventricular valve regurgitation and restrictive physiology results in atrial enlargement, which can be severe. Atrial enlargement predisposes patients to atrial arrhythmia development, particularly atrial fibrillation, which is found in almost one-third of patients with chronic EMF. Occasionally, cardiac conduction disturbances may result from progressive fibrosis, including junctional arrhythmia, heart block, and intraventricular conduction delay.[56]

Large pericardial effusions are mostly seen in right ventricular (RV) forms of EMF. Although commonly well tolerated,[57] the presence of pericardial effusion further impairs the diastolic function, already compromised by the endocardial thickening, decreasing exercise capacity, and increasing systemic venous pressures.

More than half of EMF patients show biventricular involvement (55%),[11] but most show either a right- (more commonly) or left-sided

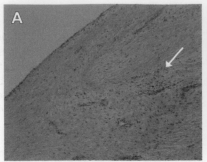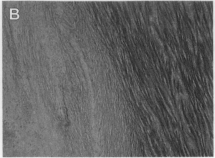

Fig. 2. (*A*) Hematoxylin-eosin staining of the thickened endocardium shows hypercellularity, foci of inflammation, and hypervascularization (*arrow*). (*B*) Van Gieson staining of the subendocardium shows myocytes entrapped in strands of fibrosis (*red*).

predominance. RV-dominant EMF results in systemic venous hypertension presenting in affected patients as elevated jugular venous pressure, facial swelling, hepatosplenomegaly, and exophthalmos.[58,59] Peripheral edema would be physiologically expected but is rarely seen except in the end stages of cardiac failure. Pulmonary hypertension secondary to chronic pulmonary thromboembolism may occur when thrombi are present in the right atrium (most commonly) or ventricle.[60,61] Left ventricular (LV)-dominant EMF is typically seen as part of biventricular disease. Cardiac auscultation shows a mitral opening snap, reflecting abnormal mitral motion, and a short systolic murmur of mitral regurgitation and loud pulmonary component of the second sound caused by pulmonary hypertension related to increase in left atrial pressure.

DIAGNOSTIC TESTING
Laboratory Testing and Serum Markers

There is no diagnostic laboratory test for EMF. Eosinophilia, most commonly seen during the early stages of EMF,[62] is an inconsistent finding (0%–70%) at time of diagnosis.[34,43,47] Hypoalbuminemia seen in advanced disease is likely multifactorial. Ascitic fluid in EMF is exudative (compared with transudative fluid typically resulting from heart failure), with elevated protein and lymphocytes, suggesting an inflammatory component.[51] Serum autoantibodies (IgG and IgM) directed against myocardial proteins have been shown in limited immunologic investigations, but their role in EMF pathogenesis is not conclusive.[24,63]

Electrocardiography

The electrocardiogram in EMF reflects the underlying distribution and severity of cardiac disease.[64] In RV-dominant EMF, there are peaked p-waves reflecting right atrial enlargement, and either a

QR pattern in V1 or a dominant R-wave in lead V2. LV EMF typically has widened p-waves reflecting left atrial enlargement, and ST depression and T-wave inversions can be seen in the lateral leads and sometimes more diffusely. Milder EMF cases are sometimes diagnosed during a general diagnostic work-up for mitral murmur. In patients with pulmonary hypertension, the electrocardiogram shows RV hypertrophy and right-axis deviation.[43]

Arrhythmias are common in patients with advanced disease. Atrial fibrillation risk seems to correlate to atrial size but may also result from inflammation.[51] Progressive fibrosis is thought to interfere with cardiac condition. Heart block can be seen, with first-degree block typical, complete heart block uncommon, and need for a pacemaker rare. Other conduction abnormalities include junctional rhythm and intraventricular conduction delays. Fatal ventricular arrhythmia has been reported.[65]

Chest Radiograph

The chest radiograph in EMF is notable for right, left, or biatrial enlargement, ranging from mild to severe abnormalities in parallel with EMF severity.[47] In RV-dominant EMF, a dilated RV outflow track can create a prominence over the left heart border, and normal or decreased vascular markings are seen (**Fig. 3**). In LV-dominant EMF there is prominence of the main pulmonary artery and evidence of pulmonary venous congestion.[66] Pleural and pericardial effusions are common, regardless of dominant chamber. Rarely, endocardial calcification is visible.[43,47]

Echocardiography

Echocardiography is the standard modality for EMF diagnosis showing a high level of agreement (82.8%) between expert echocardiographic interpretation and surgical pathology.[53] The

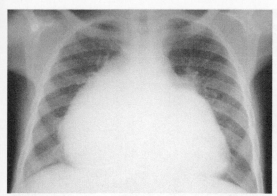

Fig. 3. Chest x-ray of a patient with RV EMF shows pronounced cardiomegaly caused by severe right atrial dilation and pericardial effusion with clear lung fields.

echocardiogram in EMF reflects global endocardial fibrosis and is characterized by thickened endocardium, severely dilated atria, commonly with mural or free thrombi (**Figs. 4** and **5**), atrioventricular valve dysfunction, and retracted ventricles—often containing apical thrombi. In 2008, diagnostic criteria and severity scoring were developed for use in prospective population-based studies of EMF (**Table 1**).[11] The diagnosis of EMF is made when 2 major or 1 major and 2 minor criteria are identified; scores determine the severity of the disease (score <8 indicates mild, 8–15 moderate, and >15 severe EMF).

Patients with EMF have varying degrees and patterns of endocardial thickening, which can be seen as echo brightness along the endocardial surface.[67] In mild EMF, this typically manifests as patchy fibrosis of the ventricular septum or along the ventricular free walls. As the disease advances, large fibrotic plaques develop in 1 or both ventricles and can obliterate a portion of the ventricular cavity, typically the trabeculated portion of the RV, the LV apex, and posterior mitral valve recess. Ventricular thrombi are commonly seen, typically early in the disease course, and are thought to determine ventricular obliteration[68,69] in combination with scarring and fibrosis. Three-dimensional echocardiography, when available, can more completely characterize the extent of RV involvement and thrombus.[70]

Fibrosis and ventricular obliteration lead to a restricted ventricular filling pattern, characterized by a tall E wave with E/A ratio greater than 2, a deceleration time less than 120 ms, and an isovolumic relaxation time less than 160 ms.[71] Fibrosis of the LV apex can lead to restricted movement and notably increased contractile force from the basal septum, the so-called Merlon sign.[67,68] On M-mode, the "septal bounce" created by rapid anterior movement in early diastole can be seen and results in a characteristic "M" pattern (**Fig. 6**).[72]

Fibrosis typically also affects the atrioventricular valves, the severity of involvement ranging from diffuse thickening to severe restriction, sometimes with complete leaflet adhesion to the endocardial surface. In right-dominant disease, severe tricuspid regurgitation results from valve retraction and fusion to the endocardium. In the most advanced forms wide noncoaptation results in an unguarded tricuspid annulus and leads to low-velocity regurgitation reflecting equalization of pressure in the right atrium and RV. LV-dominant

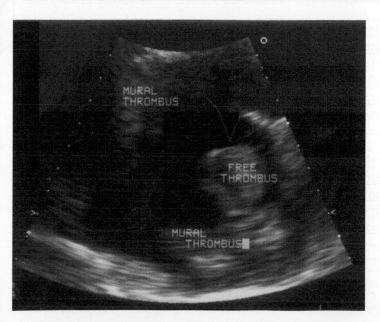

Fig. 4. Subcostal view shows mural and free right atrial thrombi in the in a patient with right EMF.

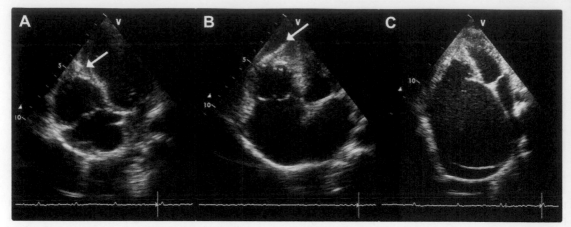

Fig. 5. The spectrum of RV EMF. (*A*) Mild: obliteration of the RV apical region (*arrow*), thickened endocardium, and dilatation of the tricuspid annulus. (*B*) Moderate: thickening of the tricuspid leaflets, obliteration and calcification of the RV apex, mild retraction of the RV apex (*arrow*), and dilatation of the tricuspid annulus with right atrium dilatation. (*C*) Severe: obliteration of the RV apex with cavity reduction, shortening of the tricuspid leaflets and tricuspid annulus dilatation, aneurysmal right atrium and compression of the left atrium, and small pericardial effusion.

EMF is characterized by restriction of the posterior mitral leaflet leading to eccentric, posteriorly directed mitral regurgitation. In the most severe cases, there is complete adhesion of the posterior mitral leaflet and papillary muscle to the endocardium, leading to massive mitral regurgitation.

Increased atrial pressure results from a combination of restricted ventricular filling and atrioventricular valve regurgitation and leads to progressive and sometimes massive atrial dilation and aneurysmal atria.[47,68] In right-dominant EMF, elevated right atrial pressure causes severe

Table 1		
Criteria for assessment of the severity of endomyocardial fibrosis		
Criterion		**Score**
Major Criteria		
Endomyocardial plaques >2 mm in thickness		2
Thin (<1 mm) endomyocardial patches affecting more than one ventricular wall		3
Obliteration of the right ventricular or left ventricular apex		4
Thrombi or spontaneous contrast without severe ventricular dysfunction		4
Retraction of the right ventricular apex (right ventricular apical notch)		4
Atrioventricular valve dysfunction owing to adhesion of the valvular apparatus to the ventricular wall		1–4[a]
Minor Criteria		
Thin endomyocardial patches localized to one ventricular wall		1
Restrictive flow pattern across mitral or tricuspid valves		2
Pulmonary valve diastolic opening		2
Diffuse thickening of the anterior mitral leaflet		1
Enlarged atrium with normal sized ventricle		2
M movement of the interventricular septum and flat posterior wall		1
Enhanced density of the moderator or other intraventricular bands		1

[a] The score is assigned according to the severity of atrioventricular regurgitation.
From Mocumbi AO, Ferreira MB, Sidi D, et al. A population study of endomyocardial fibrosis in a rural area of Mozambique. N Engl J Med 2008;359(1):46; with permission.

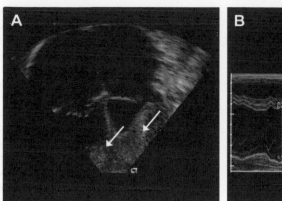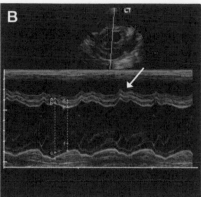

Fig. 6. (*A*) Biventricular EMF with marked LV and RV cavity reduction caused by bilateral apical obliteration (*arrows*), thickened mitral and tricuspid valve leaflets, and severe biatrial enlargement. (*B*) M-mode shows the characteristic M shape of the intraventricular septum (*white arrow*) in early diastole.

dilation of the superior and inferior vena cava and reversal of flow into the hepatic veins, which can be seen on pulsed and color Doppler interrogation.[71] In left-dominant EMF, increased left atrial pressure results in pulmonary hypertension.[47,58,68,73] Pericardial effusions are common, and can be quite large, although typically not resulting in tamponade.[23,43,68,74]

Multimodality Imaging

Multimodality imaging is not routinely conducted for EMF diagnosis but, if available, can provide complementary information. Cardiac computed tomography accurately diagnoses EMF and provides improved data on disease distribution (compared with echocardiography) by delineation and mapping endocardial fibrosis.[75] Cardiac MRI provides detailed, quantitative data on ventricular chamber size, shape, and extent of thrombosis[29,76–78] and may provide an early diagnostic advantage compared with echocardiography.[79,80] Myocardial perfusion imaging and late gadolinium enhancement identify avascular and fibrotic areas and show good histopathologic correlation.[2,81] Cardiac catheterization can be helpful when echocardiographic images are not adequate and cardiac computed tomography or MRI is not available but is relatively contraindicated because of the risk of fragmentation and embolization when thrombus is present. Additionally, challenges with the technical performance of catheterization and its interpretation can arise secondary to severe anatomic distortion. Pressure measurements show elevated end diastolic pressures in the affected chambers corresponding to severity of disease and a "dip and plateau" pattern or square root sign. Angiography outlines apical obliteration, decreased ventricular trabeculations, small

ventricular cavity size, atrioventricular valve regurgitation, and dilated atria.[47,82] Endomyocardial biopsy provides definitive diagnosis if positive, but patchy ventricular fibrosis can lead to false-negative biopsy results. Additionally, biopsy may be technically challenging or impossible in advanced disease when endocardial thickening is severe[43,47] or intracavitary thrombi are present.

DIFFERENTIAL DIAGNOSIS

EMF endemic areas also see high rates of other acquired cardiac disease. LV-dominant EMF can be difficult to distinguish from the mitral regurgitation seen in rheumatic heart disease, when apical obliteration and marked endocardial thickening are absent.[47] Moreover, there are reports of the 2 conditions occurring together.[10,26,83] Compared with patients with rheumatic heart disease and significant mitral regurgitation, patients with left-sided EMF will have lower-than-expected mitral regurgitation velocity (reflecting high left atrial/pulmonary venous pressure), less-than-expected LV dilation, and severe atrial dilation.[47] Posterior mitral leaflet restriction can be seen in both conditions, but in LV EMF there is often adhesion or complete fusion of the leaflet to the endocardial surface. EMF can also be confused on clinical evaluation with constrictive pericarditis, a common finding in areas in which tuberculosis remains endemic. EMF is distinguished in this case by ventricular apical obliteration, severely dilated atria, and normal pericardial thickness.[43] In challenging cases, and when available, MRI can be useful in distinguishing these diagnoses. Other competing diagnoses to exclude, depending on the patient's location, are restrictive cardiomyopathy, apical hypertrophic cardiomyopathy, Loeffler endocarditis, amyloidosis, hemochromatosis, sarcoidosis, and Ebstein's anomaly.[47,84,85]

MANAGEMENT
Medical Management

Historically, medical management in EMF was palliative and targeted only at symptomatic relief. However, recent advances in heart failure and arrhythmia management resulted in improved quality of life, decreased morbidity, and increased survival time for patients with EMF. Given the inflammatory component of both acute and chronic EMF,[53] steroids are often considered. However, steroids do not change the re-accumulation rate for chronic ascites[86] and have no proven survival benefit.[87] Still, some clinicians advocate for a 7- to 10-day course of steroids if acute EMF is recognized, although this must be weighted against their potential for negative side effects in a population with high rates of infectious diseases, including tuberculosis.[87]

Symptomatic heart failure is treated using a combination of diuretics, vasodilators, and β-blockers, according to the disease pattern and presentation. Among diuretics, spironolactone is preferred, as it may have additional benefit as an antifibrotic and has been found to improve survival in other forms of heart failure.[88] Oral anticoagulants are recommended for patients with atrial or ventricular thrombi, severely decreased ventricular function, or atrial fibrillation to prevent thromboembolic complications.[43] Paracentesis provides symptomatic relief in patients with severe ascites, but re-accumulation is often rapid, necessitating frequent hospitalizations and repeated procedures. Albumin replacement, if available, can mitigate protein losses.[58] Atrial fibrillation is typically managed with rate control given the high degree of reoccurrence with electrical cardioversion. Conduction delays are commonly seen but are rarely of significance to warrant pacemaker placement.[65]

Surgical Management

Surgical interventions can increase survival[89–93] but require experienced operators, well-equipped cardiac facilities, and trained intensive care teams capable of managing open-heart surgery and the often complex postoperative recovery. Surgery is recommended for all EMF patients with New York Heart Classification III or IV[94,95] and should be undertaken before the development of irreversible hepatic and cardiac damage.[87] Patients with long-standing ascites, extreme cachexia, chronic pulmonary thromboembolism, extensive endocardial fibrosis or calcification, impaired ventricular function, and extreme leaflet shortening represent high-risk surgical patients, and surgical intervention is relatively contraindicated in low-resource settings.[87,96]

Endocardectomy and atrioventricular valve repair or replacement is the most common surgical strategy. In many patients, a relatively well-defined cleavage plane allows for removal of the fibrotic endocardium and freeing of the underlying healthy myocardium. Valvular repair is favored over mechanical valve replacement given the challenges of anticoagulant managment.[23] Atrial reduction is often preformed concurrently to reduce the risk of atrial arrhythmias and thrombus formation.[97] Cavopulmonary anastomosis and "1.5 ventricle" repair may be helpful in palliating severe right-sided EMF and has been used to stabilize patients before endocardectomy and after endocardectomy when the RV cavity remains inadequately sized.[98–100]

The early postoperative mortality rate is 18% to 29%, and mortality is typically related to postoperative complications of endocardectomy including low cardiac output syndrome, pericardial effusion and tamponade, and complete atrioventricular block.[7,92,94] Late mortality is also significant but has been improving over time secondary to preference of valve repair instead of replacement and to improved myocardial protection techniques.[87] EMF can recur after surgery, but rates of reoccurrence are variable (6%–18.8%) and are not fully characterized.[101,102]

PROGNOSIS

Despite evidence of recent improvements in survival, EMF carries a poor prognosis, with high morbidity and mortality. Early data from Uganda showed an average 2-year survival after diagnosis, whereas more recent data show up to 68% 10-year survival rate.[92] Death is usually attributable to heart failure, acute thromboembolism, and arrhythmia.[43] Clinical predictors of early mortality include hemoglobin less than 10 g/dL, cyanosis, embolic episodes, QRS duration greater than 0.12 ms, and rapid clinical deterioration before diagnosis.[56] Echocardiographic assessment of diastolic function may have prognostic value. A study of 32 patients with biventricular EMF found that A' peak was an independent predictor of % Vo_2 and that EMF patients with Vo_2 less than 53% had 8.5 times the risk of mortality compared with those with more favorable indices.[103] Cardiac MRI, when available, can also aid in defining the prognosis. Increased ratio of endocardial fibrous tissue per body surface area is associated with increased probability of surgery and mortality.[81]

SUMMARY

EMF remains an important, yet poorly understood, cause of restrictive cardiomyopathy worldwide. Diagnosis is most often late, access to cardiac surgery is limited, and prognosis is poor. Clinical research on disease etiology and basic science research into disease pathogenesis are critical to identify preventative strategies and therapeutic targets that could improve outcomes. International collaboration, modern research techniques, and increased funding are needed to improve our understanding of this neglected tropical disease.

REFERENCES

1. Yacoub S, Kotit S, Mocumbi AO, et al. Neglected diseases in cardiology: a call for urgent action. Nat Clin Pract Cardiovasc Med 2008;5(4):176-7.
2. Mocumbi AO. Recent trends in the epidemiology of endomyocardial fibrosis in Africa. Paediatr Int Child Health 2012;32(2):63-4.
3. Nair DV. Endomyocardial fibrosis in Kerala. Indian Heart J 1971;23(3):182-90.
4. Kurian S, Nair DV. Ecology of endomyocardial fibrosis in Kerala State. Indian Heart J 1980;32(3):156-62.
5. Kutty VR, Abraham S, Kartha CC. Geographical distribution of endomyocardial fibrosis in south Kerala. Int J Epidemiol 1996;25(6):1202-7.
6. Yin R. Endomyocardial fibrosis in China. Chin Med Sci J 2000;15(1):55-60.
7. da Costa FD, Moraes CR, Rodriques JV, et al. Early surgical results in the treatment of endomyocardial fibrosis. A Brazilian cooperative study. Eur J Cardiothorac Surg 1989;3(5):408-13.
8. Ferreira B, Matsika-Claquin MD, Hausse-Mocumbi AO, et al. Geographic origin of endomyocardial fibrosis treated at the central hospital of Maputo (Mozambique) between 1987 and 1999. Bull Soc Pathol Exot 2002;95(4):276-9 [in French].
9. Rutakingirwa M, Ziegler JL, Newton R, et al. Poverty and eosinophilia are risk factors for endomyocardial fibrosis (EMF) in Uganda. Trop Med Int Health 1999;4(3):229-35.
10. Shaper AG, Hutt MS, Coles RM. Necropsy study of endomyocardial fibrosis and rheumatic heart disease in Uganda 1950-1965. Br Heart J 1968;30(3):391-401.
11. Mocumbi AO, Ferreira MB, Sidi D, et al. A population study of endomyocardial fibrosis in a rural area of Mozambique. N Engl J Med 2008;359(1):43-9.
12. Patel AK, Ziegler JL, D'Arbela PG, et al. Familial cases of endomyocardial fibrosis in Uganda. Br Med J 1971;4(5783):331-4.
13. Lowenthal MN. Endomyocardial fibrosis: familial and other cases from northern Zambia. Med J Zambia 1978;12(1):2-7.
14. Davies J, Spry CJ, Vijayaraghavan G, et al. A comparison of the clinical and cardiological features of endomyocardial disease in temperate and tropical regions. Postgrad Med J 1983;59(689):179-85.
15. Freers J, Mayanja-Kizza H, Ziegler JL, et al. Echocardiographic diagnosis of heart disease in Uganda. Trop Doct 1996;26(3):125-8.
16. Cilliers AM, Adams PE, Mocumbi AO. Early presentation of endomyocardial fibrosis in a 22-month-old child: a case report. Cardiol Young 2011;21(1):101-3.
17. Jatene MB, Contreras IS, Lameda LC, et al. Endomyocardial fibrosis in infancy. Arq Bras Cardiol 2003;80(4):438-45.
18. Brockington IF, Edington GM. Adult heart disease in western Nigeria: a clinicopathological synopsis. Am Heart J 1972;83(1):27-40.
19. Vijayaraghavan G, Sivasankaran S. Tropical endomyocardial fibrosis in India: a vanishing disease! Indian J Med Res 2012;136(5):729-38.
20. Akinwusi PO, Odeyemi AO. The changing pattern of endomyocardial fibrosis in South-west Nigeria. Clin Med Insights Cardiol 2012;6:163-8.
21. Kennedy N, Miller P, Adamczick C, et al. Endomyocardial fibrosis: the first report from Malawi. Paediatr Int Child Health 2012;32(2):86-8.
22. Ellis J, Martin R, Wilde P, et al. Echocardiographic, chest X-ray and electrocardiogram findings in children presenting with heart failure to a Ugandan paediatric ward. Trop Doct 2007;37(3):149-50.
23. Grimaldi A, Mocumbi AO, Freers J, et al. Tropical endomyocardial fibrosis: natural history, challenges, and perspectives. Circulation 2016;133(24):2503-15.
24. van der Geld H, Peetoom F, Somers K, et al. Immunohistological and serological studies in endomyocardial fibrosis. Lancet 1966;2(7475):1210-3.
25. Shaper AG, Kaplan MH, Foster WD, et al. Immunological studies in endomyocardial fibrosis and other forms of heart-disease in the tropics. Lancet 1967;1(7490):598-600.
26. Shaper AG. Endomyocardial fibrosis and rheumatic heart-disease. Lancet 1966;1(7438):639-41.
27. Rashwan MA, Ayman M, Ashour S, et al. Endomyocardial fibrosis in Egypt: an illustrated review. Br Heart J 1995;73(3):284-9.
28. Andy JJ. Helminthiasis, the hypereosinophilic syndrome and endomyocardial fibrosis: some observations and an hypothesis. Afr J Med Med Sci 1983;12(3-4):155-64.

29. Martin TN, Weir RA, Dargie HJ. Contrast-enhanced magnetic resonance imaging of endomyocardial fibrosis secondary to Bancroftian filariasis. Heart 2008;94(9):1116.

30. Berenguer A, Plancha E, Munoz Gil J. Right ventricular endomyocardial fibrosis and microfilarial infection. Int J Cardiol 2003;87(2–3):287–9.

31. Carneiro Rde C, Santos AL, Brant LC, et al. Endomyocardial fibrosis associated with mansoni schistosomiasis. Rev Soc Bras Med Trop 2011;44(5):644–5.

32. Jaiyesimi F. Controversies and advances in endomyocardial fibrosis: a review. Afr J Med Med Sci 1982;11(2):37–46.

33. Bukhman G, Ziegler J, Parry E. Endomyocardial fibrosis: still a mystery after 60 years. PLoS Negl Trop Dis 2008;2(2):e97.

34. Freers J, Masembe V, Schmauz R, et al. Endomyocardial fibrosis syndrome in Uganda. Lancet 2000;355(9219):1994–5.

35. Mathai A, Kartha CC, Balakrishnan KG. Serum immunoglobulins in patients with endomyocardial fibrosis. Indian Heart J 1986;38(6):470–2.

36. Brockington IF, Ikeme AC, Bohrer SP. Contributions to the diagnosis of endomyocardial fibrosis. Acta Cardiol 1973;28(3):255–72.

37. Valiathan MS, Kartha CC, Eapen JT, et al. A geochemical basis for endomyocardial fibrosis. Cardiovasc Res 1989;23(7):647–8.

38. Davies H. Endomyocardial fibrosis and the tuberous diet. Int J Cardiol 1990;29(1):3–8.

39. Connor DH, Somers K, Nelson AM, et al. The cause of endomyocardial fibrosis in Uganda. Trop Doct 2012;42(4):206–7.

40. Shaper AG. Plantain diets, serotonin, and endomyocardial fibrosis. Am Heart J 1967;73(3):432–4.

41. Ojo GO, Parratt JR. Urinary excretion of 5-hydroxyindoleacetic acid in nigerians with endomyocardial fibrosis. Lancet 1966;1(7442):854–6.

42. Sezi CL. Effect of protein deficient cassava diet on Cercopithecus aethiops hearts and its possible role in the aetiology and pathogenesis of endomyocardial fibrosis in man. East Afr Med J 1996;73(5 Suppl):S11–6.

43. Mocumbi AO, Falase AO. Recent advances in the epidemiology, diagnosis and treatment of endomyocardial fibrosis in Africa. Heart 2013;99(20):1481–7.

44. Mehrotra AN, Maheshwari HB, Khosla SN, et al. Endomyocardial fibrosis. (A report of two cases in brothers). J Assoc Physicians India 1964;12:845–50.

45. Beaton AMD, Sable CMD, Brown JP, et al. Genetic susceptibility to endomyocardial fibrosis. Glob Cardiol Sci Pract 2014;2014(4):473–81.

46. Parry EH, Abrahams DG. The natural history of endomyocardial fibrosis. Q J Med 1965;34(136):383–408.

47. Hassan WM, Fawzy ME, Al Helaly S, et al. Pitfalls in diagnosis and clinical, echocardiographic, and hemodynamic findings in endomyocardial fibrosis: a 25-year experience. Chest 2005;128(6):3985–92.

48. Andy JJ, Bishara FF, Soyinka OO. Relation of severe eosinophilia and microfilariasis to chronic African endomyocardial fibrosis. Br Heart J 1981;45(6):672–80.

49. Bolarin DM, Andy JJ. Clinical feminization and serum testosterone levels in male patients with chronic African endomyocardial fibrosis. Trop Geogr Med 1982;34(4):309–12.

50. Marijon E, Hausse AO, Ferreira B. Typical clinical aspect of endomyocardial fibrosis. Int J Cardiol 2006;112(2):259–60.

51. Freers J, Mayanja-Kizza H, Rutakingirwa M, et al. Endomyocardial fibrosis: why is there striking ascites with little or no peripheral oedema? Lancet 1996;347(8995):197.

52. Jaiyesimi F, Akinyemi OO, Falase AO. Arterial oxygen desaturation in right ventricular endomyocardial fibrosis (R.V. EMF): a re-evaluation of its pathogenesis. Afr J Med Med Sci 1977;6(4):159–63.

53. Mocumbi AO, Carrilho C, Sarathchandra P, et al. Echocardiography accurately assesses the pathological abnormalities of chronic endomyocardial fibrosis. Int J Cardiovasc Imaging 2011;27(7):955–64.

54. Ball JD, Williams AW, Davies JN. Endomyocardial fibrosis. Lancet 1954;266(6821):1049–54.

55. Frustaci A, Abdulla AK, Possati G, et al. Persisting hypereosinophilia and myocardial activity in the fibrotic stage of endomyocardial disease. Chest 1989;96(3):674–5.

56. Gupta PN, Valiathan MS, Balakrishnan KG, et al. Clinical course of endomyocardial fibrosis. Br Heart J 1989;62(6):450–4.

57. Palmer PES. The imaging of tropical disease: with epidemiology, pathology, and clinical correlation, vol. 2. New York: Springer; 2000.

58. Mocumbi AO, Yacoub S, Yacoub MH. Neglected tropical cardiomyopathies: II. Endomyocardial fibrosis: myocardial disease. Heart 2008;94(3):384–90.

59. Somers K, Brenton DP, Sood NK. Clinical features of endomyocardial fibrosis of the right ventricle. Br Heart J 1968;30(3):309–21.

60. Fernandez Vazquez E, Lacarcel Bautista C, Alcazar Navarrete B, et al. Chronic thromboembolic pulmonary hypertension associated with endomyocardial fibrosis of the right ventricle. Arch Bronconeumol 2003;39(8):370–2 [in Spanish].

61. Ribeiro PA, Muthusamy R, Duran CM. Right-sided endomyocardial fibrosis with recurrent pulmonary emboli leading to irreversible pulmonary hypertension. Br Heart J 1992;68(3):326–9.

62. Andy JJ, Ogunowo PO, Akpan NA, et al. Helminth associated hypereosinophilia and tropical endomyocardial fibrosis (EMF) in Nigeria. Acta Trop 1998;69(2):127–40.

63. Mocumbi AO, Latif N, Yacoub MH. Presence of circulating anti-myosin antibodies in endomyocardial fibrosis. PLoS Negl Trop Dis 2010; 4(4):e661.

64. Jaiyesimi F. Observations on the so-called non-specific electrocardiographic changes in endomyocardial fibrosis. East Afr Med J 1982;59(1): 56–69.

65. Tharakan JA. Electrocardiogram in endomyocardial fibrosis. Indian Pacing Electrophysiol J 2011; 11(5):129–33.

66. Ikeme AC. The diagnosis of endomyocardial fibrosis. Afr J Med Sci 1972;3(4):327–33.

67. Vijayaraghavan G, Davies J, Sadanandan S, et al. Echocardiographic features of tropical endomyocardial disease in South India. Br Heart J 1983; 50(5):450–9.

68. Berensztein CS, Pineiro D, Marcotegui M, et al. Usefulness of echocardiography and doppler echocardiography in endomyocardial fibrosis. J Am Soc Echocardiogr 2000,13(5):385–92.

69. Connor DH, Somers K, Hutt MS, et al. Endomyocardial fibrosis in Uganda (Davies' disease). 1. An epidemiologic, clinical, and pathologic study. Am Heart J 1967;74(5):687–709.

70. Kharwar RB, Sethi R, Narain VS. Right-sided endomyocardial fibrosis with a right atrial thrombus: three-dimensional transthoracic echocardiographic evaluation. Echocardiography 2013; 30(10):E322–5.

71. Mocumbi AO. Role of echocardiography in reserach into neglected cardiovascular diseases in Sub-Saharan Africa. In: Gaze DC, editor. The cardiovascular system – physiology, diagnostics and clinical implications. Rijeka (Croatia): Intech; 2012. p. 445–63.

72. Acquatella H, Puigbo JJ, Suarez C, et al. Sudden early diastolic anterior movement of the septum in endomyocardial fibrosis. Circulation 1979;59(4): 847–8.

73. Marijon E, Jani D, Ou P. Endomyocardial fibrosis: progression to restricted ventricles and giant atria. Can J Cardiol 2006;22(13):1163–4.

74. George BO, Talabi AI, Gaba FE, et al. Echocardiography in the diagnosis of right ventricular endomyocardial fibrosis. Postgrad Med J 1982; 58(682):467–72.

75. Mousseaux E, Hernigou A, Azencot M, et al. Endomyocardial fibrosis: electron-beam CT features. Radiology 1996;198(3):755–60.

76. Qureshi N, Amin F, Chatterjee D, et al. MR imaging of endomyocardial fibrosis (EMF). Int J Cardiol 2011;149(1):e36–7.

77. Genee O, Fichet J, Alison D. Images in cardiovascular medicine: cardiac magnetic resonance imaging and eosinophilic endomyocardial fibrosis. Circulation 2008;118(23):e710–1.

78. Chaosuwannakit N, Makarawate P. Cardiac magnetic resonance imaging for the diagnosis of endomyocardial fibrosis. Southeast Asian J Trop Med Public Health 2014;45(5):1142–8.

79. Leon D, Martin M, Corros C, et al. Usefulness of cardiac MRI in the early diagnosis of endomyocardial fibrosis. Rev Port Cardiol 2012;31(5):401–2.

80. Estornell J, Lopez MP, Dicenta F, et al. Usefulness of magnetic resonance imaging in the assessment of endomyocardial disease. Rev Esp Cardiol 2003; 56(3):321–4 [in Spanish].

81. Salemi VM, Rochitte CE, Shiozaki AA, et al. Late gadolinium enhancement magnetic resonance imaging in the diagnosis and prognosis of endomyocardial fibrosis patients. Circ Cardiovasc Imaging 2011;4(3):304–11.

82. Somers K, Brenton DP, D'Arbela PG, et al. Haemodynamic features of severe endomyocardial fibrosis of right ventricle, including comparison with constrictive pericarditis. Br Heart J 1968; 30(3):322–32.

83. Bohara DA, Ghogare MS, Taksande AR, et al. Predominant RV endomyocardial fibrosis masking rheumatic mitral stenosis. J Assoc Physicians India 2014;62(5):438–41.

84. Sliwa K, Damasceno A, Mayosi BM. Epidemiology and etiology of cardiomyopathy in Africa. Circulation 2005;112(23):3577–83.

85. Buturak A, Saygili O, Ulus S, et al. Right ventricular endomyocardial fibrosis mimicking Ebstein anomaly in a patient with Behcet's disease: case report and review of the literature. Mod Rheumatol 2014; 24(3):532–6.

86. Nabunnya YB, Kayima J, Longenecker CT, et al. The safety and efficacy of prednisolone in preventing reaccumulation of ascites among endomyocardial fibrosis patients in Uganda: a randomized clinical trial. BMC Res Notes 2015;8:783.

87. Mocumbi AO. Endomyocardial fibrosis: a form of endemic restrictive cardiomyopathy. Glob Cardiol Sci Pract 2012;2012(1):11.

88. Ferrario CM, Schiffrin EL. Role of mineralocorticoid receptor antagonists in cardiovascular disease. Circ Res 2015;116(1):206–13.

89. D'Arbela PG, Mutazindwa T, Patel AK, et al. Survival after first presentation with endomyocardial fibrosis. Br Heart J 1972;34(4):403–7.

90. Graham JM, Lawrie GM, Feteih NM, et al. Management of endomyocardial fibrosis: successful surgical treatment of biventricular involvement

and consideration of the superiority of operative intervention. Am Heart J 1981;102(4): 771–82.

91. Schneider U, Jenni R, Turina J, et al. Long-term follow up of patients with endomyocardial fibrosis: effects of surgery. Heart 1998;79(4):362–7.

92. Valiathan MS, Balakrishnan KG, Sankarkumar R, et al. Surgical treatment of endomyocardial fibrosis. Ann Thorac Surg 1987;43(1):68–73.

93. Metras D, Coulibaly AO, Ouattara K. The surgical treatment of endomyocardial fibrosis: results in 55 patients. Circulation 1985;72(3 Pt 2):II274–9.

94. Moraes F, Lapa C, Hazin S, et al. Surgery for endomyocardial fibrosis revisited. Eur J Cardiothorac Surg 1999;15(3):309–12 [discussion: 312–3].

95. Mocumbi AO, Carrilho C, Burke MM, et al. Emergency surgical treatment of advanced endomyocardial fibrosis in Mozambique. Nat Clin Pract Cardiovasc Med 2009;6(3):210–4.

96. Bertrand E, Chauvet J, Assamoi MO, et al. Results, indications and contra-indications of surgery in restrictive endomyocardial fibrosis: comparative study on 31 operated and 30 non-operated patients. East Afr Med J 1985;62(3):151–60.

97. Mocumbi AO, Sidi D, Vouhe P, et al. An innovative technique for the relief of right ventricular trabecular cavity obliteration in endomyocardial fibrosis. J Thorac Cardiovasc Surg 2007;134(4): 1070–2.

98. Yie K, Sung S, Kim D, et al. Bidirectional cavopulmonary shunt as a rescue procedure for right ventricular endomyocardial fibrosis. Interact Cardiovasc Thorac Surg 2004;3(1):86–8.

99. Anbarasu M, Krishna Manohar SR, Titus T, et al. One-and-a-half ventricle repair for right ventricular endomyocardial fibrosis. Asian Cardiovasc Thorac Ann 2004;12(4):363–5.

100. Mishra A, Krishna Manohar SR, Sankar Kumar R, et al. Bidirectional Glenn shunt for right ventricular endomyocardial fibrosis. Asian Cardiovasc Thorac Ann 2002;10(4):351–3.

101. Moraes CR, Buffolo E, Moraes Neto F, et al. Recurrence of fibrosis after endomyocardial fibrosis surgery. Arq Bras Cardiol 1996;67(4):297–9 [in Portuguese].

102. Tang A, Karski J, Butany J, et al. Severe mitral regurgitation in acute eosinophilic endomyocarditis: repair or replacement? Interact Cardiovasc Thorac Surg 2004;3(2):406–8.

103. Salemi VM, Leite JJ, Picard MH, et al. Echocardiographic predictors of functional capacity in endomyocardial fibrosis patients. Eur J Echocardiogr 2009;10(3):400–5.

Innovative Approaches to Hypertension Control in Low- and Middle-Income Countries

Rajesh Vedanthan, MD, MPH[a],*, Antonio Bernabe-Ortiz, MD, MPH[b],
Omarys I. Herasme, MPH[a], Rohina Joshi, MBBS, PhD, MPH[c],
Patricio Lopez-Jaramillo, MD, PhD[d], Amanda G. Thrift, PhD[e],
Jacqui Webster, PhD[c], Ruth Webster, PhD, MIPH[c], Karen Yeates, MD, MPH[f],
Joyce Gyamfi, MS[g], Merina Ieremia, PGDHS[h], Claire Johnson, MIPH[c],
Jemima H. Kamano, MBChB, MMed[i], Maria Lazo-Porras, MD[b],
Felix Limbani, MPH[j], Peter Liu, MD[k], Tara McCready, PhD, MBA[l],
J. Jaime Miranda, MD, MSc, PhD[b], Sailesh Mohan, MD, MPH, PhD[m],
Olugbenga Ogedegbe, MD, MS, MPH[g], Brian Oldenburg, PhD, MPsych[n],
Bruce Ovbiagele, MD, MSc[o], Mayowa Owolabi, MBBS, MSc, DrM[p],
David Peiris, MBBS, PhD, MIPH[c], Vilarmina Ponce-Lucero, BA[b],
Devarsetty Praveen, MBBS, MD, PhD[q], Arti Pillay, PGDPH[r],
Jon-David Schwalm, MD, MSc[l], Sheldon W. Tobe, MD, MScCH[s],
Kathy Trieu, MPH[c], Khalid Yusoff, MBBS[t], Valentin Fuster, MD, PhD[a]

Disclosure Statement: The authors have nothing to disclose.
Funded by: NIH Grant number(s): U01 HL114180; U01 HL114200; U01 NS079179. Canadian Institutes of Health Research Grant number(s): 120389. Grand Challenges Canada Grant number(s): 0069-04; 0070-04. International Development Research Center Grant number(s): 120389. Australian National Health and Medical Research Council Grant number(s): 1040147; 1041052; 1040179; 1040030; 104018. United Kingdom Medical Research Council Grant number(s): APP 1040179; APP 1041052; J01 60201. Malaysian Ministry of Higher Education Grant number(s): 600-RMI/LRGS/5/3.
Authors' Contributions: All authors were involved in the initial draft of this article, made continual input as the drafts progressed, and approved the final draft for submission. The content within is solely the responsibility of the authors and does not necessarily represent the official views of the Global Alliance for Chronic Diseases funding agencies or affiliates.

[a] Zena and Michael A. Wiener Cardiovascular Institute, Icahn School of Medicine at Mount Sinai, One Gustave L. Levy Place, New York, NY 10029, USA; [b] CRONICAS Center of Excellence in Chronic Diseases, Universidad Peruana Cayetano Heredia, Av. Armendariz 497, Lima 18, Peru; [c] The George Institute for Global Health, University of Sydney, 50 Bridge Street, Sydney, NSW 2000, Australia; [d] Research Institute FOSCAL, Bucaramanga, Colombia; [e] School of Clinical Sciences at Monash Health, Monash University, Wellington Road and Blackburn Road, Clayton, VIC 3800, Australia; [f] School of Medicine, Queens University, 15 Arch Street, Kingston, ON K7L 3N6, Canada; [g] School of Medicine, New York University, 550 1st Avenue, New York, NY 10016, USA; [h] Samoan Ministry of Health, Motootua, Ifiifi street, Apia, Samoa; [i] College of Health Sciences, School of Medicine, Moi University, PO Box 3900, Eldoret 30100, Kenya; [j] Centre for Health Policy, School of Public Health, University of the Witwatersrand, 1 Jan Smuts Avenue, Braamfontein, Johannesburg 2000, South Africa; [k] University of Ottawa, 75 Laurier Avenue East, Ottawa, ON K1N 6N5, Canada; [l] Population Health Research Institute, 237 Barton Street East, Hamilton, ON L8L 2X2, Canada; [m] Public Health Foundation of India, Plot No. 47, Sector 44, New Delhi, India; [n] School of Population and Global Health, University of Melbourne, Parkville, VC 3010, Australia; [o] Medical University of South Carolina, 171 Ashley Avenue, Charleston, SC 29425, USA; [p] University of Ibadan, Ibadan, Nigeria; [q] The George Institute for Global Health, 301 ANR Centre, Road No 1, Banjara Hills, Hyderabad 500034, India; [r] Pacific Research Centre for the Prevention of Obesity and Non-Communicable Diseases, Fiji National University, Suva, Fiji; [s] University of Toronto, 27 King's College Circle, Toronto, ON M5S 1A1, Canada; [t] Universiti Teknologi MARA, Selangor and UCSI University, Kuala Lumpur, Malaysia
* Corresponding author. Icahn School of Medicine at Mount Sinai, One Gustave L. Levy Place, Box 1030, New York, NY 10029.
E-mail address: rajesh.vedanthan@mssm.edu

cardiology.theclinics.com

KEYWORDS

- Hypertension • Low- and middle-income countries • Community engagement • mHealth
- Task redistribution • Salt reduction • Salt substitution • Polypill

KEY POINTS

- Elevated blood pressure is a major risk factor for cardiovascular disease, and it is the leading global risk for mortality.
- There is a need for novel approaches when addressing hypertension owing to its growing health and economic burden on populations in low- and middle-income countries.
- The Global Alliance for Chronic Diseases sponsored 15 research projects focused on hypertension.
- These research projects have involved the development and evaluation of several important innovative approaches to hypertension control.
- Strategies include community engagement, salt reduction, salt substitution, task redistribution, mHealth, and fixed-dose combination therapies.

INTRODUCTION

Cardiovascular disease (CVD) is the leading cause of mortality in the world, resulting in 17.3 million deaths annually, with 80% of these deaths occurring in low- and middle-income countries (LMICs).[1] Elevated blood pressure, a major risk factor for ischemic heart disease, heart failure, and stroke,[2] is the leading global risk for mortality.[1] Despite global efforts to combat hypertension, treatment and control rates are very low in LMICs.[3] Given the continued significant health and economic burden on LMIC populations, there is an urgent need to address the problem by way of novel approaches.

Founded in 2009, the Global Alliance for Chronic Diseases (GACD), funds, coordinates, and facilitates global collaborations in implementation research, focusing on the prevention and treatment of chronic noncommunicable diseases in LMICs and vulnerable populations in high-income countries.[4] The first round of GACD-sponsored research projects focused on hypertension, and included 15 research teams from around the world.[5] These research projects have involved the development and evaluation of several important innovative approaches to hypertension control, including community engagement, salt reduction, salt substitution, task redistribution, mHealth, and fixed-dose combination therapies.

In this paper, we briefly review the rationale for each of these innovative approaches, as well as summarize the experience of some of the GACD teams in these respective areas. Where relevant, we also draw on the wider literature to illustrate how these approaches to hypertension control are being implemented in LMICs.

COMMUNITY ENGAGEMENT

Health care delivery and health systems often fail to meet the needs and expectations of those who need them.[6,7] Community engagement seeks to address this problem by optimizing the appropriateness and alignment of health care to the cultural, social, economic, and environmental setting.[8,9] It encompasses participation, mobilization, and empowerment (**Fig. 1**).[10] Participation refers to the active or passive engagement of the community in health services.[10,11] Mobilization furthers this engagement through facilitation by health professionals, and empowerment involves a capacity-building process to engage communities in planning, implementing, and/or evaluating activities to achieve more sustainable health improvements.[10,11] Community engagement has shown promise in supporting interventions to improve health outcomes related to both human immunodeficiency virus infection and AIDS, as well as maternal and child health.[12,13] However, traditional methods for determining efficacy of community engagement are inadequate because there are significant challenges in teasing out the independent effects of the intervention regarding the process of community engagement itself.

Four GACD projects described herein have been conducted in Tanzania, Kenya, Colombia, Malaysia, India, and Canada. The investigators of these GACD projects have adopted a diverse range of community engagement activities, targeted at both individuals and systems, to identify

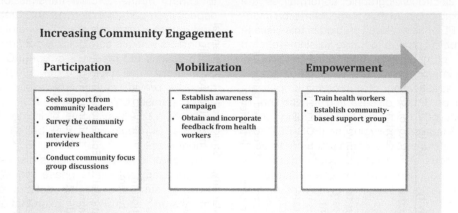

Fig. 1. Community engagement activities undertaken within Global Alliance for Chronic Diseases projects. Participation activities denote the least level of engagement while empowerment activities denote the greatest level of engagement.

barriers and facilitators for the care of hypertension, and thereby tailor the intervention to the local context (**Table 1**). Before initiating each of these studies, investigators and research staff met with community leaders, health personnel, and other relevant community stakeholders, to facilitate entry to the communities and to appropriately contextualize their approaches. Components of community engagement included (1) individual interviews with diverse stakeholders, (2) focus group discussions with hypertension patients, (3) workshops with local community health workers (CHWs) and clinicians to refine the intervention and training materials, thus enhancing the capacity of CHWs to deliver the intervention by implementing relevant and easy-to-use tools, (4) community social events and gatherings, and (5) mabaraza (singular baraza), traditional East African community gatherings, conducted among individuals with elevated blood pressure and CHWs to complement the purposive sampling inherent in focus group discussions.[14] The baraza is a unique and novel qualitative research setting that has been used as a form of participatory action research, and allows organization of a diverse and heterogeneous large group of individuals.[15] In Tanzania and Canada, the team used an adapted tool called I-RREACH (Intervention and Research Readiness Engagement and Assessment of Community Health Care).[16] This tool was developed using a community-based consensus method, and is rooted in participatory principles, equalizing the importance of the knowledge and perspectives of researchers and community stakeholders while encouraging respectful dialogue. The I-RREACH tool is an engagement and assessment tool for improving the implementation

readiness of researchers, organizations, and communities in complex interventions, and consists of 3 phases: fact finding, stakeholder dialogue, and community member/patient dialogue. Another study being conducted in Canada, Malaysia, and Colombia leveraged nonmedical community events for the purposes of screening, recruitment, intervention implementation, and follow-up. Using process evaluation, the GACD projects hope to add to our understanding of how community engagement can be used to support and strengthen programs aimed at improving hypertension control. Such an approach can be applied to more chronic diseases in low-resource settings worldwide.

The need for this research is illustrated by work elsewhere. Although it may seem self-evident that a more participatory approach will improve the acceptability, and thus the effectiveness of interventions, this is not fully supported by the evidence. Two projects conducted in Cape Town, South Africa, and El Paso, Texas, used community-based participatory research approaches to design an intervention to manage hypertension and diabetes.[17,18] Positive results included (1) improved self-efficacy to manage hypertension, (2) greater improvements in health behaviors in the intervention group than in the control group,[18] (3) the development of culturally appropriate health education materials specifically developed for low-literacy populations,[18] and (4) inclusion of learnings into local health sector planning for prevention and control of hypertension and diabetes.[17] Although the authors stated that the materials were well-received by participants in 1 study,[18] no evidence for clinical success of community engagement was provided in either study.[17,18]

Table 1
Type and target group of community engagement activities undertaken within Global Alliance for Chronic Diseases projects, including timing of engagement and materials developed through each activity

Region	Type	Target Group	Timing of Engagement	Rationale for Activity	Materials Developed
India	Community entry	Community leaders	Before the initiation of study activities within each cluster/community unit	To gain entry into the community	Protocol, specific aims, abstract
	Survey of community members	Individuals	Once at study initiation length: 60–90 min	To identify barriers to seeking health care and/or treatment	Survey
	Community focus group discussions	Individuals with hypertension	Up to 12 focus groups, each composed of up to 10 people; 60–90 min long	To identify barriers to seeking health care and/or treatment	Structured guide for discussions
	In-depth interviews	Health care providers	23 interviews with doctors, nurses, and CHWs	To identify barriers to providing health care and/or treatment	Structured guide for interviews
	Survey of medicines	Public, private, and other medicine outlets	20 public outlets, 16 private outlets, 2 other outlets selling medicines at subsidized rates to all patients	To determine availability, affordability, and acceptability of medications	Structured list of essential medicines for audit
	Consultation via a planning day	Local and state government health officials, and local experts	Once at a 4-h planning session	To ensure that the design of the intervention fit into the health system	Final design of intervention
	Working group testing of intervention materials	CHWs and local doctors	Over 5 d, CHWs and doctors participated in a pilot training program	To develop educational materials for training CHWs and to educate people with hypertension	Educational materials for training CHWs and for people with hypertension
	Training	CHWs	5 full days of training delivered by doctors and researchers	To provide skills to CHWs to enable them to conduct a peer support group and educate people with hypertension	Education materials for CHWs

Community-based support group of people with hypertension	Letter of support and encouragement from head of village (Sarpanch)	3-mo intervention composed of 6 fortnightly education sessions delivered by CHWs, locally sourced expert advisers, health care providers, and researchers	Self-management and education support group of people with hypertension	Education materials for people with hypertension, including handouts
Dissemination of study results	Communities, local health providers, medicines outlets, Ministry of Health and Welfare, National health Mission	At end of study	To build capacity and sustainability	Development of resources for use by heath care providers for assessing and treating hypertension
Kenya				
Community entry	Community leaders, health personnel, community stakeholders	Before the initiation of study activities within each cluster/community unit	To gain entry into the community	Protocol, specific aims, abstract, and PowerPoint summary
Community gatherings (Mabaraza)	Community	Six in total (until content saturation achieved); 1–2 h long	To identify the barriers and facilitators to linkage to care for hypertension and retention to care	Structured discussion guides for Mabaraza
Focus group discussions	Individuals with hypertension and CHWs	17 total (until content saturation achieved); 1–2 h long	To identify barriers to seeking and delivering health care and/or treatment	Moderator guides
Human-centered design	Design team with diverse stakeholders; content validity testing with diverse stakeholders	Occurrence: Approximately 10 design team meetings; 9 content validity focus group discussions with patients, CHWs, and clinicians; 60 min long	Design of behavioral assessment and tailored communication strategy	Final design of intervention

(continued on next page)

Table 1
(continued)

Region	Type	Target Group	Timing of Engagement	Rationale for Activity	Materials Developed
Tanzania and Canada	Community entry	Community leaders/ stakeholders	Before the initiation of study activities within each of the 2 selected communities	To gain entry into the community and gauge interest	Framework for development of the I-RREACH Tool
	Completion of 3 'consensus' cycles	Stakeholders and community-based researchers in Canada and Tanzania	At project initiation moving forward over a 1-y period in 3 cycles	To test theoretical frameworks regarding researcher's practice-based knowledge, community readiness; Indigenous approaches to research, empowerment approaches	Development of the I-RREACH Tool[16]
	Community focus group discussions	Individuals with hypertension and their families as well as local health care providers	3 focus groups were held in participating Indigenous communities in Canada and 1 in Tanzania of varying length with a total of 45 participants	To identify major factors that may impact on the effectiveness of evidence-based educational short message service (SMS) messages for people with hypertension and reduce health inequalities	Content from focus groups informed the development of the SMS messages to be used for the intervention in each country
	Training	CHWs and local health providers	In the second year, CHWs and doctors participated in country specific training programs on hypertension and cardiovascular disease as well as use of the mHealth tools/ equipment. In Tanzania there was also a pre–post evaluation of knowledge gained and an observed standardized clinical examination	To prepare CHWs and health providers to provide educational support to their communities (people with hypertension and their families)	Educational materials for training CHWs and health providers

Training	Local health providers (Tanzania only)	5 full days of training delivered by doctors and researchers in year 3 to evaluate the appropriateness of the treatment algorithm for management of hypertension (adapted from the existing Tanzanian hypertension guideline)	To provide skills to health providers to enable them to manage hypertension effectively	Treatment algorithm for hypertension that is specific to low-resource rural setting in sub-Saharan Africa
Dissemination of study results	Communities, local health providers, medicines outlets, Ministry of Health and Social Welfare, National health Mission	Will occur at end of study	To build capacity and sustainability	Dissemination of resources for use by heath care providers for assessing and treating hypertension
Colombia, Malaysia, & Canada				
Community social events or other nonclinical gatherings	NPHW attend the community events	NPHW attend events opportunistically with the permission of event organizers	Posters explaining the NPHW attendance; curated collections of local government brochures regarding cardiovascular health and other available health services; personalized healthy lifestyle counseling based on WHO recommendations (intervention only).	

Abbreviations: CHW, community health worker; I-RREACH, Intervention and Research Readiness Engagement and Assessment of Community Health Care; NPHW, nonphysician health workers; WHO, World Health Organization.

SALT REDUCTION

Evidence shows that a reduction in the consumption of sodium—found in table salt and naturally occurring foods such as milk, eggs, meat, and shellfish—decreases blood pressure in adults and diminishes the risk of CVD.[19,20] Although there is controversy about the most appropriate target for sodium intake, higher sodium intake in general is associated with poorer outcomes.[21] The World Health Organization (WHO) recommends a reduction in sodium intake to less than 2 g/d in adults.[22] In 2013, member states of the United Nations established a target to reduce the average population salt intake by 30% by 2025,[23] and 75 countries now have strategies in place to achieve this target.[24] The majority of these national programs are multifaceted and include initiatives such as industry engagement to lower salt content in foods, consumer education and awareness, and establishing front-of-pack labeling schemes and nutrition standards for foods procured in public settings.

Three of the GACD hypertension programs have implemented innovative salt reduction programs to reduce blood pressure. The first step in any program is to measure existing consumption patterns. These projects measured salt intake using 24-h urine excretion and tried to understand people's knowledge and eating behaviors through community surveys. Average daily salt excretion at baseline varied from 7 g in Samoa,[25] 11 g in Fiji, 9.5 in Andhra Pradesh, India, and 8.6 g in Delhi/Haryana, India, to 12.6 g in Shanxi, China. The information on diet was then used to inform the different intervention strategies. Based on the WHO's framework for Creating an Enabling Environment for Salt reduction,[26] the project in Fiji and Samoa used multifaceted intervention programs to reduce salt in the food supply, while concurrently implementing media and community mobilization campaigns to increase awareness (**Fig. 2**).[27] A parallel project in Andhra Pradesh and Delhi/Haryana, India, used community surveys and stakeholder mapping and established a comprehensive food composition database (based on the George Institute's leading Food-Switch innovation for monitoring the food supply and identifying healthy choices).[28] This information is being used to inform the development of a government-led salt reduction strategy for India. The Little Emperor project in China trained children to encourage their parents to reduce salt intake. Implemented in the northern province of Shanxi, the researchers taught the children about the harmful effects of a salty diet and asked them

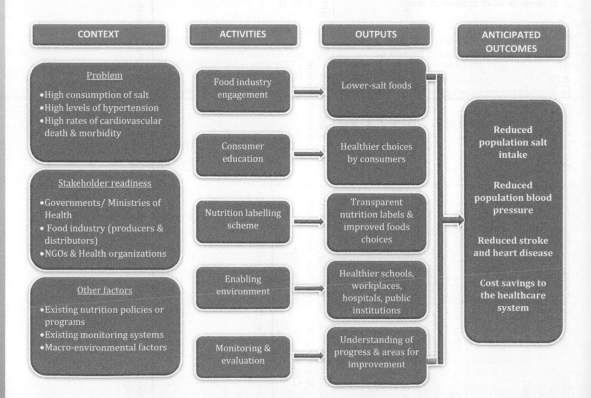

Fig. 2. Framework for salt reduction strategies, including context, activities, outputs, and anticipated outcomes.

to share the messages with adults back home. Innovative children's approaches including hiding the salt pot and making up rhymes or using their status as "Little Emperors" to refuse to eat unhealthy foods led to a 26% reduction in participants' salt intake in less than 4 months.[29] More than 270 million people currently have hypertension in China; therefore, if applied nationally, such a strategy could have substantial health and potential economic benefits.

Postintervention monitoring in Fiji and Samoa is being finalized and has been supplemented through an in-depth process evaluation to better understand how the interventions have been implemented and potential barriers to effectiveness. Some of the challenges have included the changing political environment, difficulties of multisectoral action and limited experience in engaging the food industry. Mainstreaming the agendas with the Health Ministries in the different countries has been key to overcoming some of these problems. The lessons are being documented and will be disseminated widely through the WHO Collaborating Centre for Population Salt Reduction at the George Institute for Global Health, thus supporting rapid and effective translation of research into policy and practice. These and other studies will help to elucidate and clarify the relationship between sodium reduction and CVD.

Salt Substitution

In addition to salt reduction, salt substitution is an innovative, nonpharmacologic approach to reduce blood pressure. It involves the partial replacement of sodium chloride with any combination of other salt containing potassium, magnesium, or aluminum. A meta-analysis from 6 randomized, controlled trials using different combinations of salt substitute in comparison to usual salt found, in pooled results, that a salt substitute reduced systolic blood pressure by −4.9 mm Hg (95% confidence interval, -7.3 to -2.5) and diastolic blood pressure −1.5 mm Hg (95% confidence interval, -2.7 to -0.3). However, in the subgroup analysis, the effect was significant only among individuals with hypertension.[30]

One of the GACD projects conducted in Peru[31] is using a population-wide approach to test the effect on blood pressure of replacing regular salt by an iodine-fortified substitute containing 25% potassium chloride and 75% sodium chloride. This involves a pragmatic stepped wedge trial design, in which the intervention is progressively implemented at random in 6 villages. The study has been implemented in 2 phases (**Fig. 3**). The first phase was exploratory and included (a) formative in-depth interviews and focus group discussions, (b) a triangle taste test, which found that a salt with 25% of potassium chloride was indistinguishable from regular salt,[32] and (c) the development of a social marketing campaign targeting primarily women responsible for cooking at their home, and focused on promoting consumption and adherence of participants to the potassium-enriched salt. The second phase involved implementation of the intervention. The salt substitute has progressively replaced the common salt used in households, relying heavily on the social marketing/branding campaign as well as educational entertainment delivered by trained CHWs. Salt replacement has been implemented at households, bakeries, community kitchens, and restaurants in each village.

Previous salt substitute strategies have focused on delivering the salt substitute product among participants with a diagnosis of hypertension, focusing almost exclusively on the hypertension status of the participant rather than on the product's concept. For instance, the salt substitute used in other studies were no different between intervention and control arms (ie, bags were identical in appearance; products were manufactured, packaged, and labeled by the same company).[33–35] The novelty of the Peru study relies on the implementation mechanisms that were developed and put in place, at the community level, aiming to increase the uptake of the salt substitute product as well as ensuring its sustained used over time in populations, irrespective of hypertension status. To date, acceptability of the salt substitute to participants has been successful with very low rates of adverse effects related to its use. The study is ongoing and the fourth wedge has been concluded, with expected outcomes in early 2017. If successful, this project's implementation approach may serve as a model for other LMIC settings.

TASK REDISTRIBUTION

In most countries, primary care physicians are the main providers of health care for individuals with CVD. Unfortunately, most LMICs have an inadequate number of physicians, especially in rural and remote regions where a majority of the population reside.[36,37] According to the WHO Global Health Observatory, there are 0.3 physicians available for every 1000 population in low-income countries, 1.2 physicians per 1000 population in lower-middle income countries, and 2.0 per 1000 population in upper-middle income countries.[38] In response to this physician workforce shortage,

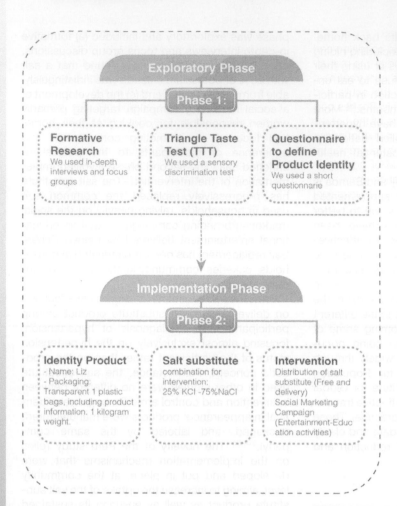

Fig. 3. Launching a salt substitute to reduce blood pressure at the population level in Peru, divided into 2 phases.

appropriate strategies for task redistribution—from doctors to a team consisting of doctors and trained nonphysician health workers (NPHWs)—have been developed and implemented, especially in the areas of maternal and child health needs[39,40] and human immunodeficiency virus infection and AIDS.[41]

Task redistribution describes a situation where a task normally performed by a physician is shared between physicians and other health workers with a different or lower level of education and training (**Fig. 4**).[42] Task redistribution may be aided by technology, clear guidelines, or close supervision by physicians, to help standardize the performance and interpretation of certain tasks, therefore allowing them to be performed by NPHWs.[43] Systematic reviews on task redistribution for CVD management[44,45] indicate that not many studies have been conducted to test the effectiveness of task redistribution, and that further operational research, including detailed

process evaluation, is required to understand the complexity, effectiveness, and cost-effectiveness of task redistribution within different country contexts. Recent studies involving task redistribution have shown that NPHWs can be trained effectively in the implementation of CVD prevention and management guidelines,[46,47] successfully screen individuals at high risk of CVD,[48,49] provide lifestyle education and adherence support to patients,[50] and support patients with acute coronary syndrome.[51] This approach has also been shown to be cost effective for chronic disease care in the LMIC context.[52,53] Although there are now some published studies concerning the effectiveness of task redistribution, there remain large evidence gaps and obstacles regarding the translation of positive research findings into routine health care delivery in LMICs, while also ensuring quality of care, safety, and patient acceptability. These shortcomings notwithstanding, task redistribution for the prevention and control of hypertension

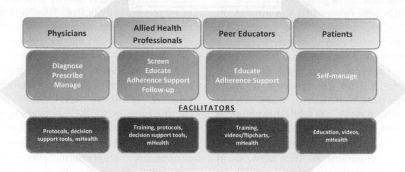

Physicians	Allied Health Professionals	Peer Educators	Patients
Diagnose Prescribe Manage	Screen Educate Adherence Support Follow-up	Educate Adherence Support	Self-manage

FACILITATORS

| Protocols, decision support tools, mHealth | Training, protocols, decision support tools, mHealth | Training, videos/flipcharts, mHealth | Education, videos, mHealth |

Fig. 4. The process of task redistribution for the management of hypertension adapted from the World Health Organization's recommendations on task shifting. (*Adapted from* World Health Organization, PEPFAR, UNAIDS. Task shifting: rational redistribution of tasks among health workforce teams: global recommendations and guidelines. 2016. Available at: http://www.who.int/healthsystems/TTR-TaskShifting.pdf. Accessed September 26, 2016.)

and other chronic diseases presents a great opportunity that could increase access to care, reduce health care costs, free up physician time for other tasks, and increase system efficiency in the long term.

Eight of the GACD projects included a component of task redistribution for the detection and management of hypertension. These include the redistribution of tasks related to hypertension screening, referral to clinicians, providing lifestyle advice, and support for adherence to medications to NPHWs. All the studies supported NPHWs by training them for 2 to 6 days, followed by retraining where required.[14,54,55] Some studies facilitated task redistribution by using mHealth technology,[14,56] whereby NPHWs used electronic decision support tools to screen individuals in the community and link them to hypertension care. Process and interim evaluations have identified that the main barriers to task redistribution include resistance from other health professionals; increasing NPHW workload owing to additional tasks; complexity of training materials; health system-related issues such as nonavailability or nonfunctioning blood pressure machines, poor drug supply, and lack of physician availability for referral; regulatory restrictions, including the inability to prescribe medications; and low remuneration of NPHWs.[57] The key enablers included an increase in the enthusiasm and motivation of NPHWs to be trained and take on new roles, as well as a reduction in the physician workload leading to improved performance. All of these studies are currently in progress and will have effectiveness and cost-effectiveness results in the near future.

mHEALTH

mHealth is the use of mobile phones to improve and support health, and can be used for a variety of purposes to connect clinicians, other health workers including CHWs, and patients or patient caregivers (**Fig. 5**). mHealth can be used to provide health education, promote behavior change, facilitate decision support in diagnosis and management of a wide variety of conditions, support diagnostic testing, or link medical records.[58] Evidence for benefits of mHealth is widespread

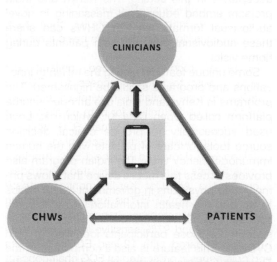

Fig. 5. Schematic illustrating the potential for mHealth to connect clinicians, community health workers, and patients. Blue arrows indicate direct interactions among individuals. Red arrows indicate interactions that are facilitated by mHealth.

among a variety of high-income country settings, and further data are emerging on the use of mHealth in LMICs with respect to the impact on clinical outcomes, processes of care, health care costs, and health-related quality of life.[59–61] There is great potential for the use of mHealth for hypertension management in LMICs, because mobile phone ownership is high and growing rapidly, even among the poor.[62] However, there remain research gaps with a relatively limited number of studies in this area, particularly in hypertension.

Five projects within the GACD research network have a mHealth component at their core, or in conjunction with other innovations, to address barriers within health systems and to optimize opportunities for the detection and management of hypertension. The projects are taking place in communities in rural Kenya,[14] rural Tanzania, both urban and rural Colombia and Malaysia, rural and remote Aboriginal communities in Canada, Nigeria,[63] and rural India. All of the projects are using either a smartphone- or tablet-based tool designed for use by CHWs to improve hypertension care; facilitate improved identification, follow-up, and tracking of patients; promote adherence to medications; and improve education of patients and CHWs. All of the programs have a component of real-time decision support. In addition, the Nigerian and Tanzanian/Canada programs also send educational, behavior change communication messages via text message directly to patients' mobile phones, whereas the India project uses interactive voice response messaging because text messaging was not acceptable in this setting. The Kenya and India projects embed educational messaging in novel audiovisual formats, so that CHWs can share these audiovisual materials with patients during home visits.

Some unique features among the mHealth innovations and programs should be highlighted. The programs in Kenya and India use an open-source platform called Open Data Kit, which has been used successfully to provide clinical decision source tools for care of patients with the human immunodeficiency virus. The Indian program also provides access to a mobile device that allows primary care physicians in government health clinics to access the health information of participants screened by CHWs; the device offers decision support for those participants identified at high CVD risk. This feature is also a component of the Tanzania-Canada program, whereby health center nurses and clinical officers can access all blood pressure measurements taken for a patient by CHWs. A substudy of the Tanzania project is also evaluating the effectiveness of a phone-based drug voucher program to ensure the authenticity of drug supply and adherence factors in hypertension control. The Nigerian program is targeting patients who have experienced a stroke and who are at high risk for another stroke. Across the programs there have been common challenges, which include both technical and human factors. Technical factors have included mobile network coverage and server issues. Human factors have included overcoming end-user challenges with the new technology, as well as implementation delays owing to government approval processes, equipment procurement delays, misalignment of incentives, competing obligations, and excessive workload for the health providers who are using these new systems.

POLYPILL: FIXED-DOSE COMBINATION THERAPY

Most patients with hypertension generally require blood pressure–lowering medication from multiple classes to achieve adequate control.[64] The need for titration of medication and addition of multiple classes of drug requires multiple physician visits and this in itself can lead to poor adherence to prescribed medication and poor attendance at scheduled visits.[65] The requirement to take multiple medications in complex regimes also encourages poor adherence.[66] For physicians, the need for repeated uptitrating or adding extra medications can lead to inertia and tacit acceptance of inadequate blood pressure control.[67,68] Initiating antihypertensive treatment with dual combination therapy not only accelerates the time taken to achieve control, but also attains a lower final target.[69,70] For the patient, improved adherence has also been demonstrated without worsening the side effect profile.[71] Further benefits in blood pressure control can also result from simplifying uptitration regimes.[70]

Use of multimodal fixed-dose combination pills (FDCs)—also known as 'polypills'—containing not only multiple low-dose blood pressure-lowering drugs, but also statins and aspirin, has the potential to reduce a person's cardiovascular risk beyond that achieved by simply lowering their blood pressure, by addressing multiple risk factors concurrently in a single pill. Multiple large clinical trials have shown that use of 'polypills' in patients at high risk of CVD improves adherence to long-term medication with consequent improvements in cholesterol and blood pressure measurements, and are highly acceptable to patients and physicians alike (**Fig. 6**).[72,73] The recently published HOPE-3 (Heart Outcomes Prevention Evaluation 3) study used a polypill type strategy in patients

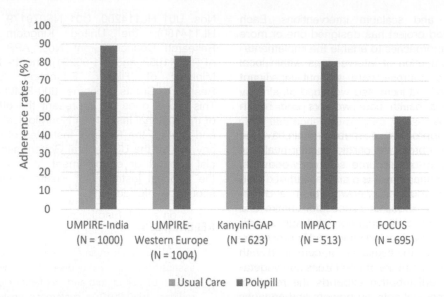

Fig. 6. Proportion of participants adherent to combination therapy at end of study in patients either with established cardiovascular disease or at high calculated risk. Adherence is defined as taking antiplatelet, statin and 2 or more blood pressure-lowering drugs at least 4 days of the last 7 at end of study in UMPIRE,[77] Kanyini-GAP,[78] and IMPACT.[79] Adherence in the FOCUS[73] trial was defined as pill count between 80% and 110% at end of study plus a score of 20/20 on the Morisky-Green questionnaire. (*Data from Refs.*[73,77-79])

at moderate CVD risk and showed a significant reduction in cardiovascular events in patients with hypertension.[74] Although reducing blood pressure was a benefit only in those in the hypertensive range, lowering cholesterol had beneficial effects in reducing fatal and nonfatal cardiovascular events overall.[75] Evidence is needed, however, on the implementation of such a strategy in real-life clinical contexts rather within the constraints of a highly regulated clinical trial.

The GACD has funded 2 projects looking at whether use of FDCs will improve management of hypertension, and also overall CVD risk, in real-life clinical contexts in several LMICs. The TRIUMPH (*TRI*ple Pill versus *U*sual care *M*anagement for *P*atients with mild-to- moderate *H*ypertension) study,[76] is a prospective, open, randomized controlled clinical trial (n = 700) of a fixed dose combination blood pressure-lowering pill ("Triple Pill")-based strategy compared with usual care among individuals with persistent mild-to-moderate hypertension on no or minimal drug therapy. The aim is to see whether early use of low-dose FDC medications will result in faster and better control of blood pressure. The HOPE-4 study, being conducted in 50 urban and rural communities in Canada, Colombia, and Malaysia is implementing and evaluating (compared with usual care) an evidence-based, contextually appropriate program for CVD risk assessment, treatment, and control involving

simplified algorithms implemented by NPHWs, supported by e-health technologies, initiation of FDC of 2 antihypertensive drugs plus 1 statin, and use of treatment supporters to optimize long-term medication and lifestyle adherence. Both studies are ongoing with outcomes anticipated in the near future.

The use of a simplified strategy using early introduction of inexpensive generic FDC pills (or 'polypills') is an approach with important potential to impact on what are currently exceedingly poor blood pressure control rates in LMICs. If found to be effective, cost-effective, and acceptable, this approach has the potential to impact the cardiovascular health of significant numbers of individuals around the world.

SUMMARY

Elevated blood pressure is the leading global risk for mortality,[1] and novel approaches for improving hypertension control are urgently required for LMICs. The GACD hypertension studies described here are beginning to disseminate outcomes, results, and lessons in relation to several different innovative approaches. In addition, they are well-poised to develop poststudy knowledge translation strategies. Finally, the GACD researchers have the potential to engage policy makers, payers, and other stakeholders, to translate the findings of individual research studies into sustainable and scalable interventions. Each GACD-funded project has designed one or more innovative approaches to enable the implementation and evaluation of interventions within local contexts, to improve care without significant disruption to, and increased workload of, already overburdened health care workers and health care systems.

All of the approaches described herein have the potential to improve the cardiovascular health of populations in low-resource settings worldwide. Community engagement is a critical part of developing and introducing any new program, and it increases the likelihood of successful uptake and implementation. Salt reduction and salt substitutes can reduce blood pressure and improve cardiovascular health, especially if combined with improved dietary intake of fresh fruits and vegetables. Task redistribution expands the reach of delegated medical acts, empowers and engages community members, improves the health literacy of communities, and improves the efficiency of the existing pool of health care providers. mHealth can additionally provide decision support, remote medical record access, and novel educational interfaces, all of which can enhance care delivery in resource-limited settings. Finally, FDC pills have the potential to transform the landscape of medical management of hypertension and CVD. The studies outlined in this report demonstrate innovative and practical methods of implementing all of these strategies for hypertension control in diverse environments and contexts worldwide.

ACKNOWLEDGMENTS

The writing group thanks Gary Parker from the GACD Secretariat for invaluable logistical and administrative support, and Drs Clara Chow, Pallab Maulik, and Martin McKee for critical review of the article. They also thank all members of the GACD Hypertension Research Program for their support and input throughout the preparation of this article. Funding for the studies described and for article submission was provided by the following GACD Hypertension Program funding agencies: Canadian Institutes of Health Research (Grant No. 120389); Grand Challenges Canada (Grant Nos. 0069-04, and 0070-04); International Development Research Centre; Canadian Stroke Network; Australian National Health and Medical Research Council (Grant Nos. ID 1040147, 1040030, 1041052, 104179, and 104018); the US National Institutes of Health (National Heart, Lung and Blood Institute and National Institute of Neurological Disorders and Stroke) (Grant Nos. U01 HL114200, U01 NS079179, and U01 HL114180); the United Kingdom Medical Research Council (Grant Nos. APP 1040179, APP 1041052, and J01 60201); and the Malaysian Ministry of Higher Education (Long-term Research Grants Scheme 600-RMI/LRGS/5/3). This report does not represent the official view of the National Institute of Neurological Disorders and Stroke, the National Institutes of Health, or any part of the US Federal Government. No official support or endorsement of this article by the National Institutes of Health is intended or should be inferred.

REFERENCES

1. Lim SS, Vos T, Flaxman AD, et al. A comparative risk assessment of burden of disease and injury attributable to 67 risk factors and risk factor clusters in 21 regions, 1990-2010: a systematic analysis for the global burden of disease study 2010. Lancet 2012; 380(9859):2224–60.
2. Lewington S, Clarke R, Qizilbash N, et al. Age-specific relevance of usual blood pressure to vascular mortality: a meta-analysis of individual data for one million adults in 61 prospective studies. Lancet 2002;360(9349):1903–13.
3. Chow CK, Teo KK, Rangarajan S, et al. Prevalence, awareness, treatment, and control of hypertension in rural and urban communities in high-, middle-, and low-income countries. JAMA 2013;310(9):959–68.
4. Global Alliance for Chronic Diseases. Available at: http://www.gacd.org/about. Accessed September 26, 2016.
5. W Tobe S, The Global Alliance for Chronic Diseases Hypertension Research Teams With the World Hypertension League. The Global Alliance for Chronic Diseases supports 15 major studies in hypertension prevention and control in low- and middle-income countries. J Clin Hypertens (Greenwich) 2016; 18(7):600–5.
6. Khatib R, Schwalm JD, Yusuf S, et al. Patient and healthcare provider barriers to hypertension awareness, treatment and follow up: a systematic review and meta-analysis of qualitative and quantitative studies. PLoS One 2014;9(1):e84238.
7. Maimaris W, Paty J, Perel P, et al. The influence of health systems on hypertension awareness, treatment, and control: a systematic literature review. PLoS Med 2013;10(7):e1001490.
8. Digiacomo M, Abbott P, Davison J, et al. Facilitating uptake of aboriginal adult health checks through community engagement and health promotion. Qual Prim Care 2010;18(1):57–64.
9. National Institute for Health and Care Excellence. Community engagement to improve health. London: National Institute for Health and Care Excellence; 2014.

Available at: https://www.nice.org.uk/guidance/lgb16/resources/community-engagement-to-improve-health-60521149786309. Accessed May 14, 2016.

10. Rosato M, Laverack G, Grabman LH, et al. Community participation: lessons for maternal, newborn, and child health. Lancet 2008;372(9642):962–71.

11. Joint United Nations Programme on HIV/AIDS (UN-AIDS). Promising practices in community engagement for elimination of new HIV infections among children by 2015 and keeping their mothers alive. Geneva (Switzerland): UNAIDS; 2012. Available at: http://www.unaids.org/sites/default/files/media_asset/20120628_JC2281_PromisingPracticesCommunity Engagements_en_0.pdf 15 May 2016.

12. Rifkin SB. Examining the links between community participation and health outcomes: a review of the literature. Health Policy Plan 2014;29(Suppl 2): ii98–106.

13. Marston C, Renedo A, McGowan CR, et al. Effects of community participation on improving uptake of skilled care for maternal and newborn health: a systematic review. PLoS One 2013;8(2):e55012.

14. Vedanthan R, Kamano JH, Naanyu V, et al. Optimizing linkage and retention to hypertension care in rural Kenya (LARK hypertension study): study protocol for a randomized controlled trial. Trials 2014;15(1):143.

15. Naanyu V, Vedanthan R, Kamano JH, et al. Barriers influencing linkage to hypertension care in Kenya: qualitative analysis from the LARK hypertension study. J Gen Intern Med 2016;31(3):304–14.

16. Maar M, Yeates K, Barron M, et al. I-RREACH: an engagement and assessment tool for improving implementation readiness of researchers, organizations and communities in complex interventions. Implement Sci 2015;10:64.

17. Bradley HA, Puoane T. Prevention of hypertension and diabetes in an urban setting in South Africa: participatory action research with community health workers. Ethn Dis 2007;17(1):49–54.

18. Balcazar HG, Byrd TL, Ortiz M, et al. A randomized community intervention to improve hypertension control among Mexican Americans: using the promotoras de salud community outreach model. J Health Care Poor Underserved 2009;20(4):1079–94.

19. He FJ, Li J, Macgregor GA. Effect of longer term modest salt reduction on blood pressure: Cochrane systematic review and meta-analysis of randomised trials. BMJ 2013;346:f1325.

20. Aburto NJ, Ziolkovska A, Hooper L, et al. Effect of lower sodium intake on health: systematic review and meta-analyses. BMJ 2013;346:f1326.

21. Reducing salt intake in populations: report of a WHO forum and technical meeting. Geneva (Switzerland): World Health Organization; 2007.

22. Guideline: sodium intake for adults and children. Geneva (Switzerland): World Health Organization; 2012.

23. World Health Organization (WHO). Monitoring framework and targets for the prevention and control of NCDs. Revised WHO discussion paper on the development of a comprehensive global monitoring framework, including indicators, and a set of voluntary global targets for the prevention and control of NCDs. 2012. Available at: http://www.who.int/nmh/events/2012/discussion_paper3.pdf. Accessed February 17, 2013.

24. Trieu K, Neal B, Hawkes C, et al. Salt reduction initiatives around the world – a systematic review of progress towards the global target. PLoS One 2015; 10(7):e0130247.

25. Webster J, Su'a SA, Ieremia M, et al. Salt intakes, knowledge, and behavior in Samoa: monitoring salt-consumption patterns through the World Health Organization's surveillance of noncommunicable disease risk factors (STEPS). J Clin Hypertens (Greenwich) 2016;18(9):884–91.

26. The World Health Organization. Creating an enabling environment for population-based salt reduction strategies. Geneva (Switzerland): World Health Organization; 2011.

27. Webster J, Snowdon W, Moodie M, et al. Cost-effectiveness of reducing salt intake in the Pacific Islands: protocol for a before and after intervention study. BMC Public Health 2014;14:107.

28. Dunford E, Trevena H, Goodsell C, et al. FoodSwitch: a mobile phone app to enable consumers to make healthier food choices and crowdsourcing of national food composition data. JMIR Mhealth Uhealth 2014;2(3):e37.

29. He FJ, Wu Y, Feng XX, et al. School based education programme to reduce salt intake in children and their families (School-EduSalt): cluster randomised controlled trial. BMJ 2015;350:h770.

30. Peng YG, Li W, Wen XX, et al. Effects of salt substitutes on blood pressure: a meta-analysis of randomized controlled trials. Am J Clin Nutr 2014;100(6): 1448–54.

31. Bernabe-Ortiz A, Diez-Canseco F, Gilman RH, et al. Launching a salt substitute to reduce blood pressure at the population level: a cluster randomized stepped wedge trial in Peru. Trials 2014;15:93.

32. Saavedra-Garcia L, Bernabe-Ortiz A, Gilman RH, et al. Applying the triangle taste test to assess differences between low sodium salts and common salt: evidence from Peru. PLoS One 2015;10(7): e0134700.

33. Salt substitution. A low-cost strategy for blood pressure control among rural Chinese. A randomized, controlled trial. J Hypertens 2007;25(10):2011–8.

34. Zhou X, Liu JX, Shi R, et al. Compound ion salt, a novel low-sodium salt substitute: from animal study to community-based population trial. Am J Hypertens 2009;22(9):934–42.

35. Zhao X, Yin X, Li X, et al. Using a low-sodium, high-potassium salt substitute to reduce blood pressure among Tibetans with high blood pressure: a patient-blinded randomized controlled trial. PLoS One 2014;9(10):e110131.

36. World Health Organization (WHO). World health report 2006: working together for health. Geneva (Switzerland): WHO; 2006.

37. Ministry of Health and Family Welfare. Rural health statistics bulletin, March 2010. New Delhi (India): Government of India; 2010.

38. World Health Organization (WHO). Density of physicians (total number per 1000 population, latest available year). Geneva (Switzerland): Global Health Observatory Data; 2016. Available at: http://www.who.int/gho/health_workforce/physicians_density_text/en/. Accessed May 13,2016.

39. Deller B, Tripathi V, Stender S, et al. Task shifting in maternal and newborn health care: key components from policy to implementation. Int J Gynecol Obstet 2015;130(Suppl 2):S25–31.

40. Dawson AJ, Buchan J, Duffield C, et al. Task shifting and sharing in maternal and reproductive health in low-income countries: a narrative synthesis of current evidence. Health Policy Plan 2014;29(3):396–408.

41. World Health Organization (WHO). Task shifting to tackle health worker shortages. Geneva (Switzerland): WHO Press; 2007.

42. Lekoubou A, Awah P, Fezeu L, et al. Hypertension, diabetes mellitus and task shifting and their management in sub-Saharan Africa. Int J Environ Res Public Health 2010;7:353–63.

43. 60th WMA general assembly. WMA resolution on task shifting from the medical profession. New Delhi: World Medical Association; 2009.

44. Joshi R, Alim M, Kengne AP, et al. Task shifting for non-communicable disease management in low and middle income countries ? A systematic review. PLoS One 2014;9(8):e103754.

45. Ogedegbe G, Gyamfi J, Plange-Rhule J, et al. Task shifting interventions for cardiovascular risk reduction in low-income and middle-income countries: a systematic review of randomised controlled trials. BMJ Open 2014;4(10):e005983.

46. Gaziano TA, Abrahams-Gessel S, Denman CA, et al. An assessment of community health workers' ability to screen for cardiovascular disease risk with a simple, non-invasive risk assessment instrument in Bangladesh, Guatemala, Mexico, and South Africa: an observational study. Lancet Glob Health 2015;3(9):e556–63.

47. Akinyemi RO, Owolabi MO, Adebayo PB, et al. Task-shifting training improves stroke knowledge among Nigerian non-neurologist health workers. J Neurol Sci 2015;359(1–2):112–6.

48. Joshi R, Chow C, Raju PK, et al. The rural Andhra Pradesh cardiovascular prevention study. J Am Coll Cardiol 2012;59(13):1188–96.

49. Kar SS, Thakur JS, Jain S, et al. Cardiovascular disease risk management in a primary health care setting of north India. Indian Heart J 2008;60(1):19–25.

50. Jafar TH, Islam M, Hatcher J, et al. Community based lifestyle intervention for blood pressure reduction in children and young adults in developing country: cluster randomised controlled trial. BMJ 2010;340:c2641.

51. Xavier D, Gupta R, Kamath D, et al. Community health worker-based intervention for adherence to drugs and lifestyle change after acute coronary syndrome: a multicentre, open, randomised controlled trial. Lancet Diabetes Endocrinol 2016;4(3):244–53.

52. Gaziano T, Abrahams-Gessel S, Surka S, et al. Cardiovascular disease screening by community health workers can be cost-effective in low-resource countries. Health Aff (Millwood) 2015;34(9):1538–45.

53. Buttorff C, Hock RS, Weiss HA, et al. Economic evaluation of a task-shifting intervention for common mental disorders in India. Bull World Health Organ 2012;90:813–21.

54. Thorogood M, Goudge J, Bertram M, et al. The Nkateko health service trial to improve hypertension management in rural South Africa: study protocol for a randomised controlled trial. Trials 2014;15:435.

55. Ogedegbe G, Plange-Rhule J, Gyamfi J, et al. A cluster-randomized trial of task shifting and blood pressure control in Ghana: study protocol. Implement Sci 2014;9:73.

56. Praveen D, Patel A, McMahon S, et al. A multifaceted strategy using mobile technology to assist rural primary healthcare doctors and frontline health workers in cardiovascular disease risk management: protocol for the SMARTHealth India cluster randomised controlled trial. Implementation Sci 2013;8:137.

57. Praveen D, Patel A, Raghu A, et al. SMARTHealth India: development and field evaluation of a mobile clinical decision support system for cardiovascular diseases in rural India. JMIR Mhealth Uhealth 2014;2(4):e54.

58. Piette JD, List J, Rana GK, et al. Mobile health devices as tools for worldwide cardiovascular risk reduction and disease management. Circulation 2015;132(21):2012–27.

59. Peiris D, Praveen D, Johnson C, et al. Use of mHealth systems and tools for non-communicable diseases in low- and middle-income countries: a systematic review. J Cardiovasc Transl Res 2014;7(8):677–91.

60. Bloomfield GS, Vedanthan R, Vasudevan L, et al. Mobile health for non-communicable diseases in Sub-Saharan Africa: a systematic review of the literature and strategic framework for research. Global Health 2014;10:49.

61. Beratarrechea A, Lee AG, Willner JM, et al. The impact of mobile health interventions on chronic disease outcomes in developing countries: a systematic review. Telemed J E Health 2014;20(1): 75–82.

62. Okoro E, Sholagberu H, Kolo P. Mobile phone ownership among Nigerians with diabetes. Afr Health Sci 2010;10(2):183–6.

63. Owolabi MO, Akinyemi RO, Gebregziabher M, et al. Randomized controlled trial of a multipronged intervention to improve blood pressure control among stroke survivors in Nigeria. Int J Stroke 2014;9(8): 1109–16.

64. Cushman WC, Ford CE, Einhorn PT, et al. Blood pressure control by drug group in the antihypertensive and lipid-lowering treatment to prevent heart attack trial (ALLHAT). J Clin Hypertens 2008; 10(10):751–60.

65. Johnston A, Stafylas P, Stergiou GS. Effectiveness, safety and cost of drug substitution in hypertension. Br J Clin Pharmacol 2010;70(3):320–34.

66. Shaw E, Anderson JG, Maloney M, et al. Factors associated with noncompliance of patients taking antihypertensive medications. Hosp Pharm 1995; 30(3):201–3.

67. Faria C, Wenzel M, Lee KW, et al. A narrative review of clinical inertia: focus on hypertension. J Am Soc Hypertens 2009;3(4).267–76.

68. Okonofua EC, Simpson KN, Jesri A, et al. Therapeutic inertia is an impediment to achieving the healthy people 2010 blood pressure control goals. Hypertension 2006;47(3):345–51.

69. Brown MJ, McInnes GT, Papst CC, et al. Aliskiren and the calcium channel blocker amlodipine combination as an initial treatment strategy for hypertension control (ACCELERATE): a randomised, parallel-group trial. Lancet 2011;377(9762):312–20.

70. Feldman RD, Zou GY, Vandervoort MK, et al. A simplified approach to the treatment of uncomplicated hypertension: a cluster randomized, controlled trial. Hypertension 2009;53(4):646–53.

71. Gupta AK, Arshad S, Poulter NR. Compliance, safety, and effectiveness of fixed-dose combinations of antihypertensive agents: a meta-analysis. Hypertension 2010;55(2):399–407.

72. Webster R, Patel A, Selak V, et al. Effectiveness of fixed dose combination medication ('polypills') compared with usual care in patients with cardiovascular disease or at high risk: a prospective, individual patient data meta-analysis of 3140 patients in six countries. Int J Cardiol 2016;205:147–56.

73. Castellano JM, Sanz G, Penalvo JL, et al. A polypill strategy to improve adherence: results from focus (Fixed-dose combination drug for secondary cardiovascular prevention) project. J Am Coll Cardiol 2014;64(20):2071–82.

74. Lonn EM, Bosch J, López-Jaramillo P, et al. Blood-pressure lowering in intermediate-risk persons without cardiovascular disease. N Engl J Med 2016;374(21):2009–20.

75. Yusuf S, Lonn E, Pais P, et al. Blood-pressure and cholesterol lowering in persons without cardiovascular disease. N Engl J Med 2016;374(21):2032–43.

76. Salam A, Webster R, Singh K, et al. TRIple pill vs Usual care Management for Patients with mild-to moderate Hypertension (TRIUMPH): study protocol. Am Heart J 2014;167(2):127–32.

77. Thom S, Poulter N, Field J, et al. Effects of a fixed-dose combination strategy on adherence and risk factors in patients with or at high risk of CVD: the umpire randomized clinical trial. JAMA 2013; 310(9):918–29.

78. Patel A, Cass A, Peiris D, et al. A pragmatic randomized trial of a polypill-based strategy to improve use of indicated preventive treatments in people at high cardiovascular disease risk. Eur J Prev Cardiol 2015;22(7):920–30.

79. Selak V, Elley CR, Bullen C, et al. Effect of fixed dose combination treatment on adherence and risk factor control among patients at high risk of cardiovascular disease: randomised controlled trial in primary care. BMJ 2014;348:g3318.

Ambulatory Blood Pressure Monitoring

A Complementary Strategy for Hypertension Diagnosis and Management in Low-Income and Middle-Income Countries

Marwah Abdalla, MD, MPH

KEYWORDS

- Ambulatory blood pressure monitoring • Resource-constrained
- Low-income and middle-income countries

KEY POINTS

- The burden of hypertension is increasing worldwide.
- Out-of-clinic blood pressure (BP) assessments, including ambulatory BP monitoring (ABPM), are recommended by several international guidelines.
- Ambulatory BP provides a better prediction of several cardiovascular (CV) outcomes compared with clinic BP.
- ABPM can be used as part of a comprehensive health care strategy to address the double burden of communicable and noncommunicable diseases and as part of task-shifting strategies in the management of hypertension within low-income and middle-income countries (LMICs).

INTRODUCTION

Worldwide, the burden of hypertension is increasing especially within LMICs.[1] Although the prevalence of hypertension within LMICs is high, awareness and control are often low.[2–5] The current burden of hypertension is greatest in populations within LMICs where approximately 1 of every 3 adults is affected by hypertension.[4] Furthermore, it is projected that LMICs will continue to bear a higher burden of the disease compared with the global average, and by 2025, 75% of individuals with hypertension will be living in LMICs.[6] Clearly, hypertension is an important public health problem within LMICs and effective

strategies to diagnose and treat hypertension are needed. The reduction of hypertension by 25% by the year 2025 is now a World Health Organization (WHO) priority.[7]

Although the diagnosis and treatment of hypertension historically have been based on the measurement of BP via automated oscillometric or manual readings taken within the clinic setting, more recently the WHO recommends that BP be recorded for several days, ideally with 2 measurements made, in the morning and evening, with additional BP measurements done outside the clinic setting to properly diagnosis hypertension.[8] Because BP is characterized by a circadian pattern over a 24-hour period with levels that are

Conflict of Interest: The author has nothing to disclose.
Funding Sources: The author is supported by HL117323-02S2 from the National Heart, Lung, and Blood Institute at the National Institutes of Health (NIH) and NIHMS-ID: 814352.
Center for Behavioral Cardiovascular Health, Division of Cardiology, Department of Medicine, Columbia University Medical Center, 622 West 168th Street, PH 9-321, New York, NY 10032, USA
E-mail address: ma2947@cumc.columbia.edu

cardiology.theclinics.com

normally highest while awake and that fall during sleep, clinic BP readings may not accurately reflect BP taken outside of the clinic setting. Although both ABPM and home BP monitoring can assess BP outside of the clinic setting,[9] ABPM is more commonly recommended within several international guidelines.[10–13] Additionally, studies have shown that ambulatory BP provides a better prediction of several CV outcomes compared with clinic BP.[13–17]

OVERVIEW OF AMBULATORY BLOOD PRESSURE MONITORING

Ambulatory BP monitors are compact automated oscillometric devices worn on a belt or pouch and connected to a sphygmomanometer cuff on the upper arm by a tube (**Fig. 1**). These monitors are typically worn for a 24-hour period and are set to obtain readings every 15 to 30 minutes throughout the day and night. During the 24-hour monitoring period, individuals are also encouraged to fill out a diary to document times of meal and medication ingestion, sleep and awakening, exercise, and any symptoms. After the 24-hour period, the monitor is returned and readings are downloaded into a computer for processing.[9]

Because ABPM can provide multiple BP measurements throughout a 24-hour period, average BP readings can be assessed over several discrete time periods, including daytime, nighttime, and 24-hour periods.[18] The daytime and nighttime periods can be defined using several different approaches, including an individual's self-report of awakening and sleeping times, fixed time periods, or actigraphy.[9,19–21] Accordingly, daytime, nighttime, and 24-hour hypertension may be diagnosed by obtaining elevated BP readings during any of these time periods. Daytime hypertension is defined as mean daytime systolic BP greater than or equal to 135 mm Hg or mean daytime diastolic BP greater than or equal to 85 mm Hg; nighttime hypertension is defined as mean nighttime systolic BP greater than or equal to 120 mm Hg or mean nighttime diastolic BP greater than or equal to 70 mm Hg; and 24-hour hypertension is defined as mean systolic BP greater than or equal to 130 mm Hg or mean diastolic BP greater than or equal to 80 mm Hg.[21]

ABPM can be used to diagnose hypertension as well as manage antihypertensive therapy among individuals with hypertension. When ambulatory BP readings are cross-classified with clinic BP readings, there are 4 BP phenotypes that can be defined (**Fig. 2**). Sustained normotension and sustained hypertension represent agreement between clinic BP and ambulatory BP readings. White coat hypertension is defined as elevated clinic BP with nonelevated ambulatory BP readings[21,22] whereas masked hypertension is defined as nonelevated clinic BP with elevated ambulatory BP readings (either in the daytime, nighttime, or throughout the 24-hour period).[21,23] Whether white coat hypertension is linked to increased CV risk and mortality has been controversial within the literature.[24–26] In contrast, several studies have shown that masked hypertension is associated with subclinical target

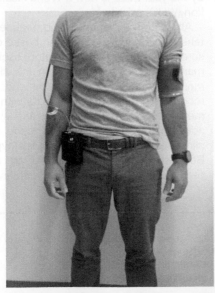
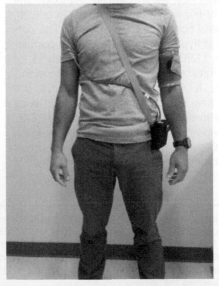

Fig. 1. The ABPM can be worn on a belt (left) or pouch (right) and is connected to a sphygmomanometer cuff on the upper arm. (*Courtesy of* Marwah Abdalla, MD, MPH, New York.)

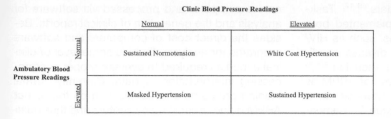

Fig. 2. The 4 blood pressure phenotypes defined by cross-classification of clinic blood pressure and ambulatory blood pressure.

organ damage, incident hypertension, and increased CV and total mortality.[16,27–29]

ABPM can also be used to identify white coat hypertension and masked hypertension among treated individuals on antihypertensive therapy.[9] Treated white coat hypertension or white coat uncontrolled hypertension can occur among individuals on antihypertensive medications who have elevated clinic BP with nonelevated ambulatory BP whereas treated masked hypertension or masked uncontrolled hypertension can occur among individuals on antihypertensive therapy who have nonelevated clinic BP with elevated ambulatory BP.

In addition to these 4 BP phenotypes, several other diurnal BP patterns and BP measures, such as nocturnal dipping, BP variability, morning surge, and orthostatic hypotension, can also be defined. During sleep, BP normally decreases, or dips, compared with awake BP. Individuals can be classified into 2 dipping groups (dipping and nondipping) as well as into 4 dipping patterns (extreme dipping, normal dipping, nondipping, and reverse dipping) based on the nighttime-daytime systolic BP ratio.[30,31] When classified into 2 dipping groups, several studies have shown that nondipping BP is associated with increased target organ damage as well as increased risk of mortality.[32–35] Likewise, studies have also shown that nondipping pattern and reverse dipping pattern are each associated with increased mortality and CV events compared with normal dipping pattern.[33,36–39] Similarly, BP normally increases (surges) on awakening compared with sleep BP. An exaggerated morning surge has been associated with an increased CV risk.[40] Thus, ABPM can provide detailed assessment of several BP phenotypes and measures, which can be helpful in the prediction of clinical outcomes.[14,18]

THE POTENTIAL APPLICABILITY AND CURRENT USE OF AMBULATORY BLOOD PRESSURE MONITORING IN LOW-INCOME AND MIDDLE-INCOME COUNTRIES

Within LMICs, health care systems are often underfunded and incur a double burden of communicable and noncommunicable diseases leading to competing health care priorities. Additionally, most health care systems in resource-constrained areas are not equipped to deal with the long-term management of chronic conditions, such as hypertension. Within certain LMICs, where communicable diseases, such as HIV and tuberculosis, are at the forefront of health care system priorities, there has been an opportunity to leverage existing communicable health care delivery systems to address noncommunicable diseases.[41] Screening for these communicable diseases has created an infrastructure for "opportunistic" screening and treatment of noncommunicable diseases, which has been shown cost effective.[41,42] Most population-wide screening initiatives to diagnose hypertension within LMICs have relied on elevated clinic BP readings. Although the use of ABPM in population-wide screening programs in LMICs has not been formerly examined, ABPM can be a complementary strategy to confirm initially elevated clinic BP readings,[43] especially among high-risk individuals who are undergoing screening or management of communicable diseases. An example of this includes individuals with HIV who have been shown at increased risk for CV diseases, including hypertension.[44] Although studies of ABPM in HIV+ individuals are limited, HIV+ individuals have an increased prevalence of nondipping BP,[45] which may put them at increased risk for CV events. Identifying the factors associated with abnormal BP phenotypes among HIV+ individuals would help elucidate the mechanisms underlying the excess CV disease risk among this population and potentially identify new targets for intervention that can mitigate this excess risk. Thus, the use of ABPM among high-risk individuals can be part of a comprehensive health care strategy to address the double burden of disease within LMICs.

Besides the double burden of communicable and noncommunicable diseases, there is also a shortage of well-trained health care providers in LMICs. As such, task shifting—the delegation of tasks to nonphysician health care providers, such as nurses and pharmacists, is now an effective strategy used in the management of several conditions within LMICs to help address the shortage of health care providers.[46,47] Task-shifting strategies have been implemented both in chronic communicable diseases, such as HIV/AIDS, and in noncommunicable disease conditions, such as diabetes and hypertension.[48–53] Few studies have examined the use of ABPM as part of task shifting strategies, however. In a recent study, James and colleagues[54] demonstrated the feasibility of a pharmacist-led hypertension management strategy using ABPM in Ireland. In both high-income countries and LMICs, pharmacists are increasingly included within the health care team. Within LMICs, pharmacists play a critical role within communities. In some areas, local pharmacies may be the only health service available.[55] The local pharmacist often has several responsibilities within resource-constrained areas that include advising individuals on the management of common conditions, prescribing and dispensing medication, and participating in basic screening and health promotion activities.[55] Local community members often develop a long-term relationship with their pharmacists who are viewed as a trusted and accessible resource. In turn, patients' engagement with their own health care is high.[56] Adoption of a pharmacist-led hypertension management strategy using ABPM within LMICs may prove effective and may increase availability of ABPM within resource-constrained areas.

Despite the utility of ABPM, there is currently underutilization of ABPM within LMICs. In a small cross-sectional survey of national and regional hypertension societies, only 36% of respondents within LMICs reported use of ABPM.[57] This may be due to various challenges both on an individual level as well as on a systematic level that may be unique to resource-constrained settings. For some individuals, use of ABPM at night may interrupt sleep.[9] Rarely, repeated inflation of the device over 24 hours can cause skin irritation. Although prior studies have shown that compared with home BP and clinic BP, ABPM is a cost-effective strategy for the diagnosis and treatment of ABPM within high-income countries,[58] the initial cost of ABPM devices is generally higher compared with other automated BP devices,[18,58] including home BP devices. This may be an additional financial burden to individuals in resource-constrained areas where often the majority of health care is paid via private spending.[41] Additionally, devices have to be returned to centers within a timely manner for processing, which may be burdensome for individuals who may have limited interaction and infrequent access to health care systems. Once an individual returns the ABPM device, the data must be downloaded onto a computer and processed via software for analysis and the generation of clinical reports. Besides the direct cost of computers and software programs for analysis, there is some level of clinical expertise required to oversee proper postprocessing interpretation of data. Currently, formal training programs and certification on the use of ABPM do not exist in many centers and thus quality standards for ABPM may vary across sites and regions.

Despite these challenges, the majority of recent guidelines, including the American Society of Hypertension/International Society of Hypertension 2014 guidelines,[12] National Institute for Clinical Excellence 2011 guidelines,[11] and the European Society of Hypertension/European Society of Cardiology 2013 guidelines,[10] have recommended the use of ABPM most commonly to exclude white coat hypertension. Most of the normality thresholds, however, for ambulatory BP published within these guidelines have been derived from European and Japanese population-based and hypertensive cohorts.[59–65] Whether normality thresholds for ambulatory BP are similar in populations with a high risk of hypertension-related adverse CV outcomes is currently unknown because some studies suggest that the risk of hypertension, BP treatment thresholds, and appropriate antihypertensive medication regimens vary with ethnic origin.[6,66–69]

Unfortunately, most of the published ABPM studies originating from investigators in LMICs are often country-specific and pooled population-based data from LMICs are currently not available. In contrast, one of the largest population-based ABPM cohorts is the International Database of Ambulatory Blood Pressure in Relation to Cardiovascular Outcome (IDACO) study,[70] which incorporates data from 12,752 participants from 12 high-income countries in Europe, Asia, and South America. Additionally, the International Ambulatory Blood Pressure Registry: Telemonitoring of Hypertension and Cardiovascular Risk Project (ARTEMIS)[71] is a large international registry of centers using ABPM in the management of hypertensive patients from 41 countries, including 12 LMICs. Studies from both IDACO and ARTEMIS have helped define the prognostic value of ABPM and ethnic differences in ambulatory BP measures.[70–72]

FUTURE AREAS OF RESEARCH

There are many important research questions related to ABPM that remain unanswered. As discussed previously, the feasibility of ABPM for large-scale hypertension screening and treatment campaigns is unknown. Defining the prevalence of ambulatory BP phenotypes and their relation to incident hypertension and target organ damage must still be elucidated within different ethnically diverse populations. It is also currently unclear whether the addition of ambulatory BP to clinic BP or home BP measurements provides further improvement on CV risk estimates.[14] Additionally, whether the initiation and titration of antihypertensive therapy based on clinic and ambulatory BP improves CV outcomes compared with clinic BP alone is unknown.[14] Lastly, data on the cost-effectiveness of ABPM are scarce and have been limited to studies mostly from the United Kingdom, the United States, Japan, and Australia.[58,73–77]

SUMMARY

Given the low awareness rates of hypertension in LMICs, most population-wide screening initiatives have relied on elevated clinic BP readings to confirm a diagnosis of hypertension.[78,79] Clinic BP, however, may not accurately capture the diurnal variation of BP over a 24-hour period. Additionally, failure to confirm elevated clinic BP readings can result in overtreatment and misdiagnosis.[43] Given the limited availability of ABPM data in LMICs, there is an urgent need for evidence-based epidemiologic and global health delivery research within this area. The use of ABPM should be considered part of a comprehensive health care approach to reduce the growing burden of hypertension within LMICs, which now mandates additional strategies beyond the traditional assessment of clinic BP.

REFERENCES

1. Yusuf S, Reddy S, Ounpuu S, et al. Global burden of cardiovascular diseases: part I: general considerations, the epidemiologic transition, risk factors, and impact of urbanization. Circulation 2001; 104(22):2746–53.

2. Chow CK, Teo KK, Rangarajan S, et al. Prevalence, awareness, treatment, and control of hypertension in rural and urban communities in high-, middle-, and low-income countries. JAMA 2013;310(9):959–68.

3. Lloyd-Sherlock P, Beard J, Minicuci N, et al. Hypertension among older adults in low- and middle-income countries: prevalence, awareness and control. Int J Epidemiol 2014;43(1):116–28.

4. Sarki AM, Nduka CU, Stranges S, et al. Prevalence of hypertension in low- and middle-income countries: a systematic review and meta-analysis. Medicine (Baltimore) 2015;94(50):e1959.

5. Mills KT, Bundy JD, Kelly TN, et al. Global disparities of hypertension prevalence and control: a systematic

analysis of population-based studies from 90 countries. Circulation 2016;134(6):441–50.

6. van de Vijver S, Akinyi H, Oti S, et al. Status report on hypertension in Africa–consultative review for the 6th Session of the African Union Conference of Ministers of Health on NCD's. Pan Afr Med J 2013;16:38.

7. WHO. NCD Global Monitoring Framework. 2011. Available at: http://www.who.int/nmh/global_monitoring_framework/en/. Accessed June 30, 2016.

8. WHO. A global brief on hypertension: silent killer, global public health crisis. 2013.

9. Shimbo D, Abdalla M, Falzon L, et al. Role of ambulatory and home blood pressure monitoring in clinical practice: a narrative review. Ann Intern Med 2015;163(9):691–700.

10. Mancia G, Fagard R, Narkiewicz K, et al. 2013 ESH/ESC practice guidelines for the management of arterial hypertension. Blood Press 2014;23(1):3–16.

11. NICE. Hypertension in adults: diagnosis and management. 2011. Available at: https://www.nice.org.uk/guidance/CG127. Accessed June 30, 2016.

12. Weber MA, Schiffrin EL, White WB, et al. Clinical practice guidelines for the management of hypertension in the community: a statement by the American Society of Hypertension and the International Society of Hypertension. J Clin Hypertens (Greenwich) 2014;16(1):14–26.

13. Shimbo D, Abdalla M, Falzon L, et al. Studies comparing ambulatory blood pressure and home blood pressure on cardiovascular disease and mortality outcomes: a systematic review. J Am Soc Hypertens 2016;10(3):224–34.e17.

14. Mancia G, Verdecchia P. Clinical value of ambulatory blood pressure: evidence and limits. Circ Res 2015;116(6):1034–45.

15. Dolan E, Stanton A, Thijs L, et al. Superiority of ambulatory over clinic blood pressure measurement in predicting mortality: the Dublin outcome study. Hypertension 2005;46(1):156–61.

16. Hansen TW, Kikuya M, Thijs L, et al. Prognostic superiority of daytime ambulatory over conventional blood pressure in four populations: a meta-analysis of 7,030 individuals. J Hypertens 2007;25(8):1554–64.

17. Schwartz CL, McManus RJ. What is the evidence base for diagnosing hypertension and for subsequent blood pressure treatment targets in the prevention of cardiovascular disease? BMC Med 2015;13:256.

18. Turner JR, Viera AJ, Shimbo D. Ambulatory blood pressure monitoring in clinical practice: a review. Am J Med 2015;128(1):14–20.

19. Booth JN 3rd, Muntner P, Abdalla M, et al. Differences in night-time and daytime ambulatory blood pressure when diurnal periods are defined by self-report, fixed-times, and actigraphy: improving the detection of hypertension study. J Hypertens 2016; 34(2):235–43.

20. Hermida RC, Ayala DE, Mojon A, et al. Influence of circadian time of hypertension treatment on cardiovascular risk: results of the MAPEC study. Chronobiol Int 2010;27(8):1629–51.

21. O'Brien E, Parati G, Stergiou G, et al. European Society of Hypertension position paper on ambulatory blood pressure monitoring. J Hypertens 2013; 31(9):1731–68.

22. Pickering TG, James GD, Boddie C, et al. How common is white coat hypertension? JAMA 1988;259(2): 225–8.

23. Pickering TG, Davidson K, Gerin W, et al. Masked hypertension. Hypertension 2002;40(6):795–6.

24. Franklin SS, Thijs L, Hansen TW, et al. Significance of white-coat hypertension in older persons with isolated systolic hypertension: a meta-analysis using the International Database on Ambulatory Blood Pressure Monitoring in Relation to Cardiovascular Outcomes population. Hypertension 2012;59(3): 564–71.

25. Mancia G, Facchetti R, Bombelli M, et al. Long-term risk of mortality associated with selective and combined elevation in office, home, and ambulatory blood pressure. Hypertension 2006;47(5):846–53.

26. Pierdomenico SD, Cuccurullo F. Prognostic value of white-coat and masked hypertension diagnosed by ambulatory monitoring in initially untreated subjects: an updated meta analysis. Am J Hypertens 2011; 24(1):52–8.

27. Abdalla M, Booth JN 3rd, Seals SR, et al. Masked hypertension and incident clinic hypertension among Blacks in the Jackson Heart Study. Hypertension 2016;68(1):220–6.

28. Bjorklund K, Lind L, Zethelius B, et al. Isolated ambulatory hypertension predicts cardiovascular morbidity in elderly men. Circulation 2003;107(9): 1297–302.

29. Redmond N, Booth JN 3rd, Tanner RM, et al. Prevalence of masked hypertension and its association with subclinical cardiovascular disease in African Americans: results from the Jackson Heart Study. J Am Heart Assoc 2016;4(3):e002284.

30. O'Brien E, Sheridan J, O'Malley K. Dippers and non-dippers. Lancet 1988;2(8607):397.

31. Kario K, Pickering TG, Matsuo T, et al. Stroke prognosis and abnormal nocturnal blood pressure falls in older hypertensives. Hypertension 2001;38(4):852–7.

32. Boggia J, Li Y, Thijs L, et al. Prognostic accuracy of day versus night ambulatory blood pressure: a cohort study. Lancet 2007;370(9594):1219–29.

33. Fagard RH, Celis H, Thijs L, et al. Daytime and night-time blood pressure as predictors of death and cause-specific cardiovascular events in hypertension. Hypertension 2008;51(1):55–61.

34. Kario K, Pickering TG, Matsuo T, et al. Stroke prognosis and abnormal nocturnal blood pressure falls in older hypertensives. Hypertension 2001;38(4):852–7.

35. Ohkubo T, Hozawa A, Yamaguchi J, et al. Prognostic significance of the nocturnal decline in blood pressure in individuals with and without high 24-h blood pressure: the Ohasama study. J Hypertens 2002; 20(11):2183–9.

36. Ben-Dov IZ, Kark JD, Ben-Ishay D, et al. Predictors of all-cause mortality in clinical ambulatory monitoring: unique aspects of blood pressure during sleep. Hypertension 2007;49(6):1235–41.

37. Fagard RH. Dipping pattern of nocturnal blood pressure in patients with hypertension. Expert Rev Cardiovasc Ther 2009;7(6):599–605.

38. Kim BK, Kim YM, Lee Y, et al. A reverse dipping pattern predicts cardiovascular mortality in a clinical cohort. J Korean Med Sci 2013;28(10):1468–73.

39. Salles GF, Reboldi G, Fagard RH, et al. Prognostic effect of the nocturnal blood pressure fall in hypertensive patients: the ambulatory blood pressure collaboration in patients with hypertension (ABC-H) meta-analysis. Hypertension 2016;67(4):693–700.

40. Kario K. Morning surge in blood pressure and cardiovascular risk: evidence and perspectives. Hypertension 2010;56(5):765–73.

41. Siddharthan T, Ramaiya K, Yonga G, et al. Noncommunicable diseases in East Africa: assessing the gaps in care and identifying opportunities for improvement. Health Aff (Millwood) 2015;34(9): 1506–13.

42. Hyle EP, Naidoo K, Su AE, et al. HIV, tuberculosis, and noncommunicable diseases: what is known about the costs, effects, and cost-effectiveness of integrated care? J Acquir Immune Defic Syndr 2014;67(Suppl 1):S87–95.

43. Piper MA, Evans CV, Burda BU, et al. Screening for high blood pressure in adults: a systematic evidence review for the U.S. Preventive Services Task Force. Rockville (MD): Agency for Healthcare Research and Quality (US); 2014. Report No.: 13-05194-EF-1.

44. Armah KA, Chang CC, Baker JV, et al. Prehypertension, hypertension, and the risk of acute myocardial infarction in HIV-infected and -uninfected veterans. Clin Infect Dis 2014;58(1):121–9.

45. Kent ST, Bromfield SG, Burkholder GA, et al. Ambulatory blood pressure monitoring in individuals with HIV: a systematic review and meta-analysis. PLoS One 2016;11(2):e0148920.

46. WHO. Task shifting to tackle health worker shortages. 2007. Available at: http://www.who.int/health systems/task_shifting_booklet.pdf. Accessed June 30, 2016.

47. Poulter NR, Prabhakaran D, Caulfield M. Hypertension. Lancet 2015;386(9995):801–12.

48. Abegunde DO, Shengelia B, Luyten A, et al. Can non-physician health-care workers assess and manage cardiovascular risk in primary care? Bull World Health Organ 2007;85(6):432–40.

49. Laurant M, Reeves D, Hermens R, et al. Substitution of doctors by nurses in primary care. Cochrane Database Syst Rev 2005;(2):CD001271.

50. Lehmann U, Van Damme W, Barten F, et al. Task shifting: the answer to the human resources crisis in Africa? Hum Resour Health 2009;7:49.

51. Lekoubou A, Awah P, Fezeu L, et al. Hypertension, diabetes mellitus and task shifting in their management in sub-Saharan Africa. Int J Environ Res Public Health 2010;7(2):353–63.

52. Morgado M, Rolo S, Castelo-Branco M. Pharmacist intervention program to enhance hypertension control: a randomised controlled trial. Int J Clin Pharm 2011;33(1):132–40.

53. Ogedegbe G, Plange-Rhule J, Gyamfi J, et al. A cluster-randomized trial of task shifting and blood pressure control in Ghana: study protocol. Implement Sci 2014;9:73.

54. James K, Dolan E, O'Brien E. Making ambulatory blood pressure monitoring accessible in pharmacies. Blood Press Monit 2014;19(3):134–9.

55. Smith F. Private local pharmacies in low- and middle-income countries: a review of interventions to enhance their role in public health. Trop Med Int Health 2009;14(3):362–72.

56. Brown D, Portlock J, Rutter P, et al. From community pharmacy to healthy living pharmacy: positive early experiences from Portsmouth, England. Res Social Adm Pharm 2014;10(1):72–87.

57. Chalmers J, Arima H, Harrap S, et al. Global survey of current practice in management of hypertension as reported by societies affiliated with the International Society of Hypertension. J Hypertens 2013; 31(5):1043–8.

58. Lovibond K, Jowett S, Barton P, et al. Cost-effectiveness of options for the diagnosis of high blood pressure in primary care: a modelling study. Lancet 2011;378(9798):1219–30.

59. Head GA, Mihailidou AS, Duggan KA, et al. Definition of ambulatory blood pressure targets for diagnosis and treatment of hypertension in relation to clinic blood pressure: prospective cohort study. BMJ 2010;340:c1104.

60. Staessen JA, O'Brien ET, Amery AK, et al. Ambulatory blood pressure in normotensive and hypertensive subjects: results from an international database. J Hypertens Suppl 1994; 12(7):S1–12.

61. Sega R, Facchetti R, Bombelli M, et al. Prognostic value of ambulatory and home blood pressures compared with office blood pressure in the general population: follow-up results from the Pressioni Arteriose Monitorate e Loro Associazioni (PAMELA) study. Circulation 2005;111(14):1777–83.

62. Mancia G, Sega R, Bravi C, et al. Ambulatory blood pressure normality: results from the PAMELA study. J Hypertens 1995;13(12 Pt 1):1377–90.

63. Rasmussen SL, Torp-Pedersen C, Borch-Johnsen K, et al. Normal values for ambulatory blood pressure and differences between casual blood pressure and ambulatory blood pressure: results from a Danish population survey. J Hypertens 1998;16(10):1415–24.

64. Pogue V, Rahman M, Lipkowitz M, et al. Disparate estimates of hypertension control from ambulatory and clinic blood pressure measurements in hypertensive kidney disease. Hypertension 2009;53(1): 20–7.

65. Sega R, Cesana G, Milesi C, et al. Ambulatory and home blood pressure normality in the elderly: data from the PAMELA population. Hypertension 1997; 30(1 Pt 1):1–6.

66. Dhillon RS, Clair K, Fraden M, et al. Hypertension in populations of different ethnic origins. Lancet 2014; 384(9939):234.

67. Yusuf S, Reddy S, Ounpuu S, et al. Global burden of cardiovascular diseases: Part II: variations in cardiovascular disease by specific ethnic groups and geographic regions and prevention strategies. Circulation 2001;104(23):2855–64.

68. Joshi P, Islam S, Pais P, et al. Risk factors for early myocardial infarction in South Asians compared with individuals in other countries. JAMA 2007; 297(3):286–94.

69. Cooper-DeHoff RM, Aranda JM Jr, Gaxiola E, et al. Blood pressure control and cardiovascular outcomes in high-risk Hispanic patients–findings from the International Verapamil SR/Trandolapril Study (INVEST). Am Heart J 2006;151(5):1072–9.

70. Asayama K, Thijs L, Li Y, et al. Setting thresholds to varying blood pressure monitoring intervals differentially affects risk estimates associated with white coat and masked hypertension in the population. Hypertension 2014;64(5):935–42.

71. Hoshide S, Kario K, de la Sierra A, et al. Ethnic differences in the degree of morning blood pressure surge and in its determinants between Japanese and European hypertensive subjects: data from the ARTEMIS study. Hypertension 2015; 66(4):750–6.

72. ARTEMIS. Available at: www.artemisnet.org. Accessed June 30, 2016.

73. Ewald B, Pekarsky B. Cost analysis of ambulatory blood pressure monitoring in initiating antihypertensive drug treatment in Australian general practice. Med J Aust 2002;176(12):580–3.

74. Fukunaga H, Ohkubo T, Kobayashi M, et al. Cost-effectiveness of the introduction of home blood pressure measurement in patients with office hypertension. J Hypertens 2008;26(4):685–90.

75. Hodgkinson J, Mant J, Martin U, et al. Relative effectiveness of clinic and home blood pressure monitoring compared with ambulatory blood pressure monitoring in diagnosis of hypertension: systematic review. BMJ 2011;342:d3621.

76. Little P, Barnett J, Barnsley L, et al. Comparison of agreement between different measures of blood pressure in primary care and daytime ambulatory blood pressure. BMJ 2002;325 (7358):254.

77. Pierdomenico SD, Mezzetti A, Lapenna D, et al. 'White-coat' hypertension in patients with newly diagnosed hypertension: evaluation of prevalence by ambulatory monitoring and impact on

cost of health care. Eur Heart J 1995;16(5): 692–7.

78. Basu S, Millett C. Social epidemiology of hypertension in middle-income countries: determinants of prevalence, diagnosis, treatment, and control in the WHO SAGE study. Hypertension 2013;62(1):18–26.

79. Pickering T. The measurement of blood pressure in developing countries. Blood Press Monit 2005; 10(1):11–2.

Ensuring Patient-Centered Access to Cardiovascular Disease Medicines in Low-Income and Middle-Income Countries Through Health-System Strengthening

Dan N. Tran, PharmD[a,1], Benson Njuguna, BPharm[a,b],
Timothy Mercer, MD, MPH[c,1], Imran Manji, BPharm[a,b],
Lydia Fischer, BA (Visual Communication Design)[c],
Marya Lieberman, PhD[d], Sonak D. Pastakia, PharmD, BCPS, MPH[a,*]

KEYWORDS

- Patient-centered access • Cardiovascular disease medicines • Availability • Accountability
- Adherence • Health-system strengthening • Low-income and middle-income countries
- Falsified and substandard medicines

KEY POINTS

- Eighty percent of deaths due to cardiovascular disease (CVD) occur in low-income and middle-inoome countries (LMICs).
- Translating available CVD prevention and treatment guidelines into practice is hampered in LMICs by inadequate supply chain systems that limit access to lifesaving medicines.
- We propose 3 barriers ("3A" challenges) to patient-centered access to essential CVD medicines: dismal *availability* of medicines, lack of *accountability* in the supply chain, and poor medication *adherence*.
- Many challenges with CVD medication access relate to on-the-ground challenges. Pilot programs demonstrated improvement in CVD medication access by standardizing supply chain management, improving human resource efficiency, and extending supply chain considerations to improve patient adherence.
- Evaluating the health impact and cost-effectiveness of these existing solutions will be crucial for scaling up and ultimately providing patient-centered access to CVD medicines in LMICs.

Disclosure Statement: The authors do not have any commercial or financial conflicts of interests, or any funding sources to declare (D.N. Tran, B. Njuguna, T. Mercer, I. Manji, L. Fischer). M. Lieberman has received funding for this project from the Bill & Melinda Gates Foundation (OPP1108078), US-AID DIV program (AID-0AA-F-15-00050), and Indiana CTSI program. S. Pastakia has previously served as a consultant for Abbott but this activity is unrelated to the work described in this article.
[a] Department of Pharmacy Practice, Purdue University College of Pharmacy, Indianapolis, IN 46202, USA;
[b] Department of Pharmacy, Moi Teaching and Referral Hospital, PO Box 3, Eldoret 30100, Kenya;
[c] Department of Medicine, Indiana University School of Medicine, 1120 West Michigan Street, Indianapolis, IN 46202, USA; [d] Department of Chemistry and Biochemistry, University of Notre Dame, 250 Nieuwland, Notre Dame, IN 46556, USA
[1] Present address: PO Box 5760, Eldoret 30100, Kenya.
* Corresponding author. PO Box 5760, Eldoret 30100, Kenya.
E-mail address: spastaki@gmail.com

Cardiol Clin 35 (2017) 125–134
http://dx.doi.org/10.1016/j.ccl.2016.08.008

INTRODUCTION

Cardiovascular disease (CVD) is the leading cause of global mortality and is expected to reach 23 million deaths by 2030.[1,2] Eighty percent of CVD deaths occur in low-income and middle-income countries (LMICs) and predominantly affects a younger population compared with high-income countries (HICs), thus having a significant impact on the economic growth of LMICs.[1,3] The mortality burden from CVD is projected to increase in LMICs alongside the lifestyle-associated epidemiologic shift favoring noncommunicable disease development.[4] The associated economic losses are also expected to reach billions of dollars over the next decade, representing yet another barrier to development for LMICs.[3] Although CVD prevention and treatment guidelines are available, translating these into practice is hampered in LMICs by inadequate health care systems with limited access to potentially lifesaving medications.[5]

Enumerating the barriers to access to CVD medicines requires an examination of both the "policy-level" barriers and "on-the-ground" issues. At the policy level, limited national funding due to competing health priorities, slow incorporation of CVD drugs into the essential medicines list (EML), and structural and financial barriers all limit access to CVD drugs and have been discussed previously with recommendations proposed.[6,7] Advocacy to create awareness among policy makers on the threat of CVDs to LMIC populations' health and economic prosperity will increase funding and foster equitable access through inclusion of more CVD drugs into the EML. Overcoming legal barriers in patent law will expedite generic availability to increase affordability with streamlined global and local procurement practices further bringing down the cost of CVD drugs in the public sector. Finally, engaging the commercial sector so as to regulate markup on CVD drugs will minimize out-of-pocket expenses for patients.[6,7]

Despite the frequent emphasis on policy-level considerations for increasing CVD medication access, the rate-limiting steps rest within the health care system's supply chain. This is the focus of our review paper.[3,8] Dismal drug availability for medicines for the prevention and treatment of CVD in public facilities in LMICs forces patients to turn to private chemists, where costs of medication are often unaffordable.[9–11] Systemic deficiencies and inefficiencies in medicine regulation and distribution have led to a rampant counterfeit medicines burden in LMICs.[12] These deficiencies together contribute to the mortality and morbidity imposed on LMIC populations.[13]

In this review article, we describe the deficiencies in the current LMIC supply chains that limit access to effective CVD medicines, and discuss existing solutions that are translatable to other low-resource settings to address these deficiencies.

CHALLENGES

We identified 3 primary barriers ("3A" challenges) in the health care system supply chain that coexist to limit access to essential CVD medicines (**Fig. 1**) The challenges are dismal *availability of* medicines, lack of *accountability* in the supply chain, and poor medication *adherence*.

Availability

A reliable supply chain system is crucial to achieve consistent availability of essential medicines.[14] Patients with CVD, or at risk for CVD, often require lifelong medicines for the treatment and prevention of CVD events. Therefore, functional CVD medicine supply chains are crucial to improve global cardiovascular health. Unfortunately, several analyses demonstrated that availability of CVD medicines across many LMIC settings is suboptimal.[7] In 2007, a cross-sectional study investigating CVD medicines in 6 LMICs revealed a less than 7.5% availability of medicines in the public sector.[10] In 2011, World Health Organization/Health Action International data of 36 countries revealed that the overall availability of these medicines was still poor, representing a mean availability of 26% in the public sector.[15] Recently, the 2016 Prospective Urban Rural Epidemiology (PURE) study showed availability of CVD medications ranged from 3% to 73% and 25% to 80% in rural and urban LMIC settings, respectively.[16]

To understand the persistently low availability rates of CVD medicines in LMICs, we analyze practical challenges with a focus on the public sector's supply chains that lead to weak supply chain design, poor operating performance, and low access for patients who need these medicines.

Within the public sector of most LMICs, the government procures medications and distributes them to other health facilities using the government Central Medical Store (CMS).[17,18] The CMS is responsible for distributing medicines to district facilities, and they, in turn, supply medicines to the subdistrict clinics.[17,18] One of the challenges faced in these settings is the unnecessary complexity of supply chain design, because most LMICs include multiple tiers of stock management before medicines can reach the intended

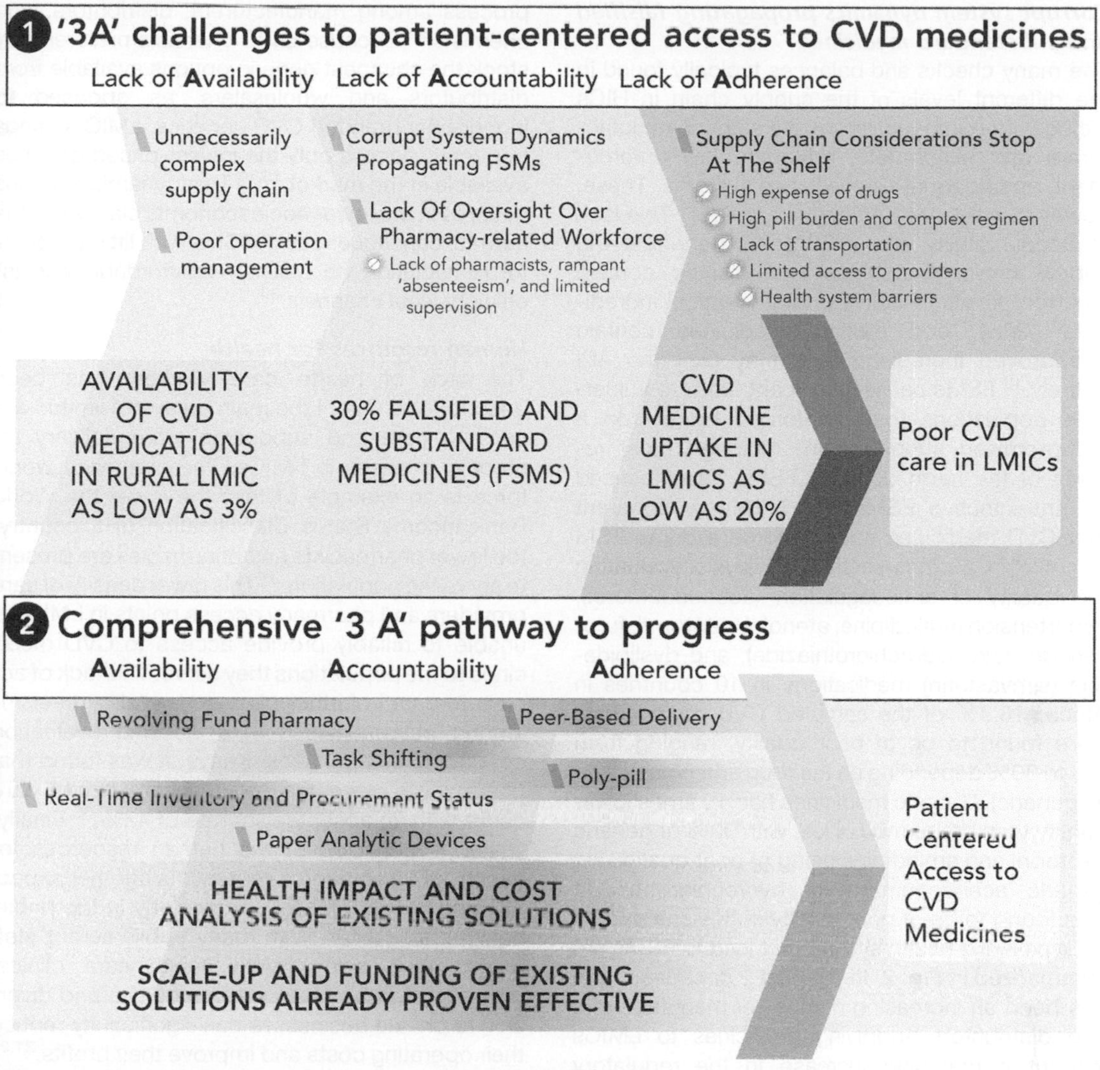

① '3A' challenges to patient-centered access to CVD medicines

Lack of **A**vailability   Lack of **A**ccountability   Lack of **A**dherence

Unnecessarily complex supply chain	Corrupt System Dynamics Propagating FSMs	Supply Chain Considerations Stop At The Shelf
Poor operation management	Lack Of Oversight Over Pharmacy-related Workforce	● High expense of drugs
	● Lack of pharmacists, rampant 'absenteeism', and limited supervision	● High pill burden and complex regimen
		● Lack of transportation
		● Limited access to providers
		● Health system barriers

AVAILABILITY OF CVD MEDICATIONS IN RURAL LMIC AS LOW AS 3%	30% FALSIFIED AND SUBSTANDARD MEDICINES (FSMS)	CVD MEDICINE UPTAKE IN LMICS AS LOW AS 20%	Poor CVD care in LMICs

② Comprehensive '3 A' pathway to progress

Availability   **A**ccountability   **A**dherence

Revolving Fund Pharmacy   Peer-Based Delivery

Task Shifting

Real-Time Inventory and Procurement Status   Poly-pill

Paper Analytic Devices

HEALTH IMPACT AND COST ANALYSIS OF EXISTING SOLUTIONS

SCALE-UP AND FUNDING OF EXISTING SOLUTIONS ALREADY PROVEN EFFECTIVE

Patient Centered Access to CVD Medicines

Fig. 1. The 3A challenges of access to CVD medicines and the comprehensive 3A pathway to progress to improve patient-centered access.

patient.[17,18] Because the CMS is responsible only for distributing medicines to district facilities, other subdistrict facilities may fall under the supervision of other departments in the Ministry of Health. Diffuse accountability, defined as "fragmentation of responsibility and governance," occurs when this supply chain structure is followed, as exemplified in countries like Ethiopia, Kenya, Mozambique, and Zambia.[17] Together with poor communication, these factors lead to long intervals between medicine resupply and distorted information about patient demand.[19]

Poor operational management also accounts for the low availability of medicines in the public sector. There is insufficient interest in investing in operating costs, such as drug distribution, leading to medicines not being delivered to designated

health facilities in a timely manner.[17,20] The inability to capture up-to-date consumption data also prohibits adequate planning for procurement and resupply.[20] Additionally, the lack of evaluation and feedback for supply chain management staff creates minimal incentives for performance improvement and requires little accountability in job performance.[17,20]

Accountability

Lack of accountability in the LMIC supply chain has hampered access to high-quality medicines for CVD.[17,21,22] In this section, we focus on (1) the corrupt system dynamics that propagate falsified and substandard medicines (FSM), and (2) the lack of oversight over pharmacy-related human resources for health.

Corrupt system dynamics propagating falsified and substandard medicines

The many checks and balances typically found in the different levels of the supply chain in HICs include adequate regulatory oversight of manufacturers and distributors, adequate law enforcement, and adequate surveillance systems. These, however, are largely absent in LMICs.[12] This lack of accountability allows FSMs to penetrate the supply chain. Substandard medicines contain incorrect levels of active pharmaceutical ingredients (APIs), and falsified medicines contain unapproved ingredients and may lack the API entirely.[12] FSMs cause significant harm to vulnerable populations that are forced to rely on a compromised supply chain. Although most reports of the harm done by FSMs have focused on anti-infective FSMs,[23–25] it is now apparent that CVD medicines have become a prime FSM target.[26] In a cross-sectional analysis evaluating the quality of anticoagulation (acenocoumarol), hypertension (amlodipine, atenolol, captopril, furosemide, and hydrochlorothiazide), and dyslipidemia (simvastatin) medications in 10 countries in Africa, 16.3% of the sampled CVD medications were found to be of poor quality, ranging from 0% to 30% depending on the drug and type (brand vs generic). Generic medicines had 10 times lower quality than brand medicines, with 30% of generic captopril and amlodipine being of poor quality. No generic acenocoumarol or hydrochlorothiazide was found to be of poor quality in this study.[26]

Gaps in the health system that lead to FSMs are summarized in **Fig. 2**. In the past 2 decades, there has been an increasing number of manufacturers and distributors supplying medicines to LMICs without a matching increase in the regulatory infrastructure in the industry. From 1995 to 2006, there was a 50% growth in spending for pharmaceuticals worldwide.[18] This increase in demand has been met with a dramatic increase in the production of medications, especially in LMICs like India, in which the pharmaceutical industry is valued at more than $24 billion.[18] Despite this, public health expenditure in sub-Saharan Africa was still below the 15% expenditure recommended by the World Health Organization's (WHO) Abuja Declaration, resulting in a constrained pool of resources allocated to regulatory activities.[27] Furthermore, as wholesalers and distributors purchase medicines from a wide variety of sources at the lowest cost, including informal suppliers who typically circumvent the registration process,[28] they risk buying medicines of compromised quality.[26] Additionally, reports have highlighted the high potential for corruption as different stakeholders try to circumvent the numerous steps involved with the procurement

process among manufacturers, distributors, and chemists.[29] Because LMIC chemists preferentially stock the cheapest generic options available from distributors and wholesalers, as opposed to higher-cost branded CVD generics, LMIC settings frequently access only the lowest-priced generics available in the market.[15,16] This dynamic exposes patients in the lower socioeconomic classes to the harmful consequences of FSMs with little potential for remediation via typically unaffordable and inefficient legal channels.[30]

Human resources for health

The lack of health care workers has been described as one of the main drivers of limited access to care and suboptimal care delivery for chronic diseases in LMICs. The pharmacy workforce is an example of this; the lower the World Bank Income Status Classification of a country, the fewer pharmacists and pharmacies are present to serve the population.[31] This lower density of care providers and pharmacy access points in LMICs is unable to reliably provide access to CVD medicines to the populations they serve. This lack of access to care is further plagued by "absenteeism" among pharmacists.[32] In a detailed evaluation conducted in Machakos, Kenya, it was found that pharmacists were the most absent health care cadre with an absenteeism rate of 42%.[33] Finally, limited supervision of the human resources for health (HRH) workforce represents another aspect of limited accountability, particularly in the public health care sector. With many public sector staff having their own private health care clinics, pilferage of public sector commodities and diversion to private businesses can significantly reduce their operating costs and improve their profits.[21,22] The lack of accountability described in this section highlights the current supply chain dynamics in which the different stakeholders consistently prioritize their own interests above the interests of the patient. As we continue to push for more impactful service delivery, we must shift to a more patient-centered approach.

Adherence

Functional medicine supply chains are fundamental to ensuring access to health care services in LMICs.[14,34] Traditionally, access has been narrowly defined as the ability or opportunity of a population to enter into the health care system and be able to obtain health care goods and services.[35,36] This defines access solely from the health-system perspective, with a focus on "supply"-side factors. In this view, a medicine supply chain may be deemed to be successful in providing access to essential medicines for a

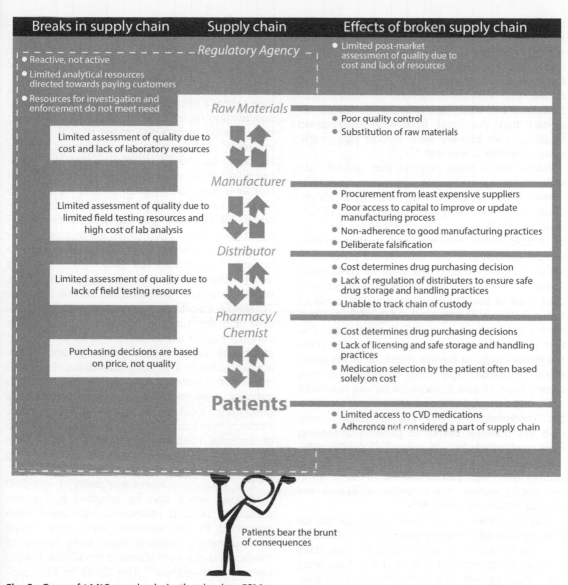

Breaks in supply chain	Supply chain	Effects of broken supply chain

Regulatory Agency
- Reactive, not active
- Limited analytical resources directed towards paying customers
- Resources for investigation and enforcement do not meet need

- Limited post-market assessment of quality due to cost and lack of resources

Raw Materials

Limited assessment of quality due to cost and lack of laboratory resources

- Poor quality control
- Substitution of raw materials

Manufacturer

Limited assessment of quality due to limited field testing resources and high cost of lab analysis

- Procurement from least expensive suppliers
- Poor access to capital to improve or update manufacturing process
- Non-adherence to good manufacturing practices
- Deliberate falsification

Distributor

Limited assessment of quality due to lack of field testing resources

- Cost determines drug purchasing decision
- Lack of regulation of distributers to ensure safe drug storage and handling practices
- Unable to track chain of custody

Pharmacy/ Chemist

Purchasing decisions are based on price, not quality

- Cost determines drug purchasing decisions
- Lack of licensing and safe storage and handling practices
- Medication selection by the patient often based solely on cost

Patients

- Limited access to CVD medications
- Adherence not considered a part of supply chain

Patients bear the brunt of consequences

Fig. 2. Gaps of LMIC supply chain that lead to FSMs.

population, by making medicines available and affordable, while ignoring a host of "demand"-side, patient-level factors including medication utilization and adherence.[35,37–39] This approach leaves the most important stakeholder, the patient, out of the picture when it comes to designing, implementing, and evaluating supply chains. If we are to reach our goals of reducing the burden of CVD in LMICs, then ensuring the uptake and adherence by patients must be part of our evaluation framework. Within this framework, the successful supply chain does not end with the delivery of essential medicines to the pharmacy or clinic; it ends with the patient actually taking those medicines consistently and realizing improved health outcomes.

Combination therapy with essential CVD medicines reduces primary and secondary coronary heart disease events by 80%.[40] Unfortunately, adherence to these medicines is low. When assessing the appropriateness of prescriptions for CVD medications from the health care provider perspective, studies have shown that there may be a low level of uptake of evidence-based recommendations by clinicians. In the WHO Prevention of Recurrences of Myocardial Infarction and Stroke (PREMISE) study, evidence-based medicines for secondary prevention of CVDs were inadequately prescribed in LMICs.[41] Aspirin was prescribed for only 79.6% of patients, beta-blockers for 44.2%, angiotensin-converting enzyme inhibitors for 39.5%, and statins for 19.6%. Another recent study found that heart failure treatment patterns in rural Kenya are poor, with only 55% of patients with dilated cardiomyopathy taking angiotensin-converting enzyme inhibitors, 45% taking beta-blockers, and 23% taking digoxin.[42] A systematic review that examined barriers to hypertension treatment by health care providers in LMICs reported that the most frequently encountered health-system barriers were lack of equipment, space, medicine, and staff.[43]

There are 5 main reasons that patients do not adhere to medication regimens: socioeconomic, medication-related, condition-related, health-system–related, and patient-related factors. In LMICs, socioeconomic factors (ie, cost of medications) and medicine-related factors (ie, pill burden and side effects) are particularly salient in determining adherence to CVD medicines.[44] Three potential costs (transportation, user fees to see the clinician, and the costs of the medicines themselves) all hinder patients from adhering to essential CVD medicines. The first and most obvious cost barrier is the price the patient pays to buy the medicine at the pharmacy. In LMICs, high prices of medicines have clearly been shown to decrease patient purchase and, therefore, uptake and adherence to essential medicines.[10,15,43,45] Transportation costs also are a major barrier to patients accessing care, particularly in rural areas.[43,46] Additionally, many patients in LMICs have to pay out-of-pocket user fees just to see clinicians, even in the public sector, which further increases the cost of accessing care.[47,48]

The complexity of the treatment regimen for primary and secondary prevention of CVDs can be overwhelming to many patients. The daily number of prescribed pills and the frequency with which patients must remember to take their medicines are recognized as factors responsible for patients' lack of adherence.[44,49] Additionally, besides availability, the side effects of medications have been found to be the most common barrier to patients' adherence to treatment. When translated to clinical significance, side effects had a twofold increased risk of nonadherence.[43]

EXISTING SOLUTIONS

To address existing deficiencies in the LMIC supply chain, programs to ensure access to CVD medicines have been established. This section highlights examples that have evaluated access to CVD and non-CVD medicines from both the supply and demand perspectives, with measurable patient-centered outcomes.

Availability

The concept of "revolving drug funds" (RDF) dates back to 1989 when an RDF project was initiated in Ghana.[50] In an RDF, seed funding is used to purchase an initial stock of medicines, which are then sold at a price point sufficient to support staff salaries and replace the initial stock. Building on the experiences and successes of RDF projects in other LMICs,[51,52] the Academic Model Providing Access To Healthcare (AMPATH) program in western Kenya created a network of revolving fund pharmacies (RFPs) in 2011 to address availability of affordable essential medicines. RFPs serve as "back-up pharmacies" when government pharmacies are unable to supply essential medicines, including CVD drugs, to patients.[53] Medicines are sold by RFPs with a small markup (10%), and the net profit earned is used to ensure an uninterrupted source of drugs. To ensure that medicines are consistently available and the patients' demand is met, RFPs conduct regular needs assessments (ie, frequent stock-take audits) to forecast usage and ensure accountability in their daily operations. They also developed a waiver system to enable access to indigent patients, and expanded to multiple geographic locations to meet patients' needs. Findings from this pilot study showed an increase of essential medicine availability to more than 90%, with 40% of sales being attributed to chronic disease medicines.

Other efforts to address availability of non-CVD medicines, which can be adopted to improve availability of CVD medicines, also have been described in the literature. New and simple communication methods have been tested to monitor and distribute stocks of medicines, specifically in rural settings.[54] The "SMS for Life" program in rural Tanzania is an example of a replicable technological advancement used to improve supply of antimalarial medicines.[54] Using widely available Short Message Service (SMS) technology, the implementers created an inventory tracking application that could geographically map medicine availability at all facilities in their network. With this system, medicine stock-outs were reduced from 78% to 26%.[54] Implementation and evaluation of health information systems to improve real-time communication of consumption rate, inventory, and procurement status should be encouraged to improve availability of medicines.

Accountability

To address the quality assurance of medicines in LMICs, several technologies have been developed to detect FSMs in these settings, including methods to analyze drug formulations.[55] Technologies suitable for LMICs allow for detection of correct API at a low cost, require no sample preparation, and can be performed outside a laboratory setting. A practical example of how these technologies may be carried out is an ongoing multi-country evaluation of Paper Analytical Devices, also known as PADs. PADs are paper cards that carry out a library of colorimetric tests to rapidly and qualitatively detect falsified medicines (**Fig. 3**). Studies using PADs to test for low-quality antimalarial, antimicrobial, and antituberculosis medicines have confirmed the high sensitivity and specificity of these devices.[56] To address the growing problems with CVD medicines, PADs have recently been formulated to test for commonly used CVD medications. Confirmatory testing with standard instrumental methods is used to follow up on suspicious products and detect FSMs.

Task shifting has been suggested as an important strategy to address the HRH shortage in LMICs that hampers CVD management.[57] Task shifting is described as the rational redistribution of tasks within the health workforce to more efficiently use the limited HRH to improve patient care.[58] To date, 4 randomized controlled trials conducted in LMICs have demonstrated the effectiveness of using nonphysician health workers to manage patients with post–acute coronary syndrome, hypertension, or diabetes.[59] These programs, led by clinically trained nurses, pharmacists, and community health workers, demonstrated an improvement in adherence to lifesaving CVD medicines, a significant reduction in blood pressure, and a reduction in glycated hemoglobin at a fraction of the cost anticipated with physician-based health care delivery.[60–63] Another study examining linkage and retention to hypertension care using community health workers in Kenya is in progress.[64]

Adherence

Holistic, patient-centered interventions have been shown to improve medication adherence. For human immunodeficiency virus, medication delivery by peer counselors was found to be more effective in improving adherence than directly observed antiretroviral therapy.[65] Similarly, in managing CVDs, the use of a multidisciplinary team of other nonphysician care providers demonstrated improved medication adherence and reduction in low-density lipoprotein cholesterol.[66]

To address adherence as one of the dimensions of supply chain management, several trials examined the effects of improved adherence on strengthening access to CVD medicines. The use of "polypills," also known as a fixed-dose, combination regimen, directly addresses the adherence barriers of regimen complexity and pill burden, and have been shown to increase patient adherence and reduce CVD events in patients with CVDs or who are at risk for CVDs.[67,68]

A few studies also showed discrepancies between evidence-based recommendations for heart failure and clinicians' prescribing patterns.[43] Strategies that have been proven to change health care professional behaviors and patient outcomes include financial incentives, audit and feedback, automated reminders, and educational outreach visits.[69] Using innovative models to address adherence from both the prescriber and patient standpoints is arguably one of the most effective solutions to improve patient-centered access to CVD medicines in LMICs.

FUTURE DIRECTIONS

CVD poses a significant public health threat to populations in LMICs that is expected to grow over the next decade.[2] CVD also imposes a significant economic burden on LMIC populations.[3] Improving access and uptake of CVD medicines is a crucial step to addressing this health and

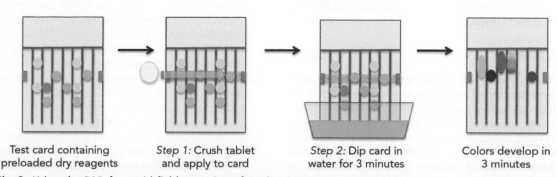

Test card containing preloaded dry reagents

Step 1: Crush tablet and apply to card

Step 2: Dip card in water for 3 minutes

Colors develop in 3 minutes

Fig. 3. Using the PAD for rapid field screening of medications.

development barrier. As discussed in this article, existing challenges in the LMIC CVD medication supply chain extend beyond previously described policy-level issues[6,7] and must include substantial "on-the-ground" deficiencies. To address these "on-the-ground" deficiencies and charter a path to improved access to CVD drugs for LMIC populations, we propose the comprehensive "3A" pathway to progress (see **Fig. 1**).

The first step is to scale up existing solutions that have already demonstrated effectiveness in addressing the "3A challenges" in the LMIC supply chain. We have highlighted examples of such context-specific solutions used in various LMIC settings and advocate that such solutions need to be scaled up to other regions and countries facing similar problems. Such solutions may need to be contextualized to address local problems and adhere to local policy frameworks so as to maximize impact, but we anticipate that the core principles and overall design will be maintained. For example, the RFP model has been demonstrated as a cost-effective solution that addresses drug availability by backing up public health facility pharmacies with affordably priced medicines.[53] Such a model may be replicated in countries facing similar problems in availability and affordability with modifications to align with local rules on pricing structures, pharmacy regulation agents, and governance of public-private partnerships.

Evaluation of the health impact and cost-effectiveness of these existing solutions is needed. A limitation of the discussed solutions is a lack of rigorous scientific evaluation to document their benefit over traditional supply chain models in LMICs. In resource-limited settings with many competing priorities, robust evidence that demonstrates clear patient-centered and economic benefits of an intervention would therefore be required to justify funding for scale up. As such, randomized and quasi-randomized trials should be conducted to identify solutions with the most significant health impact and cost-effectiveness. Although such efforts may require large resources up-front, we expect they would translate to cost savings through long-term health and economic improvements.

SUMMARY

In this review article, we described the "3A challenges," dismal *availability* to essential medicines, lack of *accountability* in the medication supply chain, and poor medication *adherence*, in the current LMIC supply chains that limit access to effective CVD care. The described existing solutions to ensure access to CVD medicines in LMIC settings can and should be applied in other

resource-limited settings; however, efforts to improve global access to CVD medicines must take into account health-system challenges. Innovation to find new patient-centered, cross-cutting, and context-specific solutions to the 3A challenges is therefore required in LMICs. Such innovations should address most or all of the 3A challenges discussed in this article, with a special emphasis on promoting patient adherence as part of the supply chain to maximize CVD outcomes.

REFERENCES

1. GBD 2013 Mortality and Causes of Death Collaborators. Global, regional, and national age-sex specific all-cause and cause-specific mortality for 240 causes of death, 1990-2013: a systematic analysis for the Global Burden of Disease Study 2013. Lancet 2015;385(9963):117–71.
2. Mathers CD, Loncar D. Projections of global mortality and burden of disease from 2002 to 2030. PLoS Med 2006;3(11):e442.
3. World Health Organization. Global status report on noncommunicable diseases 2014. Geneva (Switzerland): World Health Organization; 2014.
4. Yusuf S, Reddy S, Ounpuu S, et al. Global burden of cardiovascular diseases: part I: general considerations, the epidemiologic transition, risk factors, and impact of urbanization. Circulation 2001; 104(22):2746–53.
5. Fuster V, Kelly BB, Vedanthan R. Promoting global cardiovascular health: moving forward. Circulation 2011;123(15):1671–8.
6. Kishore SP, Kolappa K, Jarvis JD, et al. Overcoming obstacles to enable access to medicines for noncommunicable diseases in poor countries. Health Aff (Millwood) 2015;34(9):1569–77.
7. Kishore SP, Vedanthan R, Fuster V. Promoting global cardiovascular health ensuring access to essential cardiovascular medicines in low- and middle-income countries. J Am Coll Cardiol 2011;57(20): 1980–7.
8. Systems for Improved Access to Pharmaceuticals and Services (SIAPS). Enhancing health outcomes for chronic diseases in resource-limited settings by improving the use of medicines: the role of pharmaceutical care. Submitted to the U.S. Agency for International Development by the SIAPS Program. Arlington (VA): Management Sciences for Health; 2014.
9. Cameron A, Ewen M, Ross-Degnan D, et al. Medicine prices, availability, and affordability in 36 developing and middle-income countries: a secondary analysis. Lancet 2009;373(9659):240–9.
10. Mendis S, Fukino K, Cameron A, et al. The availability and affordability of selected essential medicines for chronic diseases in six low- and middle-income countries. Bull World Health Organ 2007;85(4):279–88.

11. Kankeu HT, Saksena P, Xu K, et al. The financial burden from non-communicable diseases in low- and middle-income countries: a literature review. Health Res Policy Syst 2013;11:31.

12. Almuzaini T, Choonara I, Sammons H. Substandard and counterfeit medicines: a systematic review of the literature. BMJ Open 2013;3(8):e002923.

13. Wirtz VJ, Kaplan WA, Kwan GF, et al. Access to medications for cardiovascular diseases in low- and middle-income countries. Circulation 2016; 133(21):2076–85.

14. Equitable access to essential medicines: a framework for collective action: WHO policy perspectives on medicines, No. 008, March 2004. Geneva (Switzerland): World Health Organization; 2004.

15. van Mourik MS, Cameron A, Ewen M, et al. Availability, price and affordability of cardiovascular medicines: a comparison across 36 countries using WHO/HAI data. BMC Cardiovasc Disord 2010;10:25.

16. Khatib R, McKee M, Shannon H, et al. Availability and affordability of cardiovascular disease medicines and their effect on use in high-income, middle-income, and low-income countries: an analysis of the PURE study data. Lancet 2016;387(10013): 61–9.

17. Yadav P. Health product supply chains in developing countries: diagnosis of the root causes of underperformance and an agenda for reform. Health Systems & Reform 2015;1(2):142–54.

18. Kaplan W, Mathers C. The world medicines situation 2011. 3rd edition. Geneva (Switzerland): World Health Organization; 2011.

19. Lee HL, Padmanabhan V, Whang S. The bullwhip effect in supply chains. Sloan Manage Rev 1997;38: 93–102.

20. Sarley D, Allain L, Akkihal A, et al. Estimating the global in-country supply chain costs of meeting the MDGs by 2015. Arlington (VA): USAID | DELIVER PROJECT; 2009. Task Order 1.

21. Bateman C. Drug stock-outs: inept supply-chain management and corruption. S Afr Med J 2013; 103(9):600–2.

22. Vian T. Review of corruption in the health sector: theory, methods and interventions. Health Policy Plan 2008;23(2):83–94.

23. Countering the problem of falsified and substandard drugs. Washington, DC: Institute of Medicine of the National Academies; 2013.

24. Nayyar GM, Breman JG, Newton PN, et al. Poor-quality antimalarial drugs in southeast Asia and sub-Saharan Africa. Lancet Infect Dis 2012;12(6): 488–96.

25. Newton PN, Green MD, Fernandez FM, et al. Counterfeit anti-infective drugs. Lancet Infect Dis 2006; 6(9):602–13.

26. Antignac M, Diop BI, Macquart De Terline D, et al. Quality assessment of 7 cardiovascular drugs in SubSaharan African countries: results of the seven study by drug and version of drug World Congress of Cardiology and Cardiovascular Health. Mexico City, Mexico, June 4–7, 2016.

27. Tumusiime P, Gonani A, Walker O, et al. Health systems in sub-Saharan Africa: what is their status and role in meeting the health Millennium Development Goals? African Health Monitor, Issue 14, March 2012.

28. Campos JE, Pradhan S. The many faces of corruption: tracking vulnerabilities at the sector level. Washington, DC: World Bank; 2007. License: CC BY 3.0 IGO. Available at: https://openknowledge. worldbank.org/handle/10986/6848.

29. Ho PM, Rumsfeld JS, Masoudi FA, et al. Effect of medication nonadherence on hospitalization and mortality among patients with diabetes mellitus. Arch Intern Med 2006;166(17):1836–41.

30. Fake medicines flood Kenyan market as experts warn of looming health crisis [press release]. Daily Nation; 2013.

31. Anderson C, Roy T. FIP Global Pharmacy Workforce Report. Netherlands: International Pharmaceutical Federation (FIP); 2012.

32. Chaudhury N, Hammer J, Kremer M, et al. Missing in action: teacher and health worker absence in developing countries. J Econ Perspect 2006; 20(1):91–116.

33. Deussom R, Jaskiewioz W, Dwyer S, et al. Absenteeism of health care providers in Machakos District, Kenya. Washington, DC: Institute of Policy Analysis and Research (IPAR); 2008. IPAR Policy Brief 12, no. 2.

34. Dowling P. Healthcare supply chains in developing countries: situational analysis. Arlington (VA): USAID | DELIVER PROJECT; 2011. Task Order 4.

35. Aday LA, Andersen R. A framework for the study of access to medical care. Health Serv Res 1974;9(3): 208–20.

36. Frenk J, White KL. The concept and measurement of accessibility. Washington, DC: Pan American Health Organization; 1992. p. 842–55.

37. Andersen RM. Revisiting the behavioral model and access to medical care: does it matter? J Health Soc Behav 1995;36(1):1–10.

38. Gulliford M, Figueroa-Munoz J, Morgan M, et al. What does 'access to health care' mean? J Health Serv Res Policy 2002;7(3):186–8.

39. Mooney GH. Equity in health care: confronting the confusion. Eff Health Care 1983;1(4):179–85.

40. Wald NJ, Law MR. A strategy to reduce cardiovascular disease by more than 80%. BMJ 2003; 326(7404):1419.

41. Mendis S, Abegunde D, Yusuf S, et al. WHO study on prevention of REcurrences of Myocardial Infarction and StrokE (WHO-PREMISE). Bull World Health Organ 2005;83(11):820–9.

42. Bloomfield GS, DeLong AK, Akwanalo CO, et al. Markers of atherosclerosis, clinical characteristics, and treatment patterns in heart failure: a case-control study of middle-aged adult heart failure patients in rural Kenya. Glob Heart 2016;11(1):97–107.

43. Khatib R, Schwalm JD, Yusuf S, et al. Patient and healthcare provider barriers to hypertension awareness, treatment and follow up: a systematic review and meta-analysis of qualitative and quantitative studies. PLoS One 2014;9(1):e84238.

44. Castellano JM, Copeland-Halperin R, Fuster V. Aiming at strategies for a complex problem of medical nonadherence. Glob Heart 2013;8(3):263–71.

45. Pandey KR, Meltzer DO. Financial burden and impoverishment due to cardiovascular medications in low and middle income countries: an illustration from India. PLoS One 2016;11(5):e0155293.

46. Ambaw AD, Alemie GA, W/Yohannes SM, et al. Adherence to antihypertensive treatment and associated factors among patients on follow up at University of Gondar Hospital, Northwest Ethiopia. BMC Public Health 2012;12:282.

47. Bhojani U, Thriveni B, Devadasan R, et al. Out-of-pocket healthcare payments on chronic conditions impoverish urban poor in Bangalore, India. BMC Public Health 2012;12:990.

48. McIntyre D, Thiede M, Dahlgren G, et al. What are the economic consequences for households of illness and of paying for health care in low- and middle-income country contexts? Soc Sci Med 2006;62(4):858–65.

49. Ho PM, Bryson CL, Rumsfeld JS. Medication adherence: its importance in cardiovascular outcomes. Circulation 2009;119(23):3028–35.

50. Garner P. The Bamako initiative. BMJ 1989; 299(6694):277–8.

51. Murakami H, Phommasack B, Oula R, et al. Revolving drug funds at front-line health facilities in Vientiane, Lao PDR. Health Policy Plan 2001;16(1): 98–106.

52. Uzochukwu BS, Onwujekwe OE, Akpala CO. Effect of the Bamako-Initiative drug revolving fund on availability and rational use of essential drugs in primary health care facilities in south-east Nigeria. Health Policy Plan 2002;17(4):378–83.

53. Manji I, Manyara SM, Jakait B, et al. The Revolving Fund Pharmacy Model: backing up the Ministry of Health supply chain in western Kenya. Int J Pharm Pract 2016;24:358–66.

54. Barrington J, Wereko-Brobby O, Ward P, et al. SMS for Life: a pilot project to improve anti-malarial drug supply management in rural Tanzania using standard technology. Malar J 2010;9:298.

55. Kovacs S, Hawes SE, Maley SN, et al. Technologies for detecting falsified and substandard drugs in low and middle-income countries. PLoS One 2014;9(3): e90601.

56. Paper Analytical Device Project. Available at: http://padproject.nd.edu/. Accessed June 5, 2016.

57. Joshi R, Alim M, Kengne AP, et al. Task shifting for non-communicable disease management in low and middle income countries—a systematic review. PLoS One 2014;9(8):e103754.

58. Task shifting: rational redistribution of tasks among health workforce teams. Geneva (Switzerland): World Health Organization; 2008.

59. Ogedegbe G, Gyamfi J, Plange-Rhule J, et al. Task shifting interventions for cardiovascular risk reduction in low-income and middle-income countries: a systematic review of randomised controlled trials. BMJ Open 2014;4(10):e005983.

60. Adeyemo A, Tayo BO, Luke A, et al. The Nigerian antihypertensive adherence trial: a community-based randomized trial. J Hypertens 2013;31(1): 201–7.

61. Mendis S, Johnston SC, Fan W, et al. Cardiovascular risk management and its impact on hypertension control in primary care in low-resource settings: a cluster-randomized trial. Bull World Health Organ 2010;88(6):412–9.

62. Nesari M, Zakerimoghadam M, Rajab A, et al. Effect of telephone follow-up on adherence to a diabetes therapeutic regimen. Jpn J Nurs Sci 2010;7(2): 121–8.

63. Xavier D, Gupta R, Kamath D, et al. Community health worker-based intervention for adherence to drugs and lifestyle change after acute coronary syndrome: a multicentre, open, randomised controlled trial. Lancet Diabetes Endocrinol 2016;4(3):244–53.

64. Vedanthan R, Kamano JH, Naanyu V, et al. Optimizing linkage and retention to hypertension care in rural Kenya (LARK hypertension study): study protocol for a randomized controlled trial. Trials 2014;15:143.

65. Ford N, Nachega JB, Engel ME, et al. Directly observed antiretroviral therapy: a systematic review and meta-analysis of randomised clinical trials. Lancet 2009;374(9707):2064–71.

66. Shaffer J, Wexler LF. Reducing low-density lipoprotein cholesterol levels in an ambulatory care system. Results of a multidisciplinary collaborative practice lipid clinic compared with traditional physician-based care. Arch Intern Med 1995;155(21):2330–5.

67. Lonn E, Bosch J, Teo KK, et al. The polypill in the prevention of cardiovascular diseases: key concepts, current status, challenges, and future directions. Circulation 2010;122(20):2078–88.

68. Yusuf S, Lonn E, Pais P, et al. Blood-pressure and cholesterol lowering in persons without cardiovascular disease. N Engl J Med 2016;374(21):2032–43.

69. Beran D, McCabe A, Yudkin JS. Access to medicines versus access to treatment: the case of type 1 diabetes. Bull World Health Organ 2008;86(8): 648–9.

Tuberculosis and the Heart

Arthur K. Mutyaba, MBChB, MMed, FCP(SA), Mpiko Ntsekhe, MD, PhD*

KEYWORDS

- Tuberculosis • Tuberculous pericarditis • Tuberculous myopericarditis • Tuberculous myocarditis
- Tuberculous aortitis

KEY POINTS

- Tuberculosis remains an important health problem of the developing world. Tuberculous heart disease is an important extrapulmonary manifestation of the disease.
- Tuberculous pericarditis occurs with higher frequency in individuals infected with the human immunodeficiency virus (HIV) and is characterized by differences in immune and clinical responses compared with HIV-negative individuals.
- A biomarker-based approach that uses pericardial fluid unstimulated interferon-γ, adenosine deaminase, and polymerase chain reaction offers a fast and reliable way of establishing the diagnosis.
- Four-drug antituberculous therapy is the mainstay of management for tuberculous pericarditis.
- Adjunctive steroid therapy has been shown to reduce hospitalization and progression to constrictive pericarditis, but not mortality; in HIV-positive patients, adjunctive steroids are associated with a higher incidence of malignancy.

 Video content accompanies this article at http://www.cardiology.theclinics.com.

INTRODUCTION

Recognized since antiquity, tuberculosis (TB) still contributes significantly to the global burden of disease, with an estimated 9.6 million new cases of the disease worldwide in 2014.[1] This is especially true in the developing world where human immunodeficiency virus (HIV) infection and AIDS, socioeconomic deprivation, and poor health systems infrastructure interact to make TB a significant public health problem.[2] Although it remains primarily a disease of the lungs, the classic lesion of TB—the acid fast *Mycobacterium tuberculosis* (Mtb) bacilli in a necrotic core bound by aggregates of various inflammatory cells (granuloma)—can be found in virtually any part of the body

(Fig. 1). Autopsy studies performed in the pre-HIV/AIDS era suggest that the heart is involved in approximately 2% of cases of patients who died from TB.[3] Similar studies of patients who died of TB and were coinfected with HIV demonstrate multisystemic dissemination in up to 80% of patients.[4,5] Of all the extrapulmonary manifestations of TB, involvement of the heart is second only to central nervous system TB in terms of its devastating morbidity and mortality.

It has been almost a decade since there was a comprehensive review of the main form of tuberculous heart disease.[6] That review focused on the pathogenesis, diagnosis, and management of tuberculous pericarditis and concluded by noting that there remained major gaps in our

The authors have nothing to disclose.
Division of Cardiology, Department of Medicine, Groote Schuur Hospital, University of Cape Town, E17 Cardiac Clinic, New Groote Schuur Hospital, Anzio Road, Observatory 7925, Cape Town, South Africa
* Corresponding author.
E-mail address: mpiko.ntsekhe@uct.ac.za

cardiology.theclinics.com

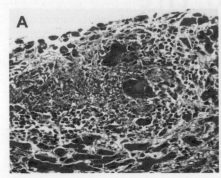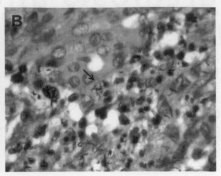

Fig. 1. *Mycobacterium tuberculosis*. Tuberculous granuloma (*A*) showing an aggregation of lymphocytes, monocytes, multinucleate giant cells with a central area of caseous necrosis. Ziehl-Neelsen stain (*B*) demonstrating acid-fast *M tuberculosis* (*arrow*). (*Courtesy of* Dr Craig Jamieson, formerly of Anatomical Pathology Department, University of Cape Town, Observatory, Cape Town, South Africa.)

understanding of the subject. The identified gaps included the need for improved diagnostic tools, a better understanding of the impact of HIV, and determination of the effectiveness of adjuvant therapy on clinical outcomes.[6] Since then, much data, predominantly from sub-Saharan Africa, have been generated to address some of these gaps. An updated comprehensive overview of TB and the heart with a summary of the new insights is therefore timely and hopefully of value to the general physician and cardiologist on the front lines of patient care.

The search strategy for this review involved a comprehensive search of MEDLINE, EMBASE and the Cochrane library of systematic reviews with the MeSH terms: "tuberculosis and the heart," "cardiac tuberculosis," "cardiovascular tuberculosis," "myopericarditis and tuberculosis," "tuberculous pericarditis," "tuberculous aortitis," and "HIV and the heart" from January 2005 to December 2015. The reference lists of selected articles were searched for articles deemed to be of relevance to the subject. Appropriate English language studies were retrieved and reviewed.

There have been a number of important advances in our understanding of tuberculous pericarditis over the last decade. Most of the new information has been generated from sub-Saharan Africa and Asia, where TB is endemic, HIV is epidemic, and the majority of patients with TB are also coinfected with HIV.[2] The *I*nvestigation of the *M*anagement of *P*ericarditis in Africa (IMPI) registry was a prospective observational cohort of consecutive patients with suspected TB pericarditis across multiple sites in sub-Saharan Africa. Important questions related to the immunopathogenesis, clinical manifestations, diagnosis, and outcomes of TB pericarditis in the HIV era were investigated in the registry.[7–18]

The IMPI immunotherapy trial was a double-blind, randomised control trial of 1400 patients with definite or probable TB pericarditis who were randomised to receive adjunctive corticosteroids or *Mycobacterium indicus pranii* versus placebo in a 2 × 2 factorial design.[19] These studies, which were conducted between 2004 and 2015, form the backbone of new insights gained since 2005.

There are 3 predominant clinical manifestations of tuberculous heart disease. In descending order of frequency, these include TB pericarditis, myocardial TB with or without aneurysm formation, and TB aortitis with or without mycotic aneurysms and pseudoaneurysms involving the aortic valve and/or sinuses of Valsalva. Important clinical, diagnostic, and management aspects of each are reviewed.

TUBERCULOUS PERICARDITIS

Tubercle bacilli access the pericardium via 3 main mechanisms. These include retrograde lymphatic spread from mediastinal, paratracheal and peribronchial lymph nodes,[20] hematogenous spread (dominant in immunocompromised hosts),[21] and, rarely, direct contiguous spread from adjacent structures such as the lungs, pleura, and spine.[20] In the presence of a competent immune system, tuberculous pericardial disease is usually localized to the pericardial space. It is typically a paucibacillary condition; tubercle proteins trigger a vigorous cell-mediated hypersensitivity response with T-helper cell (subtype 1) predominant cytokine release, leading to an inflammatory exudative effusion and its hemodynamic sequelae.[6] In patients with dysfunctional immunity as occurs in HIV/AIDS, there is evidence that mycobacterial replication is active, bacillary loads are high, and the clinical manifestations of tuberculous pericarditis are related to the impact of the infectious and virulent nature of the Mtb itself in addition to the hemodynamic sequelae.[13,21] Tuberculous pericarditis typically presents as 1 of 4 clinical syndromes, namely, acute pericarditis, effusive pericarditis and its complications, myopericarditis, and constrictive pericarditis. Although it is convenient to review them as distinct clinical entities, it is important to understand that there is much overlap in the clinical manifestations.

The triad of severe pericarditic chest pain, a pericardial friction rub, widespread ST-segment and T wave abnormalities and PR segment depression typical of acute pericarditis is an uncommon clinical presentation of tuberculous pericarditis, accounting for only 3% to 8% of patients who present with tuberculous pericarditis.[7,19] The syndrome is thought to occur soon after inoculation of tubercle bacilli into the pericardium, and is characterized pathologically by polymorphonuclear leukocytosis with abundant bacilli and granuloma formation.[3,20] The diagnosis of a tuberculous etiology depends on the presence of constitutional symptoms, lack of evidence of conventional bacterial infection, and the demonstration of concurrent TB infection elsewhere in the body; easily accessible pericardial fluid is typically absent in acute pericarditis. The resolution of symptoms with initiation of empiric antituberculous therapy in TB endemic areas is also suggestive.[6] A diagnostic index score that uses 6 clinical and laboratory variables has been developed for use in endemic areas.[22] These variables and their weighted score are outlined in **Table 1**. A summed score of 6 or more has a sensitivity of 86% and specificity of 85% for the diagnosis of tuberculous pericarditis.[22] Acute tuberculous pericarditis is managed in similar fashion to effusive tuberculous pericarditis as discussed elsewhere in this article.

Effusive pericarditis is the commonest form of pericardial TB in patients with and without HIV.[6] In the developing world, 40% to 70% of large pericardial effusions are tuberculous in origin.[18,23,24] This is in contrast with the developed world, where less than 4% of cases are tuberculous.[25] The clinical presentation of this group of patients is determined by the rate of fluid accumulation, magnitude of pericardial fluid-induced cardiac compression, and the severity of the inflammation, edema, and loss of visceral pericardial compliance.[14,26] Where cardiac compression is significant or rapid, cardiac filling and stroke volume can be compromised significantly. If hemodynamic compensatory mechanisms are adequate, the symptoms are usually those of congestive heart failure without hypotension, and the clinical signs those of a large pericardial effusion[24,27] (**Table 2**). Where pericardial fluid accumulation is relatively quick and compensatory mechanisms are inadequate, patients present with evidence of hypotension and tachycardia typical of tamponade.[26] A subset of patients may have sizable effusions with little evidence of cardiac compression, such that the constitutional symptoms of active TB predominate and the effusion may be an incidental finding (Videos 1 and 2). Where the visceral pericardium is rendered noncompliant by inflammation and postinfectious injury, patients present with a combination of the compressive hemodynamics of tamponade and the physiology of constrictive pericarditis-a syndrome aptly termed effusive constrictive pericarditis.[14,28,29] Invasive hemodynamic studies suggests that effusive constrictive pericarditis is common in patients with TB

Table 1
Tuberculous pericarditis diagnostic index

Variable	Score
Night sweats	1
Weight loss	1
Fever >38°C	2
White cell count <10 × 10⁹	3
Serum globulin > 40 g/L	3

Summed score of 6 or more is suggestive of tuberculous etiology for pericardial effusion.
Data from Reuter H, Burgess L, van Vuuren W, et al. Diagnosing tuberculous pericarditis. QJM 2006;99(12):827–39.

Table 2
Clinical signs observed in 88 patients with effusive tuberculous pericarditis

Physical Sign	Prevalence, n (%)
Sinus tachycardia	68 (77)
Pulsus paradoxus (>12 mm Hg)	32 (36)
Raised central venous pressure	74 (88)
Palpable apical impulse	53 (60)
Increased cardiac dullness	83 (94)
Muffled heart sounds	69 (78)
Pericardial friction rub	16 (18)
Hepatomegaly	84 (95)
Ascites	64 (73)
Peripheral edema	22 (25)
Tamponade	3 (3)

Data from Strang JIG. Tuberculous pericarditis in Transkei. Clin Cardiol 1984;7(12):667–70.

pericarditis occurring in up to 50% of cases.[14] The implication of a diagnosis of effusive constrictive pericarditis is not clear, although there are some observational data to suggest that long-term outcomes may be worse.[29,30] Chest radiography, an electrocardiogram, and echocardiography remain essential clinical aids in the evaluation and management of patients with suspected effusive TB pericarditis. The characteristic findings are shown in **Box 1**. Echocardiography is especially important to confirm the presence and determine the size of the effusion and its suitability for safe diagnostic or therapeutic pericardiocentesis.[31]

The early and accurate diagnosis of a tuberculous etiology of pericardial effusion has remained an important obstacle to optimal patient care. Although empiric therapy in high TB prevalence parts of the world has been advocated by some, it is important to recognize that the price to pay for missing treatable alternative causes is high.[32] Traditionally, the definitive diagnosis of tuberculous pericarditis depends on the demonstration of tubercle bacilli in the pericardial fluid or tissue by either direct examination or culture.[22,27,33] This approach yields a positive diagnosis in 57% of patients in historical series and in less than 20% of patients in contemporary series.[19,27,34] The most recent advance in the diagnosis of TB pericarditis relates to the usefulness of unstimulated gamma interferon (uIFN-γ, a pericardial fluid biomarker of TB infection) and polymerase chain reaction–based methods of identifying Mtb

genetic material in pericardial fluid. Pandie and colleagues[18] compared the accuracy of the Xpert Mtb/RIF quantitative polymerase chain reaction assay to pericardial fluid adenosine deaminase (ADA) and uIFN-γ measurement in the diagnosis of tuberculous pericarditis. Using a cutoff value of 44 pg/mL, uIFN-γ had a sensitivity and specificity of 95.7% and 96.3%, respectively, for a diagnosis of TB, making it superior to both Xpert Mtb/RIF (sensitivity, 63.8%; specificity, 100%) and ADA at a cutoff value of 35 IU/L (sensitivity, 95.7%; specificity, 84%).[18] Despite the superiority of pericardial fluid uIFN-γ over both ADA and Xpert Mtb/RIF as a diagnostic biomarker of tuberculous pericarditis, its widespread use in clinical practice is hindered by its high cost. Given the low yield from fluid culture and the proven usefulness of modern diagnostic biomarkers, the modern diagnostic strategy in patients with suspected TB pericarditis in TB endemic areas should be to (1) exclude alternative deadly causes of an inflammatory exudative effusion (eg, bacterial, malignant, and uremic pericarditis), (2) use biomarkers of TB such as pericardial fluid uIFN-γ and ADA, (3) confirm TB at sites other than the pericardium (eg, sputum, lymph nodes, pleural or ascitic fluid), and (4) have a low threshold to treat for TB where no obvious alternative is apparent and the clinical picture fits.[18,31,35]

Although the safety and efficacy of a 6-month course of 4-drug antituberculous chemotherapy in the management of effusive tuberculous pericarditis has long been established, the role of adjunctive therapies in improving survival and pericarditis-related outcomes has been unclear until recently.[36–38] The results of the adequately powered IMPI Immunotherapy trial have provided the best evidence to date that, although adjunctive steroids decrease the incidence of constrictive pericarditis and subsequent rehospitalization by close to 45%, they do not reduce mortality rates compared with placebo.[19] In patients who were infected with HIV, steroids were associated with an increase in incidence of HIV-related malignancies, making firm recommendations about their use in this subset of patients difficult.[19] Other adjunctive therapies whose efficacy has been tested include *Mycobacterium indicus pranii*, which was neutral in the IMPI immunotherapy trial[19]; intrapericardial corticosteroids, which are neutral[39]; intrapericardial thrombolysis, which has shown promising results in a small case series[40]; and routine pericardial evacuation, which is recommended by most authorities.[31,41] Given the very close association of tuberculous pericarditis and HIV,[2] patients in whom the diagnosis is suspected should undergo HIV testing with the

---

Box 1
Clinical diagnostic aids and characteristic findings in tuberculous effusive pericarditis

Chest radiograph

Cardiomegaly, pulmonary infiltrates, pleural effusion, mediastinal lymphadenopathy

Electrocardiogram

Sinus tachycardia, diffuse ST-segment and T wave changes, QRS microvoltage, QRS alternans, atrial fibrillation

Echocardiogram

Pericardial effusion (with or without fibrin stranding), pericardial thickening, caval vessel distension with diminished inspiratory collapse,[a] paradoxic septal motion,[a] right atrial/ventricular diastolic collapse,[a] exaggerated respiratory transvalvular Doppler flow,[a] expiratory diastolic hepatic vein flow reversal[a]

[a] Indicative of cardiac tamponade.

intention of starting combination antiretroviral therapy where HIV coinfection is confirmed. Although direct comparisons are practically impossible to make, it is likely that the large difference in the use of combination antiretroviral therapy in the IMPI immunotherapy trial versus the IMPI registry (>70% vs <10%)[7,19] had a significant bearing on the large differences in survival in those who were HIV infected in the 2 studies.

The natural history of patients with effusive pericarditis is variable and the clinical course in the individual patient unpredictable. Short-term complications include tamponade; the main longer term complication is fibrotic fusion of the 2 layers of the pericardium and the development of constrictive pericarditis. In the anti-TB therapy only arm of the 1400 patient IMPI Immunotherapy trial where close to 60% of participants underwent pericardiocentesis, approximately 18% of patients were dead at 12 months, 8% progressed to develop constrictive pericarditis, 4% had a reaccumulation of the pericardial effusion with the development of tamponade, and 40% to 60% recovered fully with no long-term clinical sequelae.[19] Data from the IMPI registry suggests that the disease may present more aggressively in patients who are HIV infected as this group of patients tend to have more significant dyspnea (New York Heart Association functional classes III and IV), hemodynamic instability, and more evidence of myocardial involvement compared with their HIV-uninfected age- and sex-matched controls.[8] Finally, data from the IMPI registry suggest that the incidence of constrictive pericarditis may be significantly lower in HIV-infected participants; an explanation for this observation remains to be elucidated.[10]

The diagnosis of posttuberculous constrictive pericarditis requires a combination of a high index of suspicion, meticulous clinical evaluation for what are often subtle signs (**Table 3**), and integration of data from imaging (echocardiography, computed tomography, MRI; **Fig. 2**), and, occasionally, invasive hemodynamic evaluation.[31,42] Once the diagnosis of constrictive pericarditis has been made, establishing a tuberculous etiology is less straightforward (**Fig. 3**). This is because a significant proportion of patients present for the first time with established constriction and have no prior history of TB.[15] Whether or not a course of anti-TB therapy is required in these patients who do not have evidence of active TB is not known. Where there are recent symptoms or signs of TB or microscopic evaluation of postoperative pericardial tissue reveals active inflammation, an empiric course of anti-TB therapy is reasonable.[6,38] However, where this evidence of active TB is absent, there is little evidence of any benefit.

Table 3 Clinical signs observed in 67 patients with tuberculous constrictive pericarditis	
Physical Sign	Prevalence, n (%)
Sinus tachycardia	47 (70)
Pulsus paradoxus (>12 mm Hg)	32 (48)
Increased central venous pressure	67 (100)
Palpable apical impulse	39 (58)
Increased cardiac dullness	17 (25)
Pericardial knock	14 (21)
Muffled heart sounds	51 (76)
Sudden inspiratory S2[a] split	24 (36)
Third heart sound	30 (45)
Hepatomegaly	67 (100)
Ascites	60 (89)
Peripheral edema	63 (94)

[a] S2 – Second heart sound.
Data from Strang JIG. Tuberculous pericarditis in Transkei. Clin Cardiol 1984;7(12):667–70.

The only definitive treatment for tuberculous constrictive pericarditis remains surgical pericardiectomy, even though it is associated with a perioperative mortality of between 5% and 14%.[15,43]

In some instances of tuberculous pericarditis, the underlying myocardium can become inflamed and edematous as a complication of the disease process.[44] Evidence for this myopericarditis takes the form of elevated biomarkers of myocardial injury (troponins, creatinine kinase, etc), dynamic electrocardiographic changes consistent with myocardial injury, and evidence of mild impairment of left ventricular systolic function by direct imaging.[31,44] Where cardiac MRI is available, gadolinium enhancement of both the pericardium and myocardium is characteristic of tuberculous myopericarditis (**Fig. 4**).[31] The sparse number of case reports in the literature suggests that myopericarditis is a rare complication of tuberculous pericarditis among HIV-negative, immunocompetent patients.[45–47] However, data from the IMPI registry suggests that, among HIV-infected patients with advanced immunosuppression and CD4 counts of less than 100 cells/μL, TB myopericarditis is much more common.[9] In a cross-sectional analysis of a subset of 81 patients in the registry, 53% had evidence of myopericarditis.[9] There are no data to guide the management of this specific complication of effusive pericarditis, but the diagnosis does not seem to carry a significant adverse effect on survival.[9,44]

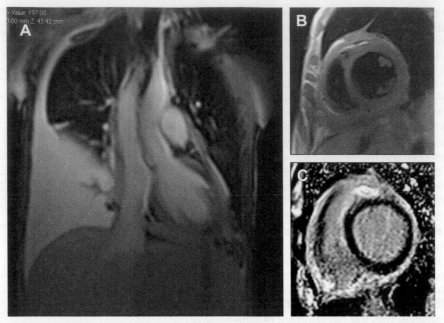

Fig. 2. Tuberculous constrictive pericarditis. A 31-year-old woman with right heart failure. Cardiac MR T1-weighted half Fourier acquisition single shot turbo spin echo image (*A*) showing large right pleural effusion, bilateral pulmonary interstitial changes, and fibrocavitatory lesions in the left lung apex and atelectasis of the right lower lobe. (*B*) Short T1 inversion recovery imaging with a normal myocardial signal intensity ratio, but a markedly thickened pericardium measuring 15 mm. (*C*) Enhancement after administration of gadolinium contrast. (*Courtesy of* Dr Ntobeko Ntusi, Division of Cardiology, Groote Schuur Hospital/University of Cape Town, Observatory, Cape Town, South Africa.)

TUBERCULOUS MYOCARDITIS

Tuberculous myocarditis (a separate entity from myopericarditis) is a very rare manifestation of cardiovascular TB with an occurrence rate of 0.14% in more than 13,000 autopsies performed over 27 years by Rose and colleagues.[48] Myocardial spread of TB is presumed to occur via mechanisms similar to those giving rise to TB pericarditis and aortitis. For reasons that are not clear, there is an apparent predilection to the right heart, particularly the right atrium.[49] Pathologically, it manifests as either nodular tuberculomas with central caseation, miliary tubercles of the heart, or a diffuse infiltrative pattern associated with pericarditis.[48] Case reports suggest that tuberculous

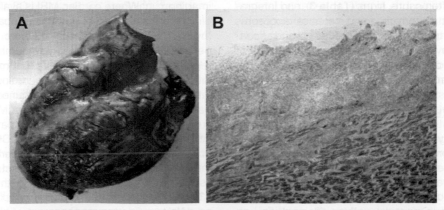

Fig. 3. Tuberculous constrictive pericarditis. (*A*) Postmortem macroscopic appearance showing pericardial thickening and adherence to myocardium. (*B*) Microscopic appearance of heart in *A* demonstrating a thickened and fibrotic pericardium with extension of fibrosis into the myocardium. (*Courtesy of* Dr Craig Jamieson, formerly of Anatomic Pathology Department, University of Cape Town, Observatory, Cape Town, South Africa.)

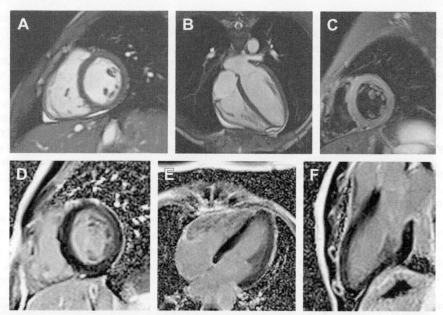

Fig. 4. A 16-year-old boy with disseminated tuberculosis (TB) with heart failure owing to TB myopericarditis. Cardiac MR steady state free precession images w (*A, B*) with short axis and horizontal long axis view showing small pericardial effusion; short T1 inversion recovery image (T2-weighted imaging) showing increased myocardial signal intensity ratio, in keeping with myocardial edema (*C*). Late gadolinium enhancement images showing midwall to subepicardial enhancement, in keeping with myocarditis (*D–F*); the pericardium also enhances. (*Courtesy of Dr Ntobeko Ntusi, Division of Cardiology, Groote Schuur Hospital/University of Cape Town, Observatory, Cape Town, South Africa.*)

myocarditis has a high case fatality rate in part because the diagnosis is difficult to make ante mortem.[50–54]

The clinical presentation of tuberculous myocarditis includes atrial and ventricular tachyarrhythmias, conduction defects, ventricular aneurysms and pseudoaneurysms, dilated cardiomyopathy with heart failure, and sudden cardiac death.[53,55–57] The diagnosis requires a high index of suspicion, an appropriate imaging modality (echocardiogram, computed tomography scan, or MRI) and demonstration of caseous granulomatous inflammation with or without Mtb bacilli in myocardial tissue obtained at endomyocardial biopsy.[53] To date, there is little to offer patients beyond the standard 4 drug anti-TB therapy.[55,56]

TUBERCULOUS AORTITIS

Tuberculous infection of the aorta is an exceedingly rare manifestation of TB with an occurrence rate of 0.004% in 22,792 postmortems examinations over 50 years.[58] Mtb bacilli can access the aortic wall via contiguous extension from an adjacent infective focus (eg, tuberculous mediastinal lymphadenitis), via the vasa vasorum as part of systemic seeding of bacilli and direct implantation of bacilli on preexisting atheromatous

plaques.[59,60] Tuberculous aortitis usually presents with mycotic aneurysms of the aorta with both the thoracic and abdominal aorta affected equally.[59] Aneurysms may be true or false and within the ascending aorta, can extend to the aortic root and involve the sinus of Valsalva.[59,61] Rarely, tuberculous aortitis can present as stenotic lesions of the aorta causing acquired aortic coarctation and hypertension.[62]

The clinical manifestations of tuberculous mycotic aneurysm relate to its mass effect on adjacent organs or the complications of rupture. Common symptoms include chest or back pain, hoarseness, and stridor. Acute aortic regurgitation and cardiac tamponade have also been reported in patients with aneurysms involving the aortic root and sinus of Valsalva.[61,63] Owing to its exceeding rarity, a high index of suspicion is required to make the diagnosis of tuberculous aortic mycotic aneurysm in patients from TB endemic areas. Where available, computed tomography angiography is a fast and sensitive modality to aid with diagnosis and is useful to delineate the size and nature of aneurysm and its relation to surrounding structures. Demonstration of contrast extravasation indicates aneurysm rupture and is an indication for emergency surgery.[61] Surgery with in situ reconstruction with prosthetic graft or extraanatomic bypass added to standard 4-drug antituberculous therapy is the current standard of care.[59] Without either form of treatment, tuberculous aortitis is uniformly fatal.[59] Confirmation of a tuberculous etiology is usually made on histology of the resected or biopsied aorta showing the typical granulomatous inflammation with caseation with or without demonstration of Mtb bacilli.

SUMMARY

TB remains a significant health problem in the developing world. Cardiovascular TB is a potentially devastating presentation of this ancient infection. The last 2 decades have witnessed tremendous progress in our understanding of the disease, including our ability to recognize and diagnose it, and our capacity to alter its natural history and improve survival through the use various therapeutic options. Most patients present with well-recognized, stereotypical clinical syndromes, and where there is timely diagnosis and prompt optimal treatment, survival has improved from a universally fatal condition before the use of 4-drug anti-TB therapy in the past century to greater than 90% in the IMPI immunotherapy trial. Despite this progress, challenges remain. Chief among them is making the evidence based interventions discussed, which should be the standard of care (such as echocardiography, pericardiocentesis kits, uIFN-γ assays, MRI for complex cases, and surgical pericardiectomy) available and accessible to the poorest and most vulnerable communities where cardiac and other forms of TB are most prevalent.

SUPPLEMENTARY DATA

Supplementary data related to this article can be found online at http://dx.doi.org/10.1016/j.ccl.2016.08.007.

REFERENCES

1. World Health Organization (WHO). Global tuberculosis report 2015. Available at: http://www.who.int/tb/publications/global_report/en/. Accessed March 16, 2016.

2. Dheda K, Barry CE, Maartens G. Tuberculosis. Lancet 2016;387(10024):1211–26.

3. Fowler NO. Tuberculous pericarditis. JAMA 1991; 266(1):99–103.

4. Rana FS, Hawken MP, Mwachari C, et al. Autopsy study of HIV-1-positive and HIV-1-negative adult medical patients in Nairobi, Kenya. J Acquir Immune Defic Syndr 2000;24(1):23–9.

5. Shafer RW, Kim DS, Weiss JP, et al. Extrapulmonary tuberculosis in patients with human immunodeficiency virus infection. Medicine (Baltimore) 1991;70(6):384–97.

6. Mayosi BM, Burgess LJ, Doubell AF. Tuberculous pericarditis. Circulation 2005;112(23):3608–16.

7. Mayosi BM, Wiysonge CS, Ntsekhe M, et al. Clinical characteristics and initial management of patients with tuberculous pericarditis in the HIV era: the Investigation of the Management of Pericarditis in Africa (IMPI Africa) registry. BMC Infect Dis 2006;6:2.

8. Mayosi BM, Wiysonge CS, Ntsekhe M, et al. Mortality in patients treated for tuberculous pericarditis in sub-Saharan Africa. S Afr Med J 2008;98(1):36–40.

9. Syed FF, Ntsekhe M, Gumedze F, et al. Myopericarditis in tuberculous pericardial effusion: prevalence, predictors and outcome. Heart 2014;100(2):135–9.

10. Ntsekhe M, Wiysonge CS, Gumedze F, et al. HIV infection is associated with a lower incidence of constriction in presumed tuberculous pericarditis: a prospective observational study. PLoS One 2008; 3(6):e2253.

11. Shenje J, Ifeoma Adimora-Nweke F, Ross IL, et al. Poor penetration of antibiotics into pericardium in pericardial tuberculosis. EBioMedicine 2015;2(11): 1640–9.

12. Matthews K, Deffur A, Ntsekhe M, et al. A compartmentalized profibrotic immune response characterizes pericardial tuberculosis, irrespective of HIV-1 infection. Am J Respir Crit Care Med 2015;192(12):1518–21.

13. Pasipanodya JG, Mubanga M, Ntsekhe M, et al. Tuberculous pericarditis is multibacillary and bacterial burden drives high mortality. EBioMedicine 2015;2(11):1634–9.

14. Ntsekhe M, Matthews K, Syed FF, et al. Prevalence, hemodynamics, and cytokine profile of effusive-constrictive pericarditis in patients with tuberculous pericardial effusion. PLoS One 2013;8(10):e77532.

15. Mutyaba AK, Balkaran S, Cloete R, et al. Constrictive pericarditis requiring pericardiectomy at Groote Schuur Hospital, Cape Town, South Africa: causes and perioperative outcomes in the HIV era (1990-2012). J Thorac Cardiovasc Surg 2014;148(6): 3058–65.

16. Matthews K, Ntsekhe M, Syed F, et al. HIV-1 infection alters CD4+ memory T-cell phenotype at the site of disease in extrapulmonary tuberculosis. Eur J Immunol 2012;42(1):147–57.

17. Matthews K, Wilkinson KA, Kalsdorf B, et al. Predominance of interleukin-22 over interleukin-17 at the site of disease in human tuberculosis. Tuberculosis (Edinb) 2011;91(6):587–93.

18. Pandie S, Peter JG, Kerbelker ZS, et al. Diagnostic accuracy of quantitative PCR (Xpert MTB/RIF) for tuberculous pericarditis compared to adenosine deaminase and unstimulated interferon-γ in a high burden setting: a prospective study. BMC Med 2014;12:101.

19. Mayosi BM, Ntsekhe M, Bosch J, et al. Prednisolone and Mycobacterium indicus pranii in tuberculous pericarditis. N Engl J Med 2014;371(12):1121–30.

20. Spodick DH. Tuberculous pericarditis. AMA Arch Intern Med 1956;98(6):737–49.

21. Ntsekhe M, Mayosi BM. Tuberculous pericarditis with and without HIV. Heart Fail Rev 2013;18(3):367–73.

22. Reuter H, Burgess L, van Vuuren W, et al. Diagnosing tuberculous pericarditis. QJM 2006;99(12):827–39.

23. Reuter H, Burgess LJ, Louw VJ, et al. The management of tuberculous pericardial effusion: experience in 233 consecutive patients. Cardiovasc J S Afr 2007;18(1):20–5.

24. Strang JIG. Tuberculous pericarditis in Transkei. Clin Cardiol 1984;7(12):667–70.

25. Khandaker MH, Espinosa RE, Nishimura RA, et al. Pericardial disease: diagnosis and management. Mayo Clin Proc 2010;85(6):572–93.

26. Shabetai R. The pathophysiology of cardiac tamponade. Cardiovasc Clin 1976;7(3):67–89.

27. Strang JI, Kakaza HH, Gibson DG, et al. Controlled clinical trial of complete open surgical drainage and of prednisolone in treatment of tuberculous pericardial effusion in Transkei. Lancet 1988;2(8614):759–64.

28. Hancock EW. Subacute effusive-constrictive pericarditis. Circulation 1971;43(2):183–92.

29. Russell JB, Syed FF, Ntsekhe M, et al. Tuberculous effusive-constrictive pericarditis. Cardiovasc J Afr 2008;19(4):200–1.

30. Ntsekhe M, Shey Wiysonge C, Commerford PJ, et al. The prevalence and outcome of effusive constrictive pericarditis: a systematic review of the literature. Cardiovasc J Afr 2012;23(5):281–5.

31. 2015 ESC Guidelines for the diagnosis and management of pericardial diseases. Available at: http://eurheartj.oxfordjournals.org/content/ehj/36/42/2921.full.pdf. Accessed May 2, 2016.

32. Mayosi BM, Volmink JA, Commerford PJ. Pericardial disease: an evidence-based approach to diagnosis and treatment. In: Yusuf S, Cairns JA, Camm JA, editors. Evidence-based cardiology. 2nd edition. United Kingdom: Blackwell Science Ltd; 2003. p. 735–48.

33. Strang G, Latouf S, Commerford P, et al. Bedside culture to confirm tuberculous pericarditis. Lancet 1991;338(8782–8783):1600–1.

34. Strang JI, Kakaza HH, Gibson DG, et al. Controlled trial of prednisolone as adjuvant in treatment of tuberculous constrictive pericarditis in Transkei. Lancet 1987;2(8573):1418–22.

35. Syed FF, Mayosi BM. A modern approach to tuberculous pericarditis. Prog Cardiovasc Dis 2007;50(3):218–36.

36. Cohn DL, Catlin BJ, Peterson KL, et al. A 62-dose, 6-month therapy for pulmonary and extrapulmonary tuberculosis. A twice-weekly, directly observed, and cost-effective regimen. Ann Intern Med 1990;112(6):407–15.

37. Ntsekhe M, Wiysonge C, Volmink JA, et al. Adjuvant corticosteroids for tuberculous pericarditis: promising, but not proven. QJM 2003;96(8):593–9.

38. Mayosi BM, Ntsekhe M, Volmink JA, et al. Interventions for treating tuberculous pericarditis. Cochrane Database Syst Rev 2002;(4):CD000526.

39. Reuter H, Burgess LJ, Louw VJ, et al. Experience with adjunctive corticosteroids in managing tuberculous pericarditis. Cardiovasc J S Afr 2006;17(5):233–8.

40. Cui H, Chen X, Cui C, et al. Prevention of pericardial constriction by transcatheter intrapericardial fibrinolysis with urokinase. Chin Med Sci J 2005;20(1):5–10.

41. Seferović PM, Ristić AD, Maksimović R, et al. Pericardial syndromes: an update after the ESC guidelines 2004. Heart Fail Rev 2013;18(3):255–66.

42. Klein Allan L, Abbara S, Agler DA, et al. American Society of Echocardiography clinical recommendations for multimodality cardiovascular imaging of patients with pericardial disease: endorsed by the Society for Cardiovascular Magnetic Resonance and Society of Cardiovascular Computed Tomography. J Am Soc Echocardiogr 2013;26(9):965–1012.

43. Bashi V, John S, Ravikumar E, et al. Early and late results of pericardiectomy in 118 cases of constrictive pericarditis. Thorax 1988;43(8):637–41.

44. Imazio M, Brucato A, Barbieri A, et al. Good prognosis for pericarditis with and without myocardial involvement: results from a multicenter, prospective cohort study. Circulation 2013;128(1):42–9.

45. Desai N, Desai S, Chaddha U, et al. Tuberculous myopericarditis: a rare presentation in an immunocompetent host. BMJ Case Rep 2013.

46. Schrire V. Experience with pericarditis at Groote Schuur Hospital, Cape Town: an analysis of one hundred and sixty cases studied over a six-year period. S Afr Med J 1959;33:810–7.

47. Rooney JJ, Crocco JA, Lyons HA. Tuberculous pericarditis. Ann Intern Med 1970;72(1):73–81.

48. Rose AG. Cardiac tuberculosis. A study of 19 patients. Arch Pathol Lab Med 1987;111(5):422–6.

49. Momtahen M, Givtaj N, Ojaghi Z, et al. Cardiac tuberculoma of the right atrium. J Card Surg 2011;26(4):367–9.

50. Hitsumoto T, Ikeda S, Miyazaki S, et al. The case of tuberculous myocarditis manifested by extensive myocardial calcification. J Card Fail 2015;21(10S):170.

51. Behr G, Palin HC, Temperly JM. Myocardial tuberculosis. Br Med J 1977;1(6066):951.

52. Silingardi E, Rivasi F, Santunione AL, et al. Sudden death from tubercular myocarditis. J Forensic Sci 2006;51(3):667–9.

53. Agarwal R, Malhotra P, Awasthi A, et al. Tuberculous dilated cardiomyopathy: an under-recognized entity? BMC Infect Dis 2005;5:29.

54. Njovane X. Intramyocardial tuberculosis–a rare under-diagnosed entity. S Afr Med J 2009;99(3):152–3.

55. Michira BN, Alkizim FO, Matheka DM. Patterns and clinical manifestations of tuberculous myocarditis: a systematic review of cases. Pan Afr Med J 2015;21:118.

56. Liu A, Hu Y, Coates A. Sudden cardiac death and tuberculosis - how much do we know? Tuberculosis (Edinb) 2012;92(4):307–13.

57. Kinare SG, Bhatia BI. Tuberculous coronary arteritis with aneurysm of the ventricular septum. Chest 1971;60(6):613–6.

58. Parkhurst GF, Dekcer JP. Bacterial aortitis and mycotic aneurysm of the aorta; a report of twelve cases. Am J Pathol 1955;31(5).821–35.

59. Long R, Guzman R, Greenberg H, et al. Tuberculous mycotic aneurysm of the aorta: review of published medical and surgical experience. Chest 1999; 115(2):522–31.

60. Gornik HL, Creager MA. Aortitis. Circulation 2008; 117(23):3039–51.

61. Pathirana U, Kularatne S, Karunaratne S, et al. Ascending aortic aneurysm caused by Mycobacterium tuberculosis. BMC Res Notes 2015;8:659.

62. Lin M-M, Cheng H-M. Images in cardiovascular medicine: tuberculous aortitis. Intern Med 2012; 51(15):1983–5. Available at: http://www.ncbi.nlm. nih.gov/pubmed/22864122. Accessed June 21, 2016.

63. Palaniswamy C, Kumar U, Selvaraj DR, et al. Tuberculous mycotic aneurysm of aortic root: an unusual cause of cardiac tamponade. Trop Doct 2009; 39(2):112–3.

Approaches to Sustainable Capacity Building for Cardiovascular Disease Care in Kenya

Felix A. Barasa, MMED[a],*, Rajesh Vedanthan, MD, MPH[b],
Sonak D. Pastakia, PharmD, BCPS, MPH[c], Susie J. Crowe, PharmD[c],
Wilson Aruasa, MMED[a], Wilson K. Sugut, MMED[a],
Russ White, MD, MPH[d,e], Elijah S. Ogola, MMED[f],
Gerald S. Bloomfield, MD, MPH[g], Eric J. Velazquez, MD[g]

KEYWORDS

- Capacity building • Low- and middle-income countries • Kenya • Sustainable cardiovascular care

KEY POINTS

- Essential quality cardiovascular care is possible and sustainable in Kenya despite resource constraints.
- Investment in skilled manpower, specialized equipment and resources, pharmacy services and clear policies are being harnessed to address this epidemic and reduce VD-related premature deaths.
- Building strong partnerships and embracing equity in service delivery coupled with primary prevention of emerging CVD should be further enhanced for best yields.

INTRODUCTION

Cardiovascular disease (CVD) is the leading cause of morbidity and mortality worldwide, with the majority of these occurring in low- and middle-income countries (LMICS).[1] By 2020, it is estimated that CVD will remain as the leading contributor to the global health burden, accounting for 73% of total global mortality and 56% of total morbidity.[2] Toward the end of last century, CVD was identified as an emerging epidemic in these countries in contrast with high-income countries (HICs), where this menace is largely being controlled via identification of major risk factors through population-based studies and effective strategies, building on investments in prevention programs, skilled manpower, and sophisticated equipment for the treatment of those with established disease.[1] Although the prevalence of traditional CVD risk

Disclosure Statement: R. Vedanthan is supported by the Fogarty International Center of the National Institutes of Health under Award Number K01 TW 009218 - 05. The content is solely the responsibility of the authors and does not necessarily represent the official views of the National Institutes of Health. Drs F.A. Barasa, S.D. Pastakia, S.J. Crowe, W.K. Sugut, W. Aruasa, R. White, G.S. Bloomfield, and E. Velazquez have nothing to disclose.
[a] Moi Teaching and Referral Hospital, Eldoret, Kenya; [b] Zena and Michael A. Wiener Cardiovascular Institute, Icahn School of Medicine at Mount Sinai, New York, NY, USA; [c] Purdue University College of Pharmacy, West Lafayette, IN, USA; [d] Tenwek Mission Hospital, Bomet, Kenya; [e] Alpert School of Medicine, Brown University, 2 Dudley Street, PO Box 39, Providence, RI 02905, USA; [f] Department of Clinical Medicine, College of Health Sciences, University of Nairobi, Nairobi, Kenya; [g] Department of Medicine, Duke Clinical Research Institute, Duke Global Health Institute, Duke University, Durham, NC, USA
* Corresponding author. Department of Cardiology, Moi Teaching and Referral Hospital, PO Box 3, Edoret 30100, Kenya.
E-mail address: barasaceo12@gmail.com

factors has been relatively low in most LMICs, epidemiologic and nutritional transitions coupled with tobacco trends have put a great proportion of individuals, especially the urban poor, at risk of early CVD-related death.[2–4]

Most LMICs are still afflicted with diseases of poverty like tuberculosis, malaria, and human immunodeficiency virus (HIV) infections.[5] Splitting the overstretched health budgets and resources between these endemic diseases and the emerging CVDs is a challenge in regions where resources are limited.[6] Moreover, HIV infection poses additional cardiovascular risks to those infected, thus complicating the picture because most antiretroviral therapy treatment programs do not currently support treatment for noncommunicable disease comorbidities.[7,8] Sustainable health care financing, therefore, calls for more innovative ways of funding for treatment for CVD and building capacity to supplement the meager resources this epidemic attracts from respective national governments, like the model recently described at a referral hospital in western Kenya, where a strong partnership between a North American university and the local hospital has positively transformed cardiovascular care in that region.[9] Developed country partnerships are also growing, providing not only the resources but also the much needed technical expertise like the *Academic Model Providing Access to Healthcare* (AMPATH) model in Kenya and the *Madaktari Africa* initiative in Tanzania.[10,11] In this review, we describe how Moi Teaching and Referral Hospital (MTRH), and Kenyatta National Hospital (KNH) and Tenwek Mission Hospital in Kenya as major public facilities offering specialized cardiac care and representatives of similar settings in other LMICS have developed the various elements toward building capacity for cardiovascular care and their experiences to date. KNH is situated in the Kenyan Capital of Nairobi and is the largest referral hospital in East and Central Africa with a bed capacity of 2500 and also serves as the teaching hospital for the University of Nairobi. MTRH is the only other public referral hospital in the country with a bed capacity of 800 and serves as the teaching hospital for Moi University in Eldoret, Western Kenya. Tenwek, in contrast, is a small mission hospital situated about 200 km west of Nairobi in the central Rift Valley with very well-established cardiovascular services.

BUILDING DIAGNOSTIC, HUMAN, AND TECHNICAL CAPACITY

Precise cardiac diagnosis is essential for quality patient care and prognostication. Echocardiography and electrocardiography are the standard initial diagnostic tools for cardiac evaluation, but they are not widely available. Access to echocardiography is particularly limited to specialized laboratories within established hospitals, not only owing to the high cost of the equipment, but also the extensive training in image acquisition and interpretation required for its application. As previously described in a recent publication, to fill these gaps, Duke University (North Carolina) and Moi University partnered to jumpstart a specialized and sustainable cardiac care program in Eldoret, Kenya.[11] A cardiology fellowship program was jointly started after the creation of a National Heart, Lung and Blood Institute–supported Center of Excellence in cardiovascular and pulmonary disease in Eldoret and ran for 5 years starting in 2009 with the support for clinical capacity building from the Hubert-Yeargan Center for Global Health at Duke University. This Center of Excellence program was a public–private partnership created with the overall goal of contributing to the reduction of cardiovascular and pulmonary disease burdens by catalyzing in-country research institutions to develop a global network of biomedical research centers that conduct collaborative research, train researchers, and advise on policy across 11 centers globally.[12,13] Senior cardiologists and an experienced ultrasonographer accompanied by echocardiogram machines (Philips CX50, Los Angeles, CA) were posted to train both the Kenyan echocardiography technicians and fellows. During this training period, the knowledge base and skills of existing technicians was greatly enhanced and the volume of echocardiogram studies doubled from about 15 to more than 30 per day as more patients and clinicians were drawn to the quality cardiac diagnostic services. Because there is no formal echocardiography training program in sub-Saharan Africa, this cardiac diagnostic unit has transformed itself into a training center in echocardiography for medical personnel from both government and missionary hospitals around the country with an increasing need for echocardiography services.

Another innovative approach of filling the needs of clinical practice in LMIC settings is the use of handheld ultrasound devices. Studies from both HICs and LIMCs support the ability of focused cardiac ultrasound imaging to provide accurate and clinically meaningful information compared with physical examination alone in intensive care units, at the bedside, and in the community.[14–16] One such device (V-scan, General Electric, Crotonville, NY) is available at MTRH for provision of point of care diagnostic value. The technology has also been found very useful in Tanzania especially in rural areas without electricity and Fiji, where school nurses have used the device for mass screening of rheumatic heart disease (RHD) among children aged 5 to 15 years.[17,18]

Accessibility to specialized physicians and cardiologists is another limiting factor in the care of cardiac patients. MTRH, for instance, serves a catchment population of about 25 million people mainly drawn from the western part of the country. It has 2 medical wards that are typically filled to capacity, a 6-bed intensive care unit, and until recently no adult cardiologist. The aforementioned cardiac fellowship program has yielded 2 cardiologists who have since been recognized by the Kenya Medical board and the third awaits certification. This program is being funded by the Moi University School of Medicine since the end of the Center of Excellence grant in 2014. As part of the capacity building, the University of Nairobi, in partnership with KNH, is also in the advanced stages of starting a similar fellowship program with international benchmarking. Once commissioned, the 2 programs will be able to train a sufficient number of cardiologists not only for the country, but also for the region.

SPECIALIZED OUTPATIENT CARDIOLOGY CLINICS

MTRH runs a busy outpatient cardiology service organized into 3 clinics: general adult cardiology, RHD clinic, and pediatric cardiology. These clinics are staffed by cardiologists with the resident medical officer attending to those patients who walk in on unofficial clinic days. The RHD clinic is projected to run alongside the cardiac disease in the pregnancy clinic with obstetricians owing to the similar needs and demographics of the 2 patient populations. Five hundred patients are seen monthly with teaching and mentorship opportunities to medical students, interns, residents, and visiting students from within and outside the region.

At KNH, another busy cardiology clinic with a waiting time of more than 3 months runs weekly with a patient turnover of over 150. Teaching and mentorship of internal medicine residents by senior cardiologists from the hospital occurs as the former prepare to do most of the cardiovascular work in the counties upon their graduation as internists.

PHARMACY SERVICES FOR CARDIOVASCULAR DISEASE

With the multifactorial needs of patients with CVD, integrated interdisciplinary care is essential to optimize health outcomes. One of the frequently underused components of this interdisciplinary team are pharmacists.[19–21] Because pharmacists tend to have frequent encounters with patients as they receive their medications, pharmacy intervention could be a particularly impactful point for improving care for patients with CVD needs. One critical role for pharmacists in LMICs is maintaining consistent availability for essential medication supplies where drug procurement systems are often inefficient, often leading to inconsistent availability of essential medications. One proposed method for combating essential medicine shortages in the public sector is the revolving fund pharmacy model, where the initial supply of essential medication is purchased or donated, and then medications are sold at a slightly higher price. Proceeds are then used to purchase additional medications and ensure sustainability of the stock. A number of studies have highlighted the impact of revolving fund pharmacies.[22–26] Availability of CVD medications particularly is a major handicap; for example, in Benin, only 26% and 57% of these medications are available in the public and private sectors, respectively.[26] It is therefore essential for pharmacists to creatively address the noncommunicable disease supply chain in LMICs to make effective CVD care possible.

In addition to managing the supply chain (See Dan and colleagues article, "Ensuring Patient Centered Access to Cardiovascular Disease Medicines in Low-Income and Middle-Income Countries Through Health-System Strengthening," in this issue), the introduction of clinical pharmacy services could greatly improve the quality of patient care by directly linking the product focused needs of CVD management with the clinical needs of patients.[27–29] Furthermore, as LMICs address the burden of CVD with scarce human resources for health, pharmacists and pharmaceutical technologists represent a highly trained workforce that can be adequately used to support clinical care.[29] Although the transition of pharmacy practice to a more patient-centered care delivery model would be of great assistance to the entire health care system, we focus on the pronounced role this service have had on anticoagulation services.

In LMICs, certain conditions, such as RHD, have a disproportionately higher prevalence than in HICs, and represent a large contributor to preventable morbidity and mortality.[30,31] Caring for RHD represents a prime example of the need for interdisciplinary care. The pharmacy component is especially vital in the management of RHD, because the consistent monthly administration of penicillin has been shown to reduce recurrence of rheumatic fever by more than 55%.[32,33] RHD patients with mitral stenosis also have an elevated risk of thromboembolism. In 1 case series, such patients had an 8% risk of embolism with the risk increasing to 31% in those having concomitant atrial fibrillation.[34] The severity of mitral stenosis, however, was unspecified in this study. The unacceptably high risk of this thromboembolic complications in this population could be greatly reduced by the introduction of organized anticoagulation monitoring services that have been shown to decrease them to 0.8% with the proper use of warfarin.[35]

In HICs, pharmacist-managed anticoagulation with warfarin has demonstrated decreases in hospitalizations, major bleeding events, and thromboembolic events when compared with usual medical care.[36] Although limited published literature is available, pharmacist-managed anticoagulation clinics exist in Southeast Asia, sub-Saharan Africa, and the Middle East. In Thailand, results from an anticoagulation clinic showed that patients receiving pharmacist-managed warfarin therapy had an increase in the time in therapeutic range with no difference in major bleeding when compared with usual care.[37] At the MTRH anticoagulation clinic, a study was conducted of patients on warfarin therapy to compare the amount of time in the therapeutic range, major bleeding events, and the risk of thromboembolism between a pharmacist-managed anticoagulation clinic and published rates of similar clinics in HICs. Patients included in the study (n = 178) had the following distribution of indications for anticoagulation: venous thromboembolism (n = 117, 65%), rheumatic atrial fibrillation (n = 33, 18.5%), mechanical heart valves (n = 15, 8.4%), and nonvalvular atrial fibrillation (n = 5, 2.8%). No differences were found in percent time in therapeutic range international normalized ratio (64.6%, $P = .76$), risk of major bleeding per year (1.25%, $P = .56$), or risk of thromboembolism (5% per year, $P = .35$) between HIC and MTRH clinics.[38] Additionally, 47.7% of patients in the first ever pharmacist-managed anticoagulation clinic in Iran reached their goal international normalized ratio on subsequent visits to the clinic.[39] These limited data show that, even with minimal resources, pharmacist-managed anticoagulation clinics can result in better outcomes than usual care with the possibility of providing similar results to clinics in HICs. In addition, a study measuring the cost-effectiveness of pharmacist-managed anticoagulation treatment in Thailand supports the use of a pharmacist in this role.[40]

At MTRH, this pharmacist-managed anticoagulation clinic has treated more than 2100 patients as of June 2016, one-half of whom are on active follow-up. Anticoagulation protocols are based on 2012 American College of Chest Physicians guidelines.[41] Through a partnership with Abbott Labs (Princeton, NJ), the clinic has been able to incorporate point of care I-stat prothrombin time/international normalized ratio tests for all patients and provides warfarin tablets in pill boxes to maximize adherence. For quality assurance, the clinic sources its warfarin from a reputable prequalified drug supplier/manufacturer while the I-Stat machine operating software is continuously updated every 6 months using an appropriate web-based program as per the manufacture's recommendations. Through the use of this portable equipment, the clinic has also established a weekly service at a distant rural district hospital to access more remote patients.

CARDIAC SURGERY

With the disproportionately higher prevalence of cardiac valve abnormalities in LMICs, there is a great need for cardiac surgery. Unfortunately, cardiac surgical capacity is not well-developed in most LMICs owing to lack of both technical personnel and infrastructure.[42–44] In Kenya, the only reliable public sector cardiac surgical program is in KNH, but it is overwhelmed with a waiting list that stretches for several years. The hospital started a cardiac surgical program in the early 1970s, mainly being staffed by expatriate surgeons. In 1979, the local team took over the program, which has continued to grow, mainly treating valve disease (two-thirds of cases) with hands-on training of general surgeons to enhance capacity. In 2014, a residency program in cardiothoracic surgery was started by the University of Nairobi and will soon start matriculating specialized personnel to meet the ever increasing needs of the region. Two private hospitals in the Kenyan capital (Mater and Karen) are also offering cardiac surgical services, but their fees preclude the majority of needy patients. At MTRH, a partnership has been forged between the Medtronic Company and the hospital to start a cardiac surgical program in early 2017 and it is envisaged that this will become an alternative to KNH for patients in western Kenya and a referral center for others from neighboring countries in East Africa.

At Tenwek hospital, a partnership with Brown University (Providence, RI) has helped the initiation of a vibrant and sustainable cardiac surgical program that has assisted many low-income patients. Initially, the focus was on pulmonary and esophageal surgeries, but with an increasing number of patients presenting with advanced RHD and no viable treatment options, cardiac surgeries were recruited. Mitral commissurotomies using a Tubbs dilator were the initial procedures before transitioning to open heart operations after the acquisition of a heart–lung machine and associated cardiopulmonary bypass expertise in 2007. Through a series of camps associated with knowledge and skills transfer, local staffs have been well-trained in critical care, perfusion, cardiac anesthesia, and echocardiography to assist the expatriate surgeon perpetuate the program. To date, nearly 300 open heart cases have been performed with a perioperative mortality rate of less than 1%. A partnership with the Medtronic Company ensures a continuous supply of surgical consumables. Additionally, a cardiothoracic surgical fellowship for African surgeons is planned to begin by 2018 to further enhance capacity.

Another strategy that is gaining popularity for dissemination of cardiovascular services to rural communities is the so-called humanitarian model. This refers to actions organized by both governmental and nongovernmental organizations from HICs with the aim of implementing humanitarian programs to support low-income patients in health systems around the world, especially in pediatrics.[45] Initially, these programs were only philanthropic and reactive to human disasters, but of late, they are becoming more regular coupled with mentorship activities and training, thus aiding skills transfer and enhancing local capacities.[46] In recognition of this potential, pediatric cardiac surgeons at the World Summit on Pediatric and Congenital Heart Surgery held in Geneva in June 2015 mobilized cardiac surgery experts from HICs to perform humanitarian missions in LMICs.[47] India, Pakistan, and Chile have previously benefited from such missions with hundreds of children undergoing world-class operations at third-world costs.[48] A similar successful experience in Rwanda mainly targeting patients with RHD has also been described with attendant skill transfers to local doctors.[49] In Kenya, a model funded by Mater Hospital provides prevention services, including secondary RHD prophylaxis, facilitation for further specialized treatment, early disease management, and increased local awareness of CVD to clinicians.[50]

TASK REDISTRIBUTION AND DISSEMINATION OF SPECIALIZED CARE TO DISTRICT HOSPITALS AND HEALTH CENTERS

In Kenya, the health care system is divided into six levels: level 1 is the community; levels 2 and 3 consist of dispensaries and health centers serving a catchment population of 5000 to 20,000 individuals, respectively; level 4 facilities include subdistrict and district hospitals that serve a catchment population of approximately 500,000 to 1,000,000; and level 5 and 6 facilities serve as regional and national referral centers. AMPATH partnership has established an HIV care system in western Kenya that has served more than 160,000 patients and has recently leveraged this infrastructure to expand its clinical scope of work to develop a comprehensive chronic disease management program, focusing initially on CVD, hypertension, and diabetes.[51–53]

Integral to this effort has been geographic decentralization and task redistribution of chronic disease care to levels 1 to 3. Alongside these 2 central pillars has been an aggressive and sustained commitment to capacity building and equipping of rural health facilities. Structured and targeted training has been provided to community health workers, nurses, and clinical officers. In addition, decision support tools (both paper based and mobile based) have been provided to rural health workers to facilitate adherence to management guidelines. Rural health facilities have been provided chronic disease-related equipment and supplies, as well as a secure, consistent supply of medications.[22] Referral networks have been established, initially focused on levels 1 to 3 and level 6.

The next phase of a system-wide approach to cardiovascular care is to target levels 4 and 5, the subdistrict and district hospitals. The same principles that have been implemented successfully in the more rural settings will be leveraged and modified as appropriate for these larger facilities. Specialized training coupled with in-person mentorship and supervision will be provided by cardiovascular subspecialists from MTRH. The levels 4 and 5 health facilities are primarily staffed by general internists (internal medicine graduates) and clinical officers (physician assistants); hence, the training will be tailored to the expertise of the clinician. An integrated electronic medical record for cardiovascular patients is already in place and will help to facilitate referral, follow-up, and continuity of care.

ADMINISTRATIVE AND LEGISLATIVES MEASURES TO ENHANCE ACCESS TO CARE FOR CARDIOVASCULAR DISEASE

Health care financing is a challenge in LMICs and a primary factor limiting accessibility to cardiovascular care for low income populations. The World Health Organization assembly in 2005, in an attempt to address this challenge, adopted a universal coverage strategy, which it defined as access to key promotive, preventive, curative, and rehabilitative health interventions for all at an affordable cost. The principle of financial risk protection was also emphasized to ensure that the cost of care is not catastrophic. A related objective of health financing policy called equity in financing was also advocated, whereby households contribute to the health system on the basis of their ability to pay.[54]

In tandem with these measures, the Kenyan government through its strategic economic plan (Vision2030) launched in 2007 came up with 3 strategies for health care reforms to make the services not only equitable and affordable, but also meet highest possible standards. The document proposed 3 pathways: provision of a functional, efficient, and sustainable health infrastructure network; building of partnerships; and promotion of equitable health financing mechanisms to help achieve these goals. Further, a purchaser provider system that would reduce bureaucracies in the procurement networks including elimination of tender boards and reduction of out-of-pocket expenditures on health care to less than 25% was proposed and subsequently implemented.[55,56] The national health insurer (National Hospital Insurance Fund), was subsequently regularized through a parliamentary act to expand its services to the unemployed and those in the informal sector as well as impose stiffer penalties to employers who default on submitting monthly dues.[57] Both KNH and MTRH, being public hospitals, have embraced these new measures and have encouraged all patients visiting the hospitals to join the fund that subsequently pays for all in-patient services, including specialized surgeries. On the partnerships front, the Kenya government has engaged GE to supply hospital electronic diagnostic equipment (including cardiac diagnostics) to all level 5 facilities to improve accessibility.

To serve patients unable to pay for any services, both KNH and MTRH social work departments ensures that all admitted patients are tracked adequately to assess their ability to pay for hospital services. The social workers have become key members of the interdisciplinary inpatient rounding teams to keep pace with the clinical decisions being made on daily basis. Because of this incorporation, they are better able to provide frequent updates to the often large networks of caregivers and relatives that patients often lean on during their hospitalization. When the social workers have determined that a patient is unable to pay, they can rely on a waiver system, which ensures that such patients get the specialized services after going through a series of checks and balances that are in place to prevent abuse of the system.

SUMMARY

Essential quality cardiovascular care is possible and sustainable in Kenya despite resource constraints. Investment in skilled manpower, specialized equipment and resources, pharmacy services and clear policies are being harnessed to address this epidemic and reduce CVD-related premature deaths. Building strong partnerships and embracing equity in service delivery coupled with primary prevention of emerging CVD should be further enhanced for best yields.

ACKNOWLEDGMENTS

The authors thank Rakhi Karwa for her for contribution to the pharmacy services section.

REFERENCES

1. Reddy KS, Yusuf S. Emerging epidemic of cardiovascular disease in developing countries. Circulation 1998;97(6):596–601.
2. Ayah R, Joshi MD, Wanjiru R, et al. A population-based survey of prevalence of diabetes and correlates in an urban slum community in Nairobi, Kenya. BMC Public Health 2013;13:371.
3. Beaglehole R, Yach D. Globalisation and the prevention and control of non-communicable disease: the neglected chronic diseases of adults. Lancet 2003; 362(9387):903–8.
4. Bloomfield GS, Barasa FA, Doll JA, et al. Heart failure in sub-Saharan Africa. Curr Cardiol Rev 2013; 9(2):157–73.
5. Mocumbi AO, Sliwa K. Women's cardiovascular health in Africa. Heart 2012;98(6):450–5.
6. Sridhar D, Batniji R. Misfinancing global health: a case for transparency in disbursements and decision making. Lancet 2008;372(9644):1185–91.
7. Bloomfield GS, Alenezi F, Barasa FA, et al. Human immunodeficiency virus and heart failure in low- and middle-income countries. JACC Heart Fail 2015;3(8):579–90.
8. Lumsden RH, Bloomfield GS. The causes of HIV-Associated Cardiomyopathy: a tale of two worlds. Biomed Res Int 2016;2016:8196560.
9. Binanay CA, Akwanalo CO, Aruasa W, et al. Building sustainable capacity for cardiovascular care at a public hospital in western Kenya. J Am Coll Cardiol 2015;66(22):2550–60.
10. Madaktari Africa. Available at: http://www.madaktari.org. Accessed June 10, 2016.
11. Ampath. Our model. 2015. Available at: http://www.ampathkenya.org/our-model. Accessed March 16, 2016.
12. A global research network for non-communicable diseases. Lancet 2014;383(9927):1446–7.

13. Engelgau MM, Sampson UK, Rabadan-Diehl C, et al. Tackling NCD in LMIC: achievements and lessons learned from the NHLBI-UnitedHealth Global Health Centers of Excellence Program. Glob Heart 2016; 11(1):5–15.

14. Beaton A, Okello E, Lwabi P, et al. Echocardiography screening for rheumatic heart disease in Ugandan schoolchildren. Circulation 2012;125(25):3127–32.

15. Kwan GF, Bukhman AK, Miller AC, et al. A simplified echocardiographic strategy for heart failure diagnosis and management within an integrated noncommunicable disease clinic at district hospital level for sub-Saharan Africa. JACC Heart Fail 2013;1(3):230–6.

16. Vignon P, Dugard A, Abraham J, et al. Focused training for goal-oriented hand-held echocardiography performed by noncardiologist residents in the intensive care unit. Intensive Care Med 2007; 33(10):1795–9.

17. Engelman D, Kado JH, Remenyi B, et al. Focused cardiac ultrasound screening for rheumatic heart disease by briefly trained health workers: a study of diagnostic accuracy. Lancet Glob Health 2016; 4(6):e386–394.

18. MUSC cardiologists foster sustainability through training at advanced cardiac care center in Tanzania. Available at: http://www.flickr.com/photos/musc-cgh/sets/72157644561258004/. Accessed May 22, 2016.

19. Gilberson S, Yoder S, Lee M. Improving patient and health system outcomes through advanced pharmacy practice: a report to the US Surgeon General. 2011. Available at: http://www.accp.com/docs/positions/misc/improving patient_and_health_system_outcomes.pdf. Accessed May 31, 2016.

20. White CM. Pharmacists need recognition as providers to enhance patient care. Ann Pharmacother 2014;48(2):268–73.

21. Rodgers GP, Conti JB, Feinstein JA, et al. ACC 2009 survey results and recommendations: Addressing the cardiology workforce crisis A report of the ACC board of trustees workforce task force. J Am Coll Cardiol 2009;54(13):1195–208.

22. Manji I, Manyara SM, Jakait B, et al. The revolving fund pharmacy model: backing up the ministry of health supply chain in western Kenya. Int J Pharm Pract 2016;24(5):358–66.

23. Uzochukwu BS, Onwujekwe OE, Akpala CO. Effect of the Bamako-Initiative drug revolving fund on availability and rational use of essential drugs in primary health care facilities in south-east Nigeria. Health Policy Plan 2002;17(4):378–83.

24. Ali GK. How to establish a successful revolving drug fund: the experience of Khartoum state in the Sudan. Bull World Health Organ 2009;87(2):139–42.

25. Umenai T, Narula IS. Revolving drug funds: a step towards health security. Bull World Health Organ 1999;77(2):167–71.

26. Agodokpessi G, Ait-Khaled N, Gninafon M, et al. Assessment of a revolving drug fund for essential asthma medicines in Benin. J Pharm Policy Pract 2015;8(1):12.

27. Mendis S, Abegunde D, Oladapo O, et al. Barriers to management of cardiovascular risk in a low-resource setting using hypertension as an entry point. J Hypertens 2004;22(1):59–64.

28. Maher D, Ford N, Unwin N. Priorities for developing countries in the global response to noncommunicable diseases. Global Health 2012;8:14.

29. Campbell J, Dussault G, Buchan J, et al. A universal truth: no health without a workforce. Geneva (Switzerland): Global Health Workforce Alliance and World Health Organization; 2013.

30. Seckeler MD, Hoke TR. The worldwide epidemiology of acute rheumatic fever and rheumatic heart disease. Clin Epidemiol 2011;3:67–84.

31. Remenyi B, Carapetis J, Wyber R, et al. Position statement of the World Heart Federation on the prevention and control of rheumatic heart disease. Nat Rev Cardiol 2013;10(5):284–92.

32. Manyemba J, Mayosi BM. Penicillin for secondary prevention of rheumatic fever. Cochrane Database Syst Rev 2002;(3):CD002227.

33. Padmavati S, Sharma KB, Jayaram O. Epidemiology and prophylaxis of rheumatic fever in Delhi—a five year follow-up. Singapore Med J 1973; 14(3):457–61.

34. Coulshed N, Epstein EJ, McKendrick CS, et al. Systemic embolism in mitral valve disease. Br Heart J 1970;32(1):26–34.

35. Fleming HA. Anticoagulants in rheumatic heart disease. Lancet 1971;2(7722):486.

36. Entezari-Maleki T, Dousti S, Hamishehkar H, et al. A systematic review on comparing 2 common models for management of warfarin therapy; pharmacist-led service versus usual medical care. J Clin Pharmacol 2016;56(1):24–38.

37. Saokaew S, Sapoo U, Nathisuwan S, et al. Anticoagulation control of pharmacist-managed collaborative care versus usual care in Thailand. Int J Clin Pharm 2012;34(1):105–12.

38. Manji I, Pastakia SD, Do AN, et al. Performance outcomes of a pharmacist-managed anticoagulation clinic in the rural, resource-constrained setting of Eldoret, Kenya. J Thromb Haemost 2011;9(11): 2215–20.

39. Fahimi FS-KB, Hossein-Ahmadi Z, Salamzadeh J, et al. The first pharmacist-based warfarin-monitoring service in Iran. J Pharm Health Serv Res 2011;2:59–62.

40. Saokaew S, Permsuwan U, Chaiyakunapruk N, et al. Cost-effectiveness of pharmacist-participated warfarin therapy management in Thailand. Thromb Res 2013;132(4):437–43.

41. Salem DN, O'Gara PT, Madias C, et al. Valvular and structural heart disease: American College of

Chest Physicians Evidence-Based Clinical Practice Guidelines (8th edition). Chest 2008;133(Suppl 6): 593s–629s.

42. Grimaldi A, Ammirati E, Karam N, et al. Cardiac surgery for patients with heart failure due to structural heart disease in Uganda: access to surgery and outcomes. Cardiovasc J Afr 2014;25(5):204–11.

43. Yankah C, Fynn-Thompson F, Antunes M, et al. Cardiac surgery capacity in sub-Saharan Africa: quo vadis? Thorac Cardiovasc Surg 2014;62(5): 393–401.

44. Zuhlke L, Engel ME, Karthikeyan G, et al. Characteristics, complications, and gaps in evidence-based interventions in rheumatic heart disease: the Global Rheumatic Heart Disease Registry (the REMEDY study). Eur Heart J 2015;36(18): 1115–1122a.

45. Elahi MM, Matata BM. Cardiac Surgery for Communities in Need - Meeting the Continuous Challenges for Delivering New Models of Global Humanitarian Health Programmes. MOJ Surg 2016; 3(1):00033.

46. Novick WM, Stidham GL, Karl TR, et al. Are we improving after 10 years of humanitarian paediatric cardiac assistance? Cardiol Young 2005;15(4): 379–84.

47. Leung R. 60 Minutes Story: vacation, adventure and surgery, elective surgeries by world-class doctors at third-world prices. CBS Broadcast 2005.

48. Lancaster J. Surgeries, Side Trips for "Medical Tourists". In: Affordable care at India's private hospitals draws growing number of foreigners. Washington Post Foreign Service, USA; 2004. p. A01.

49. Swain JD, Pugliese DN, Mucumbitsi J, et al. Partnership for sustainability in cardiac surgery to address critical rheumatic heart disease in sub-Saharan Africa: the experience from Rwanda. World J Surg 2014;38(9):2205–11.

50. Yuko-Jowi CA. African experiences of humanitarian cardiovascular medicine: a Kenyan perspective. Cardiovasc Diagn Ther 2012;2(3):231–9.

51. Bloomfield GS, Kimaiyo S, Carter EJ, et al. Chronic noncommunicable cardiovascular and pulmonary disease in sub-Saharan Africa: an academic model for countering the epidemic. Am Heart J 2011; 161(5):842–7.

52. Einterz RM, Kimaiyo S, Mengech HN, et al. Responding to the HIV pandemic: the power of an academic medical partnership. Acad Med 2007;82(8): 812–8.

53. Vedanthan R, Kamano JH, Bloomfield GS, et al. Engaging the entire care cascade in western Kenya: a model to achieve the cardiovascular disease secondary prevention roadmap goals. Glob Heart 2015; 10(4):313–7.

54. World Health Assembly Resolution 58.33. Sustainable health financing, universal coverage and social health insurance. 2005.

55. Kenya Vision 2030. Available at: http://www. vision2030.go.ke/. Accessed June 9, 2016.

56. The Public Procurement And Asset Disposal ACT No. 33 of 2015. Kenya Gazette Supplement No. 207 (Acts No. 33).

57. National Hospital Insurance Fund ACT. Chapter 255. Revised Edition 2012 [1998]. Available at: www. kenyalaw.org.

Infective Endocarditis in Low- and Middle-Income Countries

Benson Njuguna, BPharm[a,c],*, Adrian Gardner, MD, MPH[b,1],
Rakhi Karwa, PharmD, BCPS[c,1], François Delahaye, MD, PhD[d]

KEYWORDS

- Endocarditis in LMIC • Developing countries • Causes • Management • Challenges

KEY POINTS

- *Staphylococcus* is an increasingly important cause of IE in LMICs, and is the leading cause of IE in UMICs.
- RHD remains the major underlying cardiac pathology of IE in LMICs, identified in almost half of reported cases.
- The rate of microorganism nonidentification is high, reaching up to 60% of IE cases in LMICs, and hampering diagnosis and treatment.
- Rates of access to surgery in UMICs for complicated IE are as high as in HICs, but remain dismal in LMICs.

INTRODUCTION

Infective endocarditis (IE) is a rare, life-threatening disease with a significant mortality and morbidity burden. In-hospital mortality approaches 25%, increasing in patients with cardiac or extracardiac complications.[1–3] IE also frequently causes debilitating morbidities, such as heart failure, stroke, and renal failure requiring dialysis, which contribute to increased mortality and disability adjusted life-years.[3–7]

The spectrum of causative microorganisms and underlying risk factors for IE has shifted dramatically in high-income countries (HICs).[8,9] Staphylococcal IE now predominates. Degenerative valve disease (DVD), prosthetic valves, and other intracardiac devices are the leading underlying cardiac conditions, with little contribution from rheumatic heart disease (RHD) and congenital heart disease (CHD).

The epidemiology of IE in low- and middle-income countries (LMICs) has been said to resemble that seen in HIC-based studies from the mid-twentieth century, which reported a predominance of IE caused by streptococcal infection, RHD, and CHD as the leading risk factors, and minimal rates of surgical intervention.[9] Reports from LMICs that mirror this epidemiology and treatment patterns are predominantly from before the turn of this millennium and consequently may not reflect the current state of IE in LMICs.[10–14]

The prevalence of RHD remains disproportionately high in LMICs, and uncorrected CHD persists in the poorest of these settings because of limited access to cardiac surgery.[15,16] It is therefore

Disclosure Statement: The authors have nothing to disclose.
[a] Department of Pharmacy, Moi Teaching and Referral Hospital, PO Box 3, Eldoret 30100, Kenya; [b] Department of Medicine, Indiana University School of Medicine, 340 West 10th Street #6200, Indianapolis, IN 46202, USA; [c] Department of Pharmacy Practice, Purdue University College of Pharmacy, 575 Stadium Mall Dr, West Lafayette, IN 47907, USA; [d] Department of Cardiology, Hospices civils de Lyon, Université Claude Bernard, Equipe d'Accueil HESPER 7425, Hôpital Louis Pradel, 28, avenue du Doyen Lépine, Bron Cedex 69677, Lyon, France
[1] Presented address: PO Box 3, Eldoret 30100, Kenya.
* Corresponding author.
E-mail address: njugunaben1@gmail.com

Cardiol Clin 35 (2017) 153–163
http://dx.doi.org/10.1016/j.ccl.2016.08.011

expected that RHD and CHD remain significant underlying cardiac conditions for IE; however, economic improvement in LMIC and upper-middle-income countries (UMIC) has led to medical progress, which may have introduced additional IE risk factors for these populations, and altered the spectrum of causative microorganisms.

This article presents the causes and treatment of IE in LMICs as reported in contemporary studies, defined as studies that primarily report findings from 2000 to 2016. Also discussed is the prevailing challenges to the diagnosis and management of IE in LMICs, and future directions in research are suggested.

METHODS

We searched PUBMED and EMBASE using the keywords "endocarditis," "IE," "low income," "middle income," and "developing country." LMICs and HICs were based on 2016 World Bank Income groups classification.[17] Articles were considered relevant if they were original research that described IE epidemiology and management experiences from LMICs from the year 2000 to 2016. When studies reported data from both before and after the year 2000, we excluded studies if most of the experience was from before 2000. We also screened the reference list of the retrieved articles for additional relevant studies.

CAUSES OF INFECTIVE ENDOCARDITIS

Prosthetic valves, DVD and intracardiac devices have replaced RHD as the major underlying cardiac risk factors for IE in HICs.[1] Comorbidities, such as diabetes mellitus, renal failure requiring dialysis, and malignancy, contribute substantially to a growing burden of health care–associated IE (HAIE).[2,18] Consequently, growing use of long-term intravascular access devices has led to skin bacteria in the form of *Staphylococcus* being the leading cause of IE in HICs.[1,2,18]

In this section, we review the prevalent underlying cardiac conditions, place of acquisition, and microbial cause of IE in LMICs. A summary of the findings is presented in **Table 1**.

Underlying Cardiac Conditions

RHD is identified as the underlying cardiac pathology in most IE cases, ranging from 28% to 45% in most of our reviewed studies.[19–24] Nel and Naidoo,[25] however, reported a much higher (78%) prevalence of underlying RHD in their study in South Africa, a country where RHD is endemic.[26]

Overall, this range of underlying RHD in IE represents a decline from the 45% to 80% reported

in earlier (pre-2000) LMIC studies.[10,11,13,27,28] Compared with HICs, however, these findings are remarkable in that RHD is identified in only 3% of IE cases from HICs.[1] This is likely because the prevalence of RHD is disproportionately high in LMICs,[29,30] which bear 79% of the global RHD burden.[15]

Underlying CHD accounts for 5% to 23% of reported IE cases.[19,21,23–25,31,32] Math and colleagues[20] reported CHD as the leading cause of IE (39%) in northern India in a cardiac surgery center with a large pediatric population, which may account for the higher findings of CHD.

Prosthetic valve IE (PVE) and pacemakers/intracardiac defibrillators are reported in 17% to 44% and 6% to 19% of IE cases in LMICs, respectively.[19–23,31,32] UMIC studies account for the higher figures in these ranges, which reflects advances in medical technology and higher access to cardiac surgery.[21,22] Indeed, the largest report of PVE cases from an LMIC comes from Simsek-Yavuz and colleagues,[21] who reported findings from a referral center in Turkey (an UMIC) in which 141 patients (44%) among 325 IE cases had PVE. A total of 52% of the total patient cohort received surgical intervention, closely approximating the rate seen in HICs.[2]

DVD contributes little to the IE epidemiology in LMICs, accounting for less than 10% of cases.[19,21,23,32] Elbey and colleagues,[31] however, reported a high rate of DVD (23%) in a multicenter retrospective study in Turkey. Mean patient age was 47 years, higher than that typically seen in LMIC studies, which may explain the higher rate of DVD. Overall, unlike in HICs where DVD is the major underlying cardiac disease in native valve IE (NVE), a lower aged mean patient population in LMICs limits its contribution.[1,8,9,18]

Place of Infection Acquisition

The burden of HAIE is growing in HICs, reported in 30% of IE in recent studies.[1,2,18] Advances in medical technology, increased indwelling intravascular device use, and increased prevalence of comorbidities, such as end-stage renal disease, contribute to this burden.[33]

Two LMIC studies reported on the site of acquisition of IE. Simsek-Yavuz and colleagues[21] characterized 23% of IE cases as HAIE at a referral center in Turkey, whereas Damasco and colleagues[34] reported predominantly HAIE (56%) in two centers in Brazil. In the latter study, an indwelling intravenous catheter was the main source of infection in the entire patient cohort, whereas among HAIE cases, 55% had chronic renal insufficiency as a comorbidity. The authors

Table 1
Selected prospective or retrospective observational studies describing the epidemiology, management, and outcomes of infective endocarditis in low- and middle-income countries

Country	Author, Year (Ref Number)	Study Description, IE Cases[a]	Underlying Cardiac Conditions	Microbiology[b]	Management	Mortality
Lao, PDR	Mirabel et al,[19] 2015	Retrospective, 11 definite, 25 possible	RHD, 33% CHD, 19% PV, 17% DVD, 8%	Organism identified: 13 cases Streptococci, 54% Staphylococci, 15% Enterococci, 15% *Escherichia coli*, 15%	Antibiotic therapy: β-lactam alone, 28% β-lactam + AG, 64% Peptide[c] alone, 0% Peptide[c] + AG, 0% Other, 8% Hospital stay (median, days), 16 Surgical intervention, none	In-hospital, 25% 2 y, 40%
India	Gupta et al,[23] 2013	Retrospective, 61 definite	RHD, 38% PV, 31% CHD, 23% Prior IE, 8% MVP, 3% DVD, 3%	Organism identified: 42 cases Streptococci, 21% Staphylococci, 21% Gram-negative, 29% Fungi, 14% Others, 17%	Antibiotic therapy, NR Hospital stay (median, days), NR Surgical intervention, 49%	In-hospital, 7%
India	Math et al,[20] 2011	Prospective, 104 definite	CHD, 39% RHD, 30% PV, 20% Prior IE, 15%	Organism identified: 43 cases Streptococci, 19% Staphylococci, 16% *Acinetobacter*, 16% Enterococci, 12% *Pseudomonas*, 12% *Klebsiella*, 9% Other/mixed, 21%	Antibiotic therapy: β-lactam alone, NR β-lactam + AG, 27% Peptide[c] alone, NR Peptide[c] + AG, NR Other, 59% Antibiotic duration (mean, days), 36 Surgical intervention, 15%	In-hospital, 26%

(continued on next page)

Table 1
(continued)

Country	Author, Year (Ref Number)	Study Description, IE Cases[a]	Underlying Cardiac Conditions	Microbiology[b]	Management	Mortality
Turkey	Simsek-Yavuz et al,[21] 2015	Prospective-retrospective,[d] 280 definite, 45 probable	RHD, 34% PV, 44% CHD, 14% DVD, 6% Pacemaker/ICD, 6% Prior IE, 6%	Organism identified: 253 cases Staphylococci, 36% Streptococci, 19% Enterococci, 7% *Brucella*, 5% NFGNR, 5% Other, 6%	Antibiotic therapy: β-lactam alone, NR β-lactam + AG, 54% Peptide[c] alone, NR Peptide[c] + AG, 18% Hospital stay (mean, days), 37 Surgical intervention, 52%	In-hospital, 28%
Brazil	Damasco et al,[34] 2014	Prospective, 56 definite, 15 possible	Structural heart disease, 52%	Organism identified: 60 cases Staphylococci, 38% Enterococci, 27% Streptococci, 25% Other, 8%	Antibiotic therapy: AG, 62% β-lactam, 76% Peptide,[c] 33% Amphotericin B, 11% Hospital stay (mean, days): Community-acquired IE, 37 Hospital-associated IE, 59 Surgical intervention, 17%	In-hospital, 46%
South Africa	Nel & Naidoo,[25] 2014	Prospective, 77 definite	RHD, 78% CHD, 6%	Organism identified: 36 cases Staphylococci, 47% Streptococci, 20% Propionibacterium, 3%	Antibiotic therapy, NR Hospital stay (mean, days), NR Surgical intervention, 52%	Overall, 23%
Turkey	Elbey et al,[31] 2013	Retrospective, 248 definite	PV, 30% RHD, 28% DVD, 23% CHD, 7% Pacemaker, 6% MVP, 4%	Organisms identified: 152 cases Staphylococci, 48% Streptococci, 18% Enterococci, 18% Gram-negative, 16% *Candida*, 1%	Antibiotic therapy, NR Antibiotic duration (mean, days), 28 Surgical intervention, 33%	In-hospital, 33%

Brazil	Nunes et al,[22] 2010	Prospective, 49 definite, 13 possible	RHD, 40% PV, 31% Prior IE, 23% Pacemaker/ICD, 19%	Organism identified: 40 cases Staphylococci, 48% Streptococci, 20% Enterococci, 15% Fungi, 5% Other, 13%	Antibiotic therapy, NR Hospital stay (mean, days), 41 Surgical intervention, 53%	In-hospital, 31%
Tunisia	Rekik et al,[42] 2009	Retrospective, 43 definite, 5 possible	PVE, 100%	Organism identified: 23 cases Staphylococci, 30% Streptococci, 17% Gram-negative rods, 17% Bartonella, 13% Other, 22%	Antibiotic therapy, NR Hospital stay (mean, days), 38 Surgical intervention, 42%	In-hospital, 23%
Tunisia	Trabelsi et al,[24] 2008	Retrospective, 125 definite, 9 possible	RHD, 45% CHD, 16% DVD, 8% Pacemaker/ICD, 2% PV, 0% (all cases were NVE)	Organism identified: 87 cases Streptococci, 24% Staphylococci, 22% Bartonella, 8% Others, 13%	Antibiotic therapy, NR Hospital stay (mean, days), NR Surgical intervention, 51%	In-hospital, 19%
Turkey	Leblebicioglu et al,[32] 2006	Prospective, 101 definite, 11 possible	Unspecified cardiovascular pathology, 20% Past rheumatic fever, 18% PV, 17% CHD, 5%	Organism identified: 94 cases Staphylococci, 50% Streptococci, 29% Enterococci, 16% Others, 5%	Antibiotic therapy: β-lactam, 39% Peptide,[c] 47% Hospital stay (mean, days), 36 Surgical intervention, 13%	30 d, 29%

Abbreviations: AG, aminoglycoside; ICD, implantable cardioverter-defibrillator; IVDU, intravenous drug use; MVP, mitral valve prolapse; NFGNR, nonfermentative gram-negative rods; NR, not reported; NVE, native valve endocarditis; PDR, People's Democratic Republic; PV, prosthetic valve; PVE, prosthetic valve endocarditis.

[a] Cases defined by modified Dukes' criteria.

[b] Percentages are expressed as a function of only the cases where microorganisms are identified.

[c] Peptide antibiotics include vancomycin, teicoplanin, and daptomycin.

[d] Prospective for the first 5 years then retrospective for remaining period.

attributed the higher HAIE rates to advances in medical practices in Rio de Janeiro.

Microbial Etiology

Staphylococcus is now the leading causative microorganism of IE in HICs, followed by *Streptococcus* and *Enterococcus*. Together, these microorganisms account for greater than 80% of the microbial causes of IE in HICs.[1,2,18]

Describing the microbial causes of IE in LMICs is extremely challenging because limited data exist on IE as it is, and one's ability to make conclusions from the available data is further curtailed by a high rate of nonidentified microorganisms. From available data, however, *Staphylococcus* and *Streptococcus* are the leading causative microorganisms.

Staphylococcus

Staphylococcus is increasingly common, and in some instances is the leading cause of IE in LMICs (see **Table 1**). *Staphylococcus* accounts for 15% to 50% of cases with *Staphylococcus aureus* more common than coagulase negative *Staphylococcus*.[19–23,25,31,32,34] Comparison with premillennial ranges shows an increase in *Staphylococcus*, which was previously reported in less than 20% of cases.[11,13,28]

The emergence of *Staphylococcus* as a leading cause of IE in LMICs, a trend that was also previously noted in HICs, may reflect medical technology advances, increased hospital contact, and increasing comorbidities.[9,34,35] Consistent with these factors, it is noteworthy that only UMIC studies reported *Staphylococcus* as the leading cause of IE, accounting for up to 50% of cases.[21,22,25,31,32,34] In LMICs, however, *Streptococcus* still predominates.[19,20]

Streptococcus

Streptococcus causes 18% to 54% of IE cases, with viridans group streptococci predominating.[19–23,25,31,32,34] *Streptococcus* is common among younger patients, patients with community-acquired IE, and patients with rheumatic or congenital NVE[19,20,34] as demonstrated in a study from Turkey.[21]

Other organisms

Less common causes of IE in LMICs are *Enterococcus*; gram-negative bacteria; and true causative agents of blood culture–negative IE, such as *Bartonella* and *Coxiella*.[19–22] This is consistent with reports from HICs, except for *Enterococcus*, which is the third leading cause of IE in HICs after *Staphylococcus* and *Streptococcus*.

Prevalence of enterococcal IE was reported to range between 7% and 18%[19–22,31,32] in our reviewed studies. Damasco and colleagues,[34] however, reported *Enterococcus* as the second most common cause of IE, after *Staphylococcus*, accounting for 27% of cases. Furthermore, among patients aged greater than or equal to 40 years, *Enterococcus* was the most commonly isolated microorganism, indicating a predilection for increasing age, a finding supported by Simsek-Yavuz and colleagues[21] who reported increasing prevalence of *Enterococcus* in individuals greater than 50 years old.

In summary, conclusions about the microbial causes of IE in LMICs are hampered by scarce available data and a high rate of unidentified microorganisms because of widespread prior antibiotic use, limited microbiologic capacity, and inadequate sampling procedures, challenges that are discussed later. Inconsistent serologic testing for atypical microorganisms further limits etiology determination.[36] Existing data, however, highlight a prominent contribution of *Streptococcus* and a growing contribution of *Staphylococcus*, particularly in UMICs.

TREATMENT

Prompt and appropriate organism-specific antibiotic therapy is recommended to improve clinical outcomes for patients with IE, whereas surgical intervention is recommended for complicated IE.[37–40] The antimicrobial regimens used, mean hospital stay, and surgical intervention rates are summarized in **Table 1** and discussed next.

Medical Therapy

Medical therapy remains the most common treatment of IE because of limited access to cardiovascular surgery in LMICs.[16] Setting-specific treatment guidelines are nonexistent and subsequently, societal guidelines from HICs are referenced in deciding treatment.[37,38] Determination of the microbial cause of IE should be the cornerstone of selecting antibiotic therapy; however, as discussed later, this is hampered in LMICs by high rates of organism nonidentification.

In the absence of reliable microbiologic findings, antibiotic therapy in most suspected cases remains empirical. The choice of therapy varies because the guidelines for empirical therapy from HICs[41] may not be translatable to settings with different local susceptibility patterns.

In the few cases where a microbial cause is determined, antibiotics are instituted from standard guideline-based regimens.[37,38] Our reviewed studies reveal high usage of combination therapy that typically includes β-lactams or peptide antibiotics and aminoglycosides, with prolonged duration of therapy ranging between 35 and 67 days.[20,42]

Mean duration of hospital stay ranges between 16 and 38 days.[21,22,34,42] Outpatient parenteral antibiotic therapy may be considered in stable patients to decrease hospital stay.[43] Outpatient parenteral antibiotic therapy for IE, however, may not be possible in most LMIC settings because of a high rate of complications associated with late hospital presentation, and unavailability of required medical services in the outpatient setting. None of our reviewed studies reported on the rates of outpatient parenteral antibiotic therapy.

Surgical Management

Because of late presentation and/or diagnosis, patients often present with complications, such as valve abscess, systemic embolization, heart failure, and hemodynamic instability, which are indications for emergent surgical intervention. Surgical intervention rates remain low, ranging from 0% to 53% in our reviewed studies.[19–25,31,32,34,42] The higher figures in this range (42%–53%) predominantly come from UMICs.[21,22,24,25,32,42] These figures refer to surgical rates among the entire patient cohort in the given study, and not necessarily restricted to patients with indications for surgical intervention. It is therefore difficult to conclude whether intervention rates are optimal. However, in LMICs for instance, surgical intervention was less than 15%, despite more than 30% of patients with IE presenting in heart failure, an indication for surgery.[19,20] In a cardiac center in India, however, where access to surgical consult and intervention was prompt, Gupta and colleagues[23] reported a surgical intervention rate of 49%.

Among patients with complications that require emergent intervention, the optimal timing for surgery remains controversial.[44] Early surgery, however, has been shown to decrease the rate of embolic events,[40] in-hospital,[45] and 6-month mortality.[46] Two studies in our review reported on the timing of surgery. Rekik and colleagues[42] reported a mean delay to surgery of 15 days among 20 patients with PVE and indications for surgery. Similarly, Trabelsi and colleagues[24] reported a mean time between admission and surgery of 16 days among 68 patients with NVE and surgical indications.

CHALLENGES

The prevailing challenges to the diagnosis and management of IE that coexist in LMICs are illustrated in **Fig. 1** and discussed next.

High Prevalence of Rheumatic Heart Disease

The prevalence of RHD remains high and accounts for a significant portion of cardiovascular disease morbidity and mortality in LMICs (See Gene and colleagues article, "Rheumatic Heart Disease: The Unfinished Global Agenda," in this issue).[15,47] IE is a common complication of RHD and as highlighted previously, up to half of IE cases in LMICs are superimposed on RHD. A total of 79% of the 15.6 million cases of RHD in 2005 were from LMICs, driven by poor standards of living, poor nutritional status, and limited access to health care facilities and penicillin prophylaxis.[15] With recent estimates projecting that up to 80 million people worldwide have RHD, more LMIC patients are at risk for IE (See Gene and colleagues article, "Rheumatic Heart Disease: The Unfinished Global Agenda," in this issue).[48] Addressing the high burden of RHD in LMICs is therefore a key step in decreasing IE-related morbidity and mortality.

Late Hospital Presentation

Patients with IE in LMICs often present to hospital late. Median time between symptom onset and hospital presentation ranged from 15 to 36 days in our reviewed studies.[22,24,34] Consequently, patients frequently presented with IE complications, such as heart failure and stroke.[10,22] IE complications are associated with higher mortality, and require surgical intervention that is often unavailable in LMICs, further worsening clinical outcomes.

High Rate of Organism Nonidentification

Identification of causative microorganisms, mainly through blood cultures, is the cornerstone of IE diagnosis and is crucial to the initiation of effective organism-specific antimicrobial therapy.[49] The rate of organism nonidentification in IE from HIC studies is less than 5%, whereas this figure is generally greater than 35%, reaching up to 60%, in LMICs.[1,19,20,24,25,31,42] Causes of this high rate are multifactorial. First, widespread use of antibiotics before collection of blood samples for culture substantially decreases the likelihood of obtaining growth on culture media. In our reviewed studies, 35% to 74% of patients reported prior antibiotic use.[20,23,24,32,42]

Second, there is limited capacity for high-quality microbiology studies, particularly in lower-middle-income and low-income settings. Blood culture infrastructure is underdeveloped and testing reagents are often unavailable.[50] Facilities for serologic testing of atypical organisms are also unavailable in the poorest settings.[36] Serologic

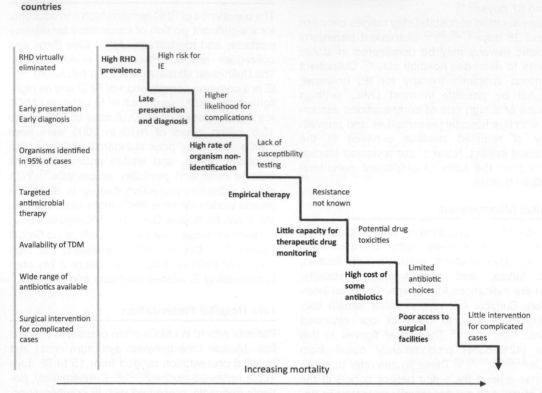

High income countries | **Low- and middle-income countries**

RHD virtually eliminated — High RHD prevalence — High risk for IE

Early presentation Early diagnosis — Late presentation and diagnosis — Higher likelihood for complications

Organisms identified in 95% of cases — High rate of organism non-identification — Lack of susceptibility testing

Targeted antimicrobial therapy — Empirical therapy — Resistance not known

Availability of TDM — Little capacity for therapeutic drug monitoring — Potential drug toxicities

Wide range of antibiotics available — High cost of some antibiotics — Limited antibiotic choices

Surgical intervention for complicated cases — Poor access to surgical facilities — Little intervention for complicated cases

Increasing mortality

Fig. 1. Prevailing challenges of IE in low- and middle-income countries. TDM, therapeutic drug monitoring.

testing increases the rate of organism identification and is particularly useful for organisms responsible for culture-negative IE, such as *Bartonella henselae*, *Brucella melitensis*, and *Coxiella burnetii*.

Third, inappropriate procedures in collecting samples for culture may occur.[51] It is recommended that at least three sets of blood culture samples are collected over a period of 12 hours, or more practically, with the first and last set obtained at least an hour apart.[49] LMIC studies, however, reported that a lower number of samples were collected, resulting in few samples fulfilling major IE criteria for blood culture.[20]

Empiric Antibiotic Therapy

Prompt identification of microorganisms and initiation of appropriate antibiotics decreases IE mortality and morbidities, such as stroke.[37,38] In the absence of organism identification in LMICs, however, antibiotic therapy in suspected cases is empirical. Choice of therapy varies among regions, hospitals, and physicians. This is because resource-poor regions often lack guidance to inform empirical therapy because local data on prevalent microorganisms and antibiotic resistance are scarce.[52]

Additional problems related to antibiotic use include cost limitations in resource-poor settings. Physicians and patients have little access to expensive regimens that may be required for drug-resistant cases.[53] Although commonly used antibiotics for IE, such as gentamicin, vancomycin, and most β-lactam antibiotics, including penicillin and ceftriaxone, are included in the World Health Organization essential medicines list, such agents as daptomycin, which may be necessary in drug-resistant IE cases, are not.[54] Antibiotic stock-outs may also occur during the course of treatment, leading to missed drug doses or unnecessary regimen changes.

Little Capacity for Therapeutic Drug Monitoring

Therapeutic drug monitoring services are frequently unavailable in LMICs.[55] Therapeutic drug monitoring is recommended for antibiotics used to manage IE, especially vancomycin and aminoglycosides, to ensure adequate drug levels are reached to maximize efficacy, decrease risk of resistance development, and avoid nephrotoxicity.[56,57] Furthermore, among patients with heart failure that commonly complicates IE, the risk of nephrotoxicity is heightened.[58]

Dismal Access to Surgery

Early surgery decreases mortality among patients with IE complications.[39,45] In HICs, approximately half of patients with IE in reported prospective series undergo surgical intervention,[1,2,59] with up to 75% of patients with indications for surgery receiving it.[59] In our reviewed studies, although UMIC studies reported surgical intervention rates close to HICs, two LMIC studies reported low rates of 0% and 15%.[19,20] We, however found no information on the rates of surgical intervention among patients with indications for surgery in LMICs. Given the high rate of complications among patients with IE in our reviewed studies, we surmise that this rate was low. Only a few referral facilities in Sub-Saharan Africa have the physical and human resource infrastructure to perform cardiovascular surgery,[16,60] and the few with such capacity often have long waiting lists, making emergent intervention difficult. Furthermore, where such opportunities are available, high costs remain an insurmountable barrier for most patients.[14]

FUTURE DIRECTIONS IN RESEARCH

A research agenda is urgently required around IE in LMICs. Our review reveals a scarcity of studies documenting clinical experience since the new millennium. In low-income countries, for instance, we found no studies meeting our search criteria. A high RHD prevalence in lower income settings, coupled with medical progress in improving economies where new IE risk factors for the population emerge, implies that IE will remain an important cardiovascular disease in LMICs. In addition, challenges in IE diagnosis and management result in higher IE-related morbidity and mortality in LMICs compared with HICs.[61] Setting-specific data are therefore required to track the clinical characteristics, diagnostic and management practices, and outcomes for patients with IE to foster investment in improving microbiologic, echocardiographic, and cardiovascular surgery capacity.

We propose the following steps to stimulate research and further understanding of IE in LMICs. First, where there is a critical lack of published data, such as in the low-income countries, retrospective reviews should be conducted based on existing records. This would serve as a first step to provide critical expeditious updates on the state of IE, while building capacity in research, and providing preliminary data that can be used to justify larger prospective studies.

Second, prospective IE registries in LMICs need to be established. Current studies are limited by few patient numbers in single health care centers, which hampers generalizability. Experiences from contemporary registries, such as the International Collaboration on Endocarditis, have effectively improved understanding of IE.[1,62] This registry, however, has predominantly included sites from HICs and UMICs, and to date has not included a site from a low-income country.[1] Experiences from International Collaboration on Endocarditis should be leveraged to build capacity in LMICs to enable them to form rigorous registries documenting experiences in their settings.

LIMITATIONS OF REVIEW

Our review has several strengths. Our focus on studies reporting findings from 2000 to 2016 provides a contemporary update on the causes of IE in LMICs, and the challenges yet to be addressed. Where possible, we have also described the differences in the IE profile between different LMIC economies.

Our review also has several limitations. We found few LMIC studies on IE, with most of them from UMICs and none from low-income countries. Therefore, this review may not adequately reflect findings from the lowest resource settings. Available studies have few patients, mostly from single centers, and are heterogeneous in nature, limiting our ability to form generalizable conclusions. Finally, most of the available data come from referral centers and thus our findings are subject to referral bias.

SUMMARY

Staphylococcus is an increasingly important cause of IE in LMICs, particularly in UMICs, although the rate of organism nonidentification is high. RHD remains the major underlying cardiac pathology, with a growing contribution of PVE. Rates of access to surgery in UMICs for complicated IE are as high as in HICs, but remain dismal in LMICs. Publication of retrospective findings in low-income settings and the formation of collaborative registries to improve understanding of contemporary IE in LMICs must be encouraged.

REFERENCES

1. Murdoch DR, Corey GR, Hoen B, et al. Clinical presentation, etiology, and outcome of infective endocarditis in the 21st century: the International Collaboration on Endocarditis-Prospective Cohort Study. Arch Intern Med 2009;169(5):463–73.
2. Selton-Suty C, Celard M, Le Moing V, et al. Preeminence of *Staphylococcus aureus* in infective endocarditis: a 1-year population-based survey. Clin Infect Dis 2012;54(9):1230–9.

3. Thuny F, Avierinos JF, Tribouilloy C, et al. Impact of cerebrovascular complications on mortality and neurologic outcome during infective endocarditis: a prospective multicentre study. Eur Heart J 2007; 28(9):1155–61.

4. Ferraris L, Milazzo L, Ricaboni D, et al. Profile of infective endocarditis observed from 2003-2010 in a single center in Italy. BMC Infect Dis 2013;13:545.

5. Nadji G, Rusinaru D, Remadi JP, et al. Heart failure in left-sided native valve infective endocarditis: characteristics, prognosis, and results of surgical treatment. Eur J Heart Fail 2009;11(7):668–75.

6. San Roman JA, Lopez J, Vilacosta I, et al. Prognostic stratification of patients with left-sided endocarditis determined at admission. Am J Med 2007; 120(4):369.e1-7.

7. Murray CJ, Vos T, Lozano R, et al. Disability-adjusted life years (DALYs) for 291 diseases and injuries in 21 regions, 1990-2010: a systematic analysis for the Global Burden of Disease Study 2010. Lancet 2012;380(9859):2197–223.

8. Coffey S, Cairns BJ, Iung B. The modern epidemiology of heart valve disease. Heart 2016;102(1): 75–85.

9. Yew HS, Murdoch DR. Global trends in infective endocarditis epidemiology. Curr Infect Dis Rep 2012; 14(4):367–72.

10. Bennis A, Zahraoui M, Azzouzi L, et al. Bacterial endocarditis in Morocco. Ann Cardiol Angeiol (Paris) 1995;44(7):339–44 [in French].

11. Garg N, Kandpal B, Garg N, et al. Characteristics of infective endocarditis in a developing country-clinical profile and outcome in 192 Indian patients, 1992-2001. Int J Cardiol 2005;98(2):253–60.

12. Ifere OA, Masokano KA. Infective endocarditis in children in the Guinea savannah of Nigeria. Ann Trop Paediatr 1991;11(3):233–40.

13. Koegelenberg CF, Doubell AF, Orth H, et al. Infective endocarditis in the Western Cape Province of South Africa: a three-year prospective study. QJM 2003; 96(3):217–25.

14. Tariq M, Alam M, Munir G, et al. Infective endocarditis: a five-year experience at a tertiary care hospital in Pakistan. Int J Infect Dis 2004;8(3):163–70.

15. Carapetis JR, Steer AC, Mulholland EK, et al. The global burden of group A streptococcal diseases. Lancet Infect Dis 2005;5(11):685–94.

16. Mocumbi AO. The challenges of cardiac surgery for African children. Cardiovasc J Afr 2012;23(3): 165–7.

17. World Bank Country and Lending Groups. Available at: https://datahelpdesk.worldbank.org/knowledgebase/articles/906519. Accessed June 1, 2016.

18. Sy RW, Kritharides L. Health care exposure and age in infective endocarditis: results of a contemporary population-based profile of 1536 patients in Australia. Eur Heart J 2010;31(15):1890–7.

19. Mirabel M, Rattanavong S, Frichitthavong K, et al. Infective endocarditis in the Lao PDR: clinical characteristics and outcomes in a developing country. Int J Cardiol 2015;180:270–3.

20. Math RS, Sharma G, Kothari SS, et al. Prospective study of infective endocarditis from a developing country. Am Heart J 2011;162(4):633–8.

21. Simsek-Yavuz S, Sensoy A, Kasikcioglu H, et al. Infective endocarditis in Turkey: aetiology, clinical features, and analysis of risk factors for mortality in 325 cases. Int J Infect Dis 2015;30:106–14.

22. Nunes MCP, Gelape CL, Ferrari TCA. Profile of infective endocarditis at a tertiary care center in Brazil during a seven-year period: prognostic factors and in-hospital outcome. Int J Infect Dis 2010;14(5): e394–8.

23. Gupta A, Gupta A, Kaul U, et al. Infective endocarditis in an Indian setup: are we entering the 'modern' era? Indian J Crit Care Med 2013;17(3):140–7.

24. Trabelsi I, Rekik S, Znazen A, et al. Native valve infective endocarditis in a tertiary care center in a developing country (Tunisia). Am J Cardiol 2008; 102(9):1247–51.

25. Nel SH, Naidoo DP. An echocardiographic study of infective endocarditis, with special reference to patients with HIV. Cardiovasc J Afr 2014;25(2):50–7.

26. Zuhlke LJ, Engel ME, Watkins D, et al. Incidence, prevalence and outcome of rheumatic heart disease in South Africa: a systematic review of contemporary studies. Int J Cardiol 2015;199:375–83.

27. Cetinkaya Y, Akova M, Akalin HE, et al. A retrospective review of 228 episodes of infective endocarditis where rheumatic valvular disease is still common. Int J Antimicrob Agents 2001;18(1):1–7.

28. Letaief A, Boughzala E, Kaabia N, et al. Epidemiology of infective endocarditis in Tunisia: a 10-year multicenter retrospective study. Int J Infect Dis 2007;11(5):430–3.

29. Remenyi B, Carapetis J, Wyber R, et al. Position statement of the World Heart Federation on the prevention and control of rheumatic heart disease. Nat Rev Cardiol 2013;10(5):284–92.

30. Seckeler MD, Hoke TR. The worldwide epidemiology of acute rheumatic fever and rheumatic heart disease. Clin Epidemiol 2011;3:67–84.

31. Elbey MA, Akdag S, Kalkan ME, et al. A multicenter study on experience of 13 tertiary hospitals in Turkey in patients with infective endocarditis. Anadolu kardiyol Derg 2013;13(6):523–7.

32. Leblebicioglu H, Yilmaz H, Tasova Y, et al. Characteristics and analysis of risk factors for mortality in infective endocarditis. Eur J Epidemiol 2006;21(1): 25–31.

33. Cahill TJ, Prendergast BD. Infective endocarditis. Lancet 2016;387(10021):882–93.

34. Damasco PV, Ramos JN, Correal JC, et al. Infective endocarditis in Rio de Janeiro, Brazil: a 5-year

experience at two teaching hospitals. Infection 2014;42(5):835–42.

35. Fowler VG Jr, Miro JM, Hoen B, et al. *Staphylococcus aureus* endocarditis: a consequence of medical progress. JAMA 2005;293(24):3012–21.

36. Rattanavong S, Fournier PE, Chu V, et al. *Bartonella henselae* endocarditis in Laos - 'the unsought will go undetected'. PLoS Negl Trop Dis 2014;8(12):e3385.

37. Baddour LM, Wilson WR, Bayer AS, et al. Infective endocarditis in adults: diagnosis, antimicrobial therapy, and management of complications: a scientific statement for healthcare professionals from the American Heart Association. Circulation 2015; 132(15):1435–86.

38. Habib G, Lancellotti P, Antunes MJ, et al. 2015 ESC guidelines for the management of infective endocarditis: the task force for the management of infective endocarditis of the European Society of Cardiology (ESC) Endorsed by: European Association for Cardio-Thoracic Surgery (EACTS), the European Association of Nuclear Medicine (EANM). Eur Heart J 2015;36(44):3075–128.

39. Kiefer T, Park L, Tribouilloy C, et al. Association between valvular surgery and mortality among patients with infective endocarditis complicated by heart failure. JAMA 2011;306(20):2239–47.

40. Kang DH, Kim YJ, Kim SH, et al. Early surgery versus conventional treatment for infective endocarditis. N Engl J Med 2012;366(26):2466–73.

41. Gould FK, Denning DW, Elliott TS, et al. Guidelines for the diagnosis and antibiotic treatment of endocarditis in adults: a report of the working party of the British Society for Antimicrobial Chemotherapy. J Antimicrob Chemother 2012;67(2):269–89.

42. Rekik S, Trabelsi I, Znazen A, et al. Prosthetic valve endocarditis: management strategies and prognosis: a ten-year analysis in a tertiary care centre in Tunisia. Neth Heart J 2009;17(2):56–60.

43. Tice AD, Rehm SJ, Dalovisio JR, et al. Practice guidelines for outpatient parenteral antimicrobial therapy. Clin Infect Dis 2004;38(12):1651–71.

44. Bannay A, Hoen B, Duval X, et al. The impact of valve surgery on short- and long-term mortality in left-sided infective endocarditis: do differences in methodological approaches explain previous conflicting results? Eur Heart J 2011;32(16):2003–15.

45. Lalani T, Cabell CH, Benjamin DK, et al. Analysis of the impact of early surgery on in-hospital mortality of native valve endocarditis: use of propensity score and instrumental variable methods to adjust for treatment-selection bias. Circulation 2010;121(8):1005–13.

46. Vikram HR, Buenconsejo J, Hasbun R, et al. Impact of valve surgery on 6-month mortality in adults with complicated, left-sided native valve endocarditis: a propensity analysis. JAMA 2003;290(24):3207–14.

47. Celermajer DS, Chow CK, Marijon E, et al. Cardiovascular disease in the developing world: prevalences,

patterns, and the potential of early disease detection. J Am Coll Cardiol 2012;60(14):1207–16.

48. Paar JA, Berrios NM, Rose JD, et al. Prevalence of rheumatic heart disease in children and young adults in Nicaragua. Am J Cardiol 2010;105(12):1809–14.

49. Li JS, Sexton DJ, Mick N, et al. Proposed modifications to the Duke criteria for the diagnosis of infective endocarditis. Clin Infect Dis 2000;30(4):633–8.

50. Archibald LK, Reller LB. Clinical microbiology in developing countries. Emerg Infect Dis 2001;7(2): 302–5.

51. Mermel LA, Maki DG. Detection of bacteremia in adults: consequences of culturing an inadequate volume of blood. Ann Intern Med 1993;119(4):270–2.

52. Alsan M, Schoemaker L, Eggleston K, et al. Out-of-pocket health expenditures and antimicrobial resistance in low-income and middle-income countries: an economic analysis. Lancet Infect Dis 2015; 15(10):1203–10.

53. Uganda SURE. 2014. Securing Ugandans' Right to Essential Medicines Program: Final Report (2009-2014). Submitted to the US Agency for International Development by the Uganda SURE Program. Arlington, VA: Management Sciences for Health.

54. 19th WHO model list of essential medicines (April 2015). Available at: http://www.who.int/medicines/publications/essentialmedicines/EML2015_8-May-15.pdf. Accessed August 9, 2016.

55. Nwobodo N. Therapeutic drug monitoring in a developing nation: a clinical guide. JRSM Open 2014;5(8). 2054270414531121.

56. Cosgrove SE, Vigliani GA, Fowler VG Jr, et al. Initial low dose gentamicin for *Staphylococcus aureus* bacteremia and endocarditis is nephrotoxic. Clin Infect Dis 2009;48(6):713–21.

57. Burgess LD, Drew RH. Comparison of the incidence of vancomycin-induced nephrotoxicity in hospitalized patients with and without concomitant piperacillin-tazobactam. Pharmacotherapy 2014;34(7):670–6.

58. Sarraf M, Masoumi A, Schrier RW. Cardiorenal syndrome in acute decompensated heart failure. Clin J Am Soc Nephrol 2009;4(12):2013–26.

59. Chu VH, Park LP, Athan E, et al. Association between surgical indications, operative risk, and clinical outcome in infective endocarditis: a prospective study from the International Collaboration on Endocarditis. Circulation 2015;131(2):131–40.

60. Zühlke L, Mirabel M, Marijon E. Congenital heart disease and rheumatic heart disease in Africa: recent advances and current priorities. Heart 2013;99(21):1554–61.

61. Thuny F, Grisoli D, Collart F, et al. Management of infective endocarditis: challenges and perspectives. Lancet 2012;379(9819):965–75.

62. Cabell CH, Abrutyn E. Progress toward a global understanding of infective endocarditis. Lessons from the International Collaboration on Endocarditis. Cardiol Clin 2003;21(2):147–58.

Rheumatic Heart Disease
The Unfinished Global Agenda

Shanti Nulu, MD, MPH[a], Gene Bukhman, MD, PhD[b,c], Gene F. Kwan, MD, MPH[c,d,*]

KEYWORDS

- Rheumatic heart disease • Rheumatic fever • Global health • Noncommunicable disease

KEY POINTS

- Rheumatic heart disease (RHD) is a neglected chronic disease of poverty.
- RHD affects an estimated 33 million people worldwide and causes 275,000 deaths annually.
- Although RHD has been eradicated from high-income countries, endemic regions of low-income and middle-income countries continue to struggle with preventive, diagnostic, and management strategies.
- Further research is needed to better understand RHD pathophysiology, epidemiology, and health system responses.

INTRODUCTION

Rheumatic heart disease (RHD) is a neglected chronic disease primarily affecting the poorest people worldwide and is the most common form of acquired heart disease among children and young adults in low-income and middle-income countries. RHD affects an estimated 33 million people worldwide by Global Burden of Disease study estimates.[1] However, up to 80 million people may have asymptomatic RHD.[2] Annually, RHD accounts for approximately 275,000 deaths, and is a major cause of premature mortality and morbidity among children and young adults in low-income and middle-income countries.[1,3]

RHD was a prioritized subject of active investigation in developed countries in the first half of the twentieth century; however, RHD was largely eradicated in developed countries by mid-century, and subsequent research endeavors investigating RHD diminished. Thus, most of our current knowledge of RHD pathophysiology and treatment is largely based on decades-old studies

that lack the modern investigative standards of today. Over the past 2 decades, there has been renewed interest in RHD in a global health context given its predominance as a major cause of cardiovascular morbidity and mortality in low-income and middle-income countries. Recently, an emerging global health equity movement has increased the awareness among global health practitioners, researchers, and policy makers to the disparity in RHD care. A growing body of new clinical research has emerged from endemic countries, to inform evidence-based interventions for RHD diagnosis and management.

This review provides an overview of the current diagnosis and treatment gaps for RHD as embedded within a historical context. First, we look back at the history of RHD as a subject of study in medicine and public health. Then, we review the evolution of RHD diagnosis as new technologies have emerged. Third, we will review the current epidemiologic data on RHD at a global level and its limitations. We next discuss current

The authors have nothing to disclose.
a Section of Cardiovascular Medicine, Yale School of Medicine, 789 Howard Avenue, New Haven, CT 06519, USA; b Division of Global Health Equity, Brigham and Women's Hospital, 641 Huntington Avenue, Boston, MA 02115, USA; c Department of Global Health and Social Medicine, Harvard Medical School, 641 Huntington Avenue, Boston, MA 02115, USA; d Section of Cardiovascular Medicine, Boston University Medical Center, Boston University School of Medicine, 88 East Newton Street, D8, Boston, MA 02118, USA
* Corresponding author. Boston University Medical Center, 88 East Newton Street, D8, Boston, MA 02118.
E-mail address: genekwan@bu.edu

management principles and gaps in knowledge. Finally, we survey current advocacy efforts to improve RHD awareness and care.

HISTORICAL OVERVIEW: WHERE WE LEFT OFF

A century ago, acute rheumatic fever (ARF) was the leading cause of death among school-age children in the United States, and was second to tuberculosis among young adults aged 20 to 30 years.[4] In New England, half of adult heart disease was caused by childhood rheumatic disease, and 8% of autopsies from New York's Presbyterian Hospital in 1938 showed evidence of "rheumatism."[5,6]

In 1927, a special research unit was established at the House of Good Samaritan in Boston where Dr T. Duckett Jones began a lifelong study of ARF. He ultimately published the first set of "Jones criteria" in 1944, systematizing the diagnosis of ARF based on the presence of discrete clinical signs.[7] In his seminal paper, Jones described ARF as "one of the important soluble medical problems of our day."[7] Indeed, such a common source of morbidity among young adults had significant social repercussions, especially in a wartime setting. During World War II it was estimated that approximately 100,000 men were rejected from military service because of RHD.[8] Crowded air bases provided an ideal setting for ARF outbreaks, with up to 25 to 100 per 1000 troops reported ARF at some bases.[9]

The high prevalence of the ARF among armed forces personnel served as an impetus for increased national attention to the disease. Experiments involving antimicrobial therapy were conducted among army recruits with good results.[5] Health service–based studies in the early penicillin era targeting high-prevalence populations showed the important role that improvements in health care access can play in diminishing disparities in ARF care.[10]

Although tempting to credit the increased access to antibiotics for the decline of RHD in the United States, it is notable that the start of the decline of ARF and RHD well preceded the antibiotic era by several decades. In addition, researchers noted that only a small percentage (<3%) of those with streptococcal infections went on to develop ARF, suggesting that other host factors played an important role in pathogenesis.[10] The decline of RHD at a societal level has been linked broadly to "primordial" factors related to the environment and host, such as living conditions, sanitation, and hygiene. Even today, RHD is more common in poor communities, and among children attending lower socioeconomic schools, those who have low formal education, lack formal employment, or live in crowded conditions.[11–15] For example, RHD is 60 times more common among poor indigenous people of Australia than nonindigenous.[16]

By the 1950s, there was waning public interest in RHD given its decline in the civilian population and the end of World War II. Further investigation into the complex determinants of ARF and RHD were not continued.[10] Speaking in 1985 when RHD had all but disappeared from the medical consciousness, the renowned epidemiologist Leon Gordis[10] ominously reminded his audience of the persistently high prevalence among children and young adults in developing countries and called urgently for renewed research on biological, host, and social determinants of disease. His call remained essentially unheeded until several decades later when increasing awareness of neglected disease among the global poor and the rise of a global health equity platform would begin to revive and reprioritize the disease.

PATHOPHYSIOLOGY AND GAPS IN SCIENCE

The pathophysiology of RHD remains incompletely understood, with host, bacterial, environmental, and genetic factors all implicated in its pathogenesis. Although Group A β-hemolytic Streptococcus (GAS) infection is undoubtedly involved, the disease has strong heritability and significant variation in natural history and severity according to host factors and geography.

Classically, ARF usually occurs 2 to 6 weeks after an episode of untreated GAS pharyngitis in approximately 0.4% to 3.0% of patients.[17,18] In patients with an active episode of ARF, the throat culture may be negative for GAS and antibody titers for streptococcal enzymes, such as streptolysin O and DNase, should be elevated. Rheumatic carditis is classically described as a pancarditis, involving the pericardium, myocardium, and endocardium.[19] Histopathologically, rheumatic myocarditis is characterized by the presence of focal perivascular inflammation, termed Aschoff bodies.[20,21]

The development of RHD occurs in some patients with ARF as a result of valvular damage from an immune-mediated process after one or repeated infections. Among Brazilian children with ARF, 72% developed chronic valvular disease and 16% developed severe mitral and/or aortic disease.[22] A prevailing theory is that cross-reactivity between moieties in the GAS strain and cardiac antigens are responsible for immunologic activation and eventual tissue destruction.[17] The streptococcal M protein and sarcomeric proteins, especially certain "rheumatogenic" M types (1, 5, 6, 14, 18, and 24) are considered likely candidates due to their similarity with intramyocellular proteins.[23] However, anti–group A carbohydrate antibodies have been implicated in the pathogenesis of valvulitis, with titer levels falling after surgical removal of inflamed valves.[24] Endothelial activation is also a necessary component of this theory of pathogenesis, as the cardiac antigens are intracellular. Antibody-mediated endothelial damage leads ultimately to T-cell activation, infiltration, and scarring.[25,26]

However, some researchers have noted that the M-protein cross-reactivity theory does not adequately explain the multisystem nature of the disease, or the characteristic pattern of cardiac involvement with propensity for valvular tissue and sparing of the myocardium.[27] Although interstitial infiltration and perivascular Aschoff nodules are commonly seen, myocardial necrosis is rarely observed, with a lack of elevation of cardiac biomarkers.[28,29] An alternative mechanism for immune activation and molecular mimicry has been suggested, involving collagen autoimmunity similar to other collagen-mediated autoimmune disease.[27] Surface components of rheumatogenic streptococcal strains have been shown to form a complex with human collagen type IV in subendothelial basement membranes, which may serve as the starting point of the immunologic cascade.[30,31]

That ARF incidence may be clustered by family genetics, occurring more commonly in patients with a family history of ARF, has been noted since 1889.[32] HLA type II molecules have been more closely associated with ARF; however, no specific HLA type has yet been implicated.[33] A meta-analysis of 435 twin pairs with ARF revealed a high degree of heritability, estimated at 60%.[34] Indeed, there is considerable geographic variability in the natural history and phenotypes of RHD across the globe, pointing to the important role of genetic factors in pathogenesis of disease. For example, African patients rarely present with ARF, and are usually diagnosed with RHD at later stages of disease.[18] Data from the Global Rheumatic Heart Disease Registry (REMEDY) show that only 22% of registered patients with RHD in low-income countries reported a prior history of ARF, compared with 49% in upper-middle-income countries.[35]

There is clearly a need for more basic science research into the pathophysiology of ARF and RHD, including genetic and environmental studies of endemic populations. A better understanding of the disease may yield insights leading to future preventive or therapeutic strategies.

THE EVOLUTION OF DIAGNOSTIC CRITERIA: FROM DIAGNOSIS OF ACUTE RHEUMATIC FEVER TO SCREENING FOR RHEUMATIC HEART DISEASE

Acute Rheumatic Fever Diagnosis and the Jones Criteria: from 1944 to 2015

Given the systemic nature of the disease, patients with ARF display a diversity of symptoms across multiple organ systems. The professed aim of T. Duckett Jones in publishing in 1944 the first "Jones" criteria for ARF diagnosis, was to systematize the wide range of previously described clinical features to avoid overdiagnosis and to facilitate ongoing research.[7] The Jones criteria have undergone 3 revisions over the decades, the last in 2015, and include both major and minor criteria (**Table 1**).[36–38] In general, the major criteria comprise 5 characteristic clinical features: carditis, migratory polyarthritis, chorea, erythema marginatum, and subcutaneous nodules. Carditis was defined more specifically in the 1965 revision as the presence of a murmur (apical systolic, mid-diastolic, or basal diastolic), cardiomegaly, pericarditis, or congestive heart failure. The apical murmur of ARF is generally thought to correlate with pathologic mitral regurgitation, which is the most common early cardiac manifestation of ARF. Since its inception until only recently, the Jones criteria relied solely on clinical bedside and laboratory findings as diagnostic criteria. The latest 2015 revision of the Jones criteria differs from prior iterations in 3 significant aspects. First, the revision now includes subclinical carditis (SCC), defined as the presence of echocardiographic valvular lesions in the absence of a murmur, as a sufficient qualification for carditis. The addition of SCC, long overdue, was in response to the large body of evidence spanning 2 decades demonstrating significantly greater detection rates for valvulitis by echocardiography as compared with auscultation alone. Second, the 2015 criteria now differentiate 2 sets of diagnostic criteria based on population risk, as a means to increase sensitivity in higher-risk populations without leading to false positives among low-risk populations. Aseptic monoarthritis may occur in up to 18% of patients as the initial presentation of ARF in high-risk populations.[39–42] Subsequently, the third modification specifies aseptic monoarthritis as a major criterion only for moderate/high-risk populations.

Table 1
The Jones criteria for diagnosis of acute rheumatic fever, and its revisions through the decades

Year (revision)	Major Criteria	Minor Criteria	Diagnosis	New Changes
1944 (Original)[7]	Carditis Arthralgia Chorea Subcutaneous nodules Recurrence	Fever Abdominal pain precordial pain Rash (most commonly erythema marginatum) epistaxis "Pulmonary findings" nonspecific laboratory findings (eg, elevated ESR)	"Any single major criterion in combination with 2 minor criteria"	
1956 (Modified)	Carditis Polyarthritis Chorea Subcutaneous nodules Erythema marginatum	Fever Arthralgia Prolonged PR Elevated ESR, WBC, or CRP Evidence of preceding streptococcal infection Prior history of ARF or RHD	2 major OR 1 major and 2 minor	Specification of "polyarthritis" rather than "arthralgia" for major criteria; specification of "carditis"
1965 (First Revision)[36]	Carditis Polyarthritis Chorea Subcutaneous nodules Erythema marginatum	Prior ARF or RHF Fever Arthralgia Elevated ESR, WBC, or CRP Prolonged PR	Evidence of prior GAS (elevated ASO titers or positive throat culture) AND 2 major OR 1 major and 2 minor	Requirement of evidence of prior GAS infection

			Evidence of prior streptococcal infection (elevated ASO titers, positive throat culture, or positive rapid antigen test) AND	Addition of exceptions
1992 (Second Revision)[37]	Carditis Polyarthritis Chorea Subcutaneous nodules Erythema marginatum	Fever Arthralgia Elevated ESR, WBC, or CRP Prolonged PR	2 major OR 1 major and 2 minor	1. Chorea as sole manifestation 2. Carditis alone if late presentation 3. In recurrence, only need 1 major or "several" minor criteria
2015 (Third Revision)[38]	Low-risk Carditis (clinical or subclinical) Polyarthritis Chorea Subcutaneous nodules Erythema marginatum Moderate/high risk Carditis (clinical or subclinical) Arthritis (monoarthritis, polyarthritis or polyarthralgia) Chorea Subcutaneous nodules Erythema marginatum	Low-risk Polyarthralgia Fever (38.5°C) ESR >60 mm CRP >3 mg/dL Prolonged PR Moderate/high risk Monoarthralgia Fever >38°C ESR >30 mm CRP >3 mg/dL Prolonged PR	Evidence of preceding GAS infection AND Initial ARF: 2 major OR 1 major and 2 minor Recurrent ARF: 2 major OR 1 major and 2 minor OR 3 minor	Differentiation of criteria by population risk category; Addition of specific values for fever, ESR, CRP cutoffs

Abbreviations: ARF, acute rheumatic fever; ASO, antistreptolysin O; CRP, C-reactive protein. ESR, erythrocyte sedimentation rate; GAS, Group A β-hemolytic Streptococcus; RHD, rheumatic heart disease; WBC, white blood cell.

From Subclinical Carditis to Rheumatic Heart Disease: the Evolution of Echocardiographic Applications

The presence of carditis in the absence of a clinical murmur was first suggested from early autopsy studies showing the presence of Aschoff nodules in patients without a known antemortem murmur.[43] However, it was only with the advent of echocardiography that clinically silent disease could be detected in the living patient. Although echocardiography became widely available in developed countries in the 1970s, it was the development of Doppler echocardiography in the 1980s, with its ability to detect regurgitation even in the absence of a murmur, which led to widespread recognition that valvular pathology may be subclinical.[44] Several studies starting in 1987 showed the utility of echocardiography in improving the identification of patients with ARF-related carditis.[45,46] In the mid-1990s, specific criteria were refined to distinguish pathologic versus physiologic regurgitation.[47,48] Studies using 2-dimensional echocardiography of valvular morphology of RHD found that mitral valve "prolapse" (or excessive leaflet motion), chordal elongation, and valvular and subvalvular thickening were common morphologic features of RHD.[49,50] A systematic review of 23 studies, using heterogeneous Doppler-based definitions of SCC, found the pooled prevalence of SCC was approximately 16.8% among patients with ARF but without clinical evidence of carditis.[51] In 2004, a joint National Institutes of Health–World Health Organization (WHO) working group developed standard surveillance protocols for GAS disease, and included for the first time echocardiography into the diagnostic criteria for RHD.[12] However, the use of echocardiography was limited to Doppler methods to detect pathologic regurgitation, with pathologic regurgitation defined as a regurgitant jet greater than 1 cm in length, in at least 2 planes, with peak velocity of greater than 2.5 m/s.

The establishment of SCC as a potential antecedent for future RHD among asymptomatic children, along with the development of new portable echocardiography technologies, led to a wave of screening studies in endemic regions. In many resource-poor settings, weak health systems present a barrier to adequate diagnosis and treatment during the initial phases of ARF, leading to a potentially larger burden of undiagnosed chronic RHD. The advent of portable echocardiography now enables community-based screening and increased detection of subclinical disease. One of the early research applications of portable echocardiography was in a landmark study by Marijon and colleagues,[52] which was based in 2 endemic sites (Mozambique and Cambodia). The study was one of the first to use a combination of Doppler (any mitral or aortic regurgitation) and morphologic echocardiographic criteria (restricted leaflet mobility, valvular and subvalvular thickening) for diagnosis of RHD. Echocardiography-based screening identified 10 times more patients with RHD than auscultation alone. A subsequent study by the same group compared the WHO Doppler-based criteria with the "combined" criteria, including morphologic findings, and found a much greater sensitivity for detection with the addition of morphologic criteria.[53] Numerous other large-scale echocardiography-based RHD screening programs in several countries have also revealed a significant burden of subclinical RHD.[54–56] It is important to distinguish the larger screening studies, which aimed to detect latent or asymptomatic RHD in the absence of ARF, from the earlier studies, which aimed at improving detection of SCC during a clinical presentation of ARF.

In response to the increasing reliance of echocardiography for diagnosis and screening of RHD, as well as greater international concern for the neglected burden of RHD among the global poor, the World Heart Federation (WHF) issued the first guidelines for echocardiographic diagnosis or RHD in 2012 (**Tables 2** and **3**).[57] The purpose of WHF guidelines is for screening of asymptomatic or mild cases of latent RHD to facilitate secondary prophylaxis to prevent disease progression. As there are normal physiologic valvular changes with aging, 2 sets of criteria were developed: one for those patients younger than 20 years and another for patients older than 20 years, which are further divided into "definite" and "borderline." In addition, given the propensity of the aortic valve to develop pathologic regurgitation with age in response to factors such as hypertension, the aortic valve criteria do not apply to those older than 35 years. In general, the criteria for "definite RHD" are an extension of the combination criteria used by the aforementioned studies (pathologic regurgitation or mitral or aortic valves with the presence of 2 morphologic features), with the additional inclusion of significant mitral stenosis with a mean gradient of greater than 4 mm Hg. The presence of both Doppler and morphologic criteria, as in the "definite" RHD category, has been shown to be associated with a greater risk for persistence or progression as compared with Doppler criteria alone.[58] "Borderline" disease is defined as either regurgitation or morphologic findings in isolation of each other and is intended to increase sensitivity among the

Table 2
2012 World Heart Federation criteria for echocardiographic diagnosis of RHD

Age <20	Definite RHD (A, B, C, or D)	A. Pathologic MR and at least 2 morphologic features of RHD of the MV
		B. MS with mean gradient >4 mm Hg
		C. Pathologic AR and at least 2 morphologic features of RHD of the AV
		D. Borderline disease of both the AV and MV
	Borderline RHD (A, B, or C)	A. At least 2 morphologic features of RHD of the MV without MR or MS
		B. Pathologic MR
		C. Pathologic MS
Age >20	Definite RHD (A, B, C, or D)	A. Pathologic MR and at least 2 morphologic features of RHD of the MV
		B. MS with mean gradient >4 mm Hg
		C. Pathologic AR and at least 2 morphologic features of RHD of the AV, only for age <35
		D. Pathologic AR and at least 2 morphologic features of the MV

Abbreviations: AR, aortic regurgitation; AV, aortic valve; MR, mitral regurgitation; MS, mitral stenosis; MV, mitral valve; RHD, rheumatic heart disease.

Data from Remenyi B, Wilson N, Steer A, et al. World Heart Federation criteria for echocardiographic diagnosis of rheumatic heart disease-an evidence based guideline. Nat Rev Cardiol 2012;9:297–309.

younger than 20 age group (see **Tables 2** and **3**). Interobserver agreement is only moderate for "borderline RHD," with kappa values of approximately 0.5 to 0.7, whereas it is better for definite RHD, with kappa values of approximately 0.8.[59,60] The clinical relevance of borderline and definite RHD diagnostic categories is discussed in a later section.

GLOBAL EPIDEMIOLOGY: EXTRAPOLATION AND UNCERTAINTY

One of the first systematic attempts at ascertaining the global prevalence of RHD used population-based data from 57 studies to estimate a total global prevalence of 15.6 million cases of RHD with 282,000 new cases and 233,000 deaths per year.[3] Most of the studies included were of school-age children using echocardiography for diagnosis. Statistical methods were used to extrapolate the prevalence to older children and young adults, and estimate the burden in regions from where there are no data.

The 2013 iteration of the Global Burden of Disease (GBD) study is based on systematic reviews including vital registration and verbal autopsy data.[1] Statistical modeling using country-level variables, such as income, education, and risk factor distribution, are used to generate estimates where data are lacking. RHD is estimated to affect 36 million people and cause 275,000 deaths (crude, all ages) annually. However, most of the RHD burden is among the global poor, with an estimated 183 disability-adjusted life years per 100,000 in low-income countries. The GBD study estimates suffer from an urban bias and lack of

Table 3
2012 World Heart Federation–specific criteria for pathologic regurgitation and morphologic features of rheumatic heart disease

Criteria for Pathologic Regurgitation		Morphologic Criteria	
Mitral	**Aortic**	**Mitral**	**Aortic**
Seen in 2 views	Seen in 2 views	AMVL thickening >3 mm*	Irregular or focal thickening
Jet length >2 cm	Jet length >1 cm	Chordal thickening	Coaptation defect
Velocity >3 m/s for 1 complete envelope	Velocity >3 m/s in early diastole	Restricted leaflet motion	Restricted leaflet motion
Pansystolic jet in at least 1 envelope	Pandiastolic jet in at least 1 envelope	Excessive leaflet tip motion during systole	Prolapse

Abbreviation: AMVL, anterior mitral valve leaflet.

* Abnormal thickening of the AMVL is age-specific and defined as follows: ≥3 mm for individuals aged ≤20 years; ≥4 mm for individuals aged 21–40 years; ≥5 mm for individuals aged >40 years.

Data from Remenyi B, Wilson N, Steer A, et al. World Heart Federation criteria for echocardiographic diagnosis of rheumatic heart disease-an evidence based guideline. Nat Rev Cardiol 2012;9:297–309.

robust representative input data, resulting in wide uncertainty intervals particularly in low-income countries. In sub-Saharan Africa, fewer than 5% of deaths, mostly in urban centers, are recorded.[61] Only 9 sub-Saharan African countries contributed cause-of-death data for GBD mortality estimates. Further, there is substantial subnational heterogeneity with respect to poverty and disease morbidity. RHD prevalence is much higher in rural areas with lower socioeconomic status than urban centers.[62] For example, southern Ghana is more representative of a middle-income country, whereas northern Ghana is much more impoverished.[63] In the GBD study, subnational estimates are now available for only a few of countries. Further, the GBD study estimates the prevalence of RHD causing morbidity, and does not include subclinical RHD.

School-based echocardiography screening studies have identified otherwise healthy children with subclinical RHD as defined by the WHF criteria. Including borderline RHD, a higher than expected prevalence was noted of 20 to 37 cases per 1000 in Uganda, Ethiopia, and South Africa.[62,64] Through extrapolation, the worldwide prevalence of subclinical RHD is estimated to be as high as 80 million, at least double that reported in the 2013 GBD study.[2,55]

In general, the regions of the world with high RHD prevalence are those with the weakest health infrastructure to support robust population-based epidemiologic studies. As such, data from endemic regions are often sparse, of poorer quality, and urban-based, despite evidence that RHD may be more prevalent in rural areas. Subsequently, many estimates of the global prevalence of RHD rely on studies with an urban bias and involve statistical extrapolation. Zuhlke and Steer[65] highlighted several key areas of uncertainty affecting the validity of the global estimates. First, the lack of representative data is highly problematic, with some data lacking entirely for specific countries or subnational regions, or limited to only urban areas. As studies comparing urban and rural prevalence have shown higher prevalence of RHD in rural areas, the reliance or largely urban-based data likely results in underestimation. Second, the heavy reliance on extrapolation to fill in gaps for non–school-age groups also may lead to underestimation, as the multiplication factors for extrapolation were from areas in which access and quality to care may be higher. Only 15% to 20% of all RHD cases are among children 5 to 14 years of age.[66] However, most screening studies are performed among school-age children. Some recent studies including young adults and pregnant women have uncovered higher than predicted prevalence of asymptomatic disease, as high as 22 per 100,000 in Nicaragua and 23 per 100,000 in Eritrea.[55,67]

MANAGEMENT OF RHEUMATIC HEART DISEASE: GAPS IN KNOWLEDGE

RHD management approaches rely on a combination of preventive and therapeutic strategies. Preventive efforts can avert the initial GAS infection (primordial prevention), impede progression from GAS infection or ARF to valvular disease (primary prevention), or hinder worsening of valvular disease among those with existing RHD (secondary prevention). Patients with symptomatic chronic valvular disease have limited therapeutic options with medical therapy, but if necessary can benefit from lifesaving surgery or percutaneous interventions.

Primordial and Primary Prevention

Primordial prevention broadly refers to societal improvements in sanitation, hygiene, and living conditions that prevent the transmission of GAS infection. Such environmental change requires substantial infrastructure investment at the country level, but is the most effective way to alter the trajectory of the disease at the population level.[11,12] In fact, deteriorating living standards following the economic decline within the former Soviet Union has led to an increase in RHD prevalence.[68]

Primary prevention with early antimicrobial treatment of streptococcal pharyngitis should avert the cascade of immunologic activation that leads to ARF. Primary prevention requires access to penicillin, and ideally to diagnostic tests such as rapid streptococcal testing and microbiology lab services. Such access at a population level depends on a well-functioning decentralized health system free of financial and physical barriers to care, trained health care workers, and a ready supply of good-quality penicillin, which are often lacking in endemic regions.[69] The use of clinical decision rules to selectively treat patients with pharyngitis without throat culture can be cost-effective at reducing RHD burden.[70]

Secondary Prevention

Secondary prevention refers to the prevention of recurrent attacks of ARF through the administration of long-term suppressive antibiotics, thus halting or delaying the progression of valvular disease. It requires both diagnostic capability, which necessitates access to echocardiography and specialist care, as well as capacity for chronic care for antibiotic therapy distribution and disease progression monitoring. With supportive care programs, retention in care for patients with RHD can be high in low-income countries.[71]

Although secondary prophylaxis has long been recommended and remains a central component of most international guidelines for RHD management, the evidence to support its efficacy is not robust. The initial basis for secondary prophylaxis guidelines are historically based on a 1972 prospective study of 115 patients with documented ARF who received monthly benzathine penicillin prophylaxis followed for a median of 10 years.[72] There were no patients in the series who exhibited clinical disease progression to valvular stenosis or congestive heart failure, and 70% of those with acute mitral regurgitation had regression of their murmur. In contrast, among 1000 patients with ARF in an earlier series from the pre-antimicrobial era, 30% died (80% of deaths from RHD and 10% from bacterial endocarditis), and 20% had regression of mitral regurgitation murmur after 20 years of follow-up.[73] Although compelling, the small-scale noncontrolled study showing improved outcomes for patients treated with penicillin would not pass today's strict standards for treatment efficacy. Even more, there have been many case reports of treatment failures of patients who, despite clear documentation of penicillin adherence, still progress to develop severe valvular disease.[74]

Additionally, the natural history of latent RHD remains unclear. Both regression and progression of valvular lesions and regurgitation are known to be common. In early follow-up studies of patients identified with SCC during episodes of ARF (n = 35–53), 23% to 40% of patients were found at 2-year to 5-year follow-up to have persistence or progression of disease.[75–77] Two recent large prevalence studies from India and Nicaragua with short-term follow-up suggest that of asymptomatic children with latent RHD by echocardiography, 30% to 40% may have disease regression or resolution, with the remaining having persistence or progression of RHD.[55,78]

It is also unclear whether patients with "borderline" or minor echo findings carry the same risk for progression as patients with "definite" RHD. According to a recent study of patients with borderline RHD, up to 52% may have regression of their valvular changes on echocardiogram by 5 years of follow-up.[60] Another recent prospective study of Aboriginal children found the risk of progression, compared with matched controls, to be 8.2-fold higher for borderline RHD valve abnormalities, whereas only 1.5-fold higher for minor nonspecific valve abnormalities.[79]

The uncertain efficacy of penicillin prophylaxis has implications for the value of echocardiography-based screening programs.[80] Such programs may uncover large numbers of patients with latent RHD. However, until the true efficacy of secondary prophylaxis is established, the estimated reduction in morbidity and mortality cannot be precisely determined. The recently launched multisite REMEDY study will provide crucial data on clinical features, risks, and outcomes for patients with RHD from endemic regions, and will hopefully provide evidence to fill in some of the gaps in knowledge regarding secondary prophylaxis.[35]

Medical Therapies

Rheumatic valvular stenosis or regurgitation may progress over time. Although mitral regurgitation is the most common form of RHD among the young,[81–83] the most common cause of mitral stenosis globally is RHD.[84] Rheumatic aortic valve disease is usually comorbid with mitral disease, although isolated aortic regurgitation can occur.[85] RHD of the tricuspid and pulmonary valves is rare in isolation, and is almost always in addition to mitral disease.[86] The subsequent hemodynamic abnormalities may eventually lead to symptomatic heart failure with ventricular remodeling and dilation, progression to valvular cardiomyopathy, and end-stage heart failure.

Although, in general, valvular cardiomyopathy is considered a surgical disease, there is some evidence that medical therapy may be helpful. Several studies have demonstrated the benefits for left ventricular remodeling with angiotensin-converting enzyme inhibitors (ACEIs). For example, in a placebo-controlled study of 47 patients with minimal or mild symptoms and moderate to severe mitral regurgitation from either RHD or mitral valve prolapse, treatment with enalapril was associated with a significant reduction in left ventricular diastolic diameter (by 0.3 cm) and 25% reduction in mitral regurgitation volume after 12 months.[87] Another study using enalapril and nicoradil was associated with a significant reduction in left ventricular end-systolic index and improvement in ejection fraction at 6 months compared with baseline.[88] In addition, low-dose ACEIs may have benefit in severe rheumatic mitral stenosis. A study of patients with significant symptomatic mitral stenosis (mitral valve orifice <1.5 cm^2) who were given low-dose enalapril showed not only its safety (with no worsening of symptoms or hypotension) but also significant improvements in symptoms and functional capacity.[89]

Percutaneous mitral balloon valvuloplasty (PMBV) is the standard first-line therapy for cases of rheumatic mitral stenosis in the absence of concomitant regurgitation and left atrial thrombus. Good intermediate and long-term outcomes with PMBV have been reported, but are limited to those patients with favorable valve morphology and the lack of postprocedural significant mitral regurgitation.[90,91] Echocardiography-based favorability scoring, which evaluates specific structural features of the mitral apparatus, such as leaflet thickening, calcification, and subvalvular thickening, has been useful in candidate selection for PMBV procedure.[92] In general, patients referred for intervention early in their disease course will tend to meet favorability criteria and can benefit most from PMBV. In the global health context, most endemic regions have few or no catheterization laboratories for referral, with most patients presenting late in the course of disease, often with mixed regurgitant and stenotic disease that is not amenable to PMBV intervention.

Surgical Therapies: Valve Repair Versus Replacement

Well-timed surgical intervention at the early symptomatic stages of rheumatic valvular cardiomyopathy is lifesaving, often representing the only curative option. Operative management entails either valve repair or replacement, with either mechanical or bioprosthetic valves. The improved durability of mechanical valves makes their use preferable in young patients. However, long-term systemic anticoagulation for thromboembolic prophylaxis is required. Warfarin therapy may be problematic for patients of childbearing age. Further, medication supply and laboratory monitoring may not be consistently available in resource-limited settings. The limited data suggest that patients in endemic regions receiving mechanical valves may do worse overall than those with bioprosthetic valves. Among New Zealand women of reproductive age, mechanical valves were associated with much higher rates of mortality, thromboembolism, and hemorrhage, despite better valve patency and lower reoperation rates as compared with bioprosthetic valves.[93] The relative risk of death was notably 6 to 8 times higher among Maori and Pacific Islander patients as compared with white women. Improved health systems to care for patients with valve replacement are needed in RHD endemic regions. Nurse-led or pharmacist-led anticoagulation programs in low-income countries can be effective.[94,95]

A repair-based operative strategy avoids such complications and logistical challenges. Experience in the 1980s to 1990s with repair of rheumatic mitral valves showed poor outcomes, with a mortality rate of 15% and reoperation rate of 27% at 5 years.[96,97] As such, mitral valve replacement (MVR) was the favored surgical approach for nearly a decade. However, recent reports from surgical centers from endemic regions reveal good outcomes with mitral valve repair when performed by experienced surgeons trained in modern rheumatic repair techniques.[98,99] A retrospective study of 81 patients at a New Zealand center showed a survival advantage with mitral valve repair compared with MVR (14-year survival of 90% vs 44%) as well as absence of thrombotic, embolic, and hemorrhagic complications compared with MVR (100% vs 45% at 14 years).[100] Indeed, mitral valve repair is now recommended over replacement by many surgeons from experienced centers.[101] Several repair strategies tailored to the pathologic rheumatic valve are currently being used at surgical centers in endemic regions and include peeling of thickened layers off the posterior leaflet, shortening the primary chordae of the anterior leaflet, and extending the posterior chordae that are retracting the leaflet, among others.[101] However, many endemic regions in low-resource settings may rely on junior surgeons without extensive training in repair techniques and may still favor valve replacement due to its relative operative simplicity with shorter cardiopulmonary bypass times.

Rheumatic Heart Disease and Maternal Health

Preexisting severe valvular disease increases the risk of pregnancy and requires specialized care to avert maternal morbidity and mortality.[102] The 2011 European Society of Cardiology (ESC) guidelines recommend that women with preexisting cardiac disease should undergo a modified WHO risk assessment to guide antenatal care.[103] According to the ESC guidelines, patients with severe mitral stenosis, severe symptomatic aortic stenosis, valve lesions associated with severe left ventricular dysfunction, or significant pulmonary hypertension are at highest risk, and pregnancy is contraindicated. Regurgitant valvular disease is better tolerated in pregnancy but may still increase the overall risk of pregnancy, requiring frequent monitoring and coordination of care among a multidisciplinary team.[104]

There is increasing recognition of untreated RHD, and cardiac disease in general, as a hidden source of maternal mortality among the global poor.[105] However, systemic deficiencies in reporting and classification of maternal deaths, as well as low levels of diagnosis by maternal health providers working in low-resource environments, have resulted in a dearth of data on cardiac causes of maternal mortality.[105,106] A few studies emphasize the interplay between cardiac disease and pregnancy. A recent study from South Africa found that of 118 cases of maternal deaths, 25% were related to preexisting RHD, with mitral stenosis as the most important contributor.[107] Importantly, the investigators found that both patient and provider factors contributed to the maternal deaths, including late presentation (>50%) and lack of expertise by the medical staff (30%). In the REMEDY study, of the 3343 registered patients with RHD across 14 countries, 55% were women of childbearing age and 4% of women were pregnant at enrollment.[35] Perhaps most alarming were the low rate of contraception (3.6%) among women of childbearing age, and the use of warfarin, a known teratogen, in 21% of pregnant women. Further research is required to uncover the reasons for such poor care among pregnant women with RHD, and to devise strategies for intervention.

Management in Low-Resource Settings

RHD management in high-prevalence regions must also account for the challenges of weak health systems. The lack of adequately trained medical providers, poor availability of diagnostic technologies, and presence of substantial patient level barriers to care must be addressed for the provision of effective care in endemic regions.

The advent of portable echocardiography has enabled screening to be performed in remote endemic areas, and remains an area of growing interest and innovation.[108] New handheld ultrasound devices at even lower cost promise even more affordability and accessibility. The human resource problem, with an inadequate force of trained physicians, especially specialists, has resulted in task-shifting efforts with customized training programs.[109] For RHD, task-shifting includes screening echocardiography and initial management by a specially trained nurse or general physician. Health workers from Fiji receiving brief training can diagnose subclinical RHD using the WHF criteria with up to 89% accuracy.[110,111]

ADVOCACY EFFORTS IN THE GLOBAL ARENA

Increasing recognition of both the immense burden of RHD globally as well as the advancement of global health equity platforms has led to greater prioritization of RHD in global agendas. The WHF has set the ambitious goal of "25 × 25 < 25" to achieve a 25% reduction in premature deaths from RHD in those younger than 25 years by 2025. The WHF has also identified specific targets pertaining to the creation of comprehensive national control programs, ensuring availability of high-quality benzathine penicillin G and testing a GAS vaccine in phase III trials.[112] In addition, the WHF, together with Medtronic Foundation and RhEACH, have launched RHD Action, a platform for resources providing technical assistance for those working in the field, as well as funding for a limited number of country-wide coordinated research and implementation projects. Further, there are a number of RHD registries that will be able to facilitate both long-term follow-up for patients and prospective research endeavors. The REMEDY study, mentioned previously, is a multicenter international hospital-based prospective registry of patients with RHD that should yield important local data from endemic regions on risk factors, determinants, and outcomes, hopefully filling in some of the knowledge gaps.[35] In sub-Saharan Africa, the African Union Commission and the Pan-African Society of Cardiology have held annual meetings for the past 4 years, where expert health leaders from 18 countries across the continent gathered to formulate a strategy to solve the RHD crisis. The group issued the Addis Ababa Communique, which lists "7 key actions" for intervention for RHD in Africa, based in turn on 7 key barriers to RHD eradication.[70] The key actions address structural barriers, such as lack of surveillance programs, overcentralization of services, and lack of national RHD programs, as well as specific deficits, such as the supply of quality benzathine penicillin, poor integration with reproductive health services, and a lack of access to cardiac surgical services.

Despite advocacy efforts, RHD remains vastly underfunded and underrecognized as a priority on the global agenda. RHD is not specifically addressed in the 2012 WHO noncommunicable disease (NCD) Action Plan.[113] The plan broadly addresses the global burden of cardiovascular disease, but limits the discussion to behavioral risk factors related to ischemic heart disease and stroke. Although NCDs are increasingly prioritized, most NCD programs target lifestyle risk factors related atherosclerotic disease, such as smoking, lack of physical activity, and obesity. However, RHD is related to an entirely different set of poverty-related determinants.[114] In addition, there is uneven attention given to certain important deficiencies in RHD control and treatment. For example, there has been much focus on identifying people with subclinical RHD through echocardiography-based screening in many endemic regions. However, there has been less attention to primordial prevention and the design of health systems interventions to treat people with RHD after identification. Further effort is needed to integrate RHD screening and care into other longitudinal chronic care programs or with maternal health services. Cardiovascular disease care in low-income countries deserves the enthusiasm with which chronic infectious diseases has been met.[115] Access to cardiac surgical services is severely lacking in many high-prevalence regions and will require concerted health systems and human resource investment.

SUMMARY

We are embarking on a new chapter in the history of RHD, with a re-invigoration of attention and resources within the medical and public health communities toward its eradication. Revised global estimates of disease burden highlight RHD as a disease of the poor. The emergence of portable echocardiography enables providers to detect disease in endemic regions with better efficiency. Our review documents key knowledge gaps relating to our understanding of disease pathophysiology, global epidemiology, and care practices for RHD management. Developing and studying equitable and resource-effective RHD prevention and management programs through multifaceted contextualized strategies will be the next frontier.

REFERENCES

1. GBD 2013 Mortality and Causes of Death Collaborators. Global, regional, and national age–sex specific all-cause and cause-specific mortality for 240 causes of death, 1990–2013: a systematic analysis for the Global Burden of Disease Study 2013. Lancet 2015;385:117–71.
2. Weinberg J, Beaton A, Aliku T, et al. Prevalence of rheumatic heart disease in African school-aged population: extrapolation from echocardiography screening using the 2012 World Heart Federation Guidelines. Int J Cardiol 2015;202:238–9.
3. Carapetis JR, Steer AC, Mulholland EK, et al. The global burden of group A streptococcal diseases. Lancet Infect Dis 2005;5:685–92.
4. Armstrong DB, Wheatley GM. Studies in rheumatic fever. New York: Metropolitan Life Ins Co; 1944.
5. Bland EF. Rheumatic fever: the way it was. Circulation 1987;76:1190–5.
6. Coburn AF. The factor of infection in the rheumatic state. Baltimore (MD): Williams and Wilkins; 1931.
7. Jones TD. The diagnosis of rheumatic fever. JAMA 1944;126:481–4.
8. Rowntree LJ. Rheumatic heart disease and the physician fitness of the nation as seen by selective service. J Pediatr 1945;26:220–9.
9. Holbrook WP. The Army-Air Force rheumatic fever control program. JAMA 1944;126:84–7.
10. Gordis L. The virtual disappearance of rheumatic fever in the United States: lessons in the rise and fall of disease. T. Duckett Jones Memorial Lecture. Circulation 1985;72:1155–62.
11. Labarthe D. Epidemiology and prevention of cardiovascular diseases: a global challenge. 2nd edition. Sudbury (MA): Jones and Bartlett Publishers; 2011.
12. World Health Organization Joint WHO/ISFC Meeting on Rheumatic Fever/Rheumatic Heart Disease Control, with Emphasis on Primary Prevention. Geneva (Switzerland): 1994. Available at: https://extranet.who.int/iris/restricted/handle/10665/60727. Accessed July 1, 2016.
13. Beaton A, Okello E, Lwabi P, et al. Echocardiography screening for rheumatic heart disease in Ugandan schoolchildren. Circulation 2012;125:3127–32.
14. Zhang W, Mondo C, Okello E, et al. Presenting features of newly diagnosed rheumatic heart disease patients in Mulago Hospital: a pilot study: cardiovascular topics. Cardiovasc J Afr 2013;24:28–33.
15. Mirabel M, Fauchier T, Bacquelin R, et al. Echocardiography screening to detect rheumatic heart disease. Int J Cardiol 2015;188:89–95.
16. Lawrence JG, Carapetis JR, Griffiths K, et al. Acute rheumatic fever and rheumatic heart disease: incidence and progression in the Northern Territory of Australia, 1997 to 2010. Circulation 2013;128:492–501.
17. Marijon E, Mirabel M, Celermajer DS, et al. Rheumatic heart disease. Lancet 2012;379(9819):953–64.
18. Mocumbi AO. Rheumatic heart disease in Africa: is there a role for genetic studies? Cardiovasc J Afr 2015;26:S21–6.
19. Virmani R, Farb A, Burke AP, et al. Pathology of acute rheumatic carditis. In: Narula J, Virmani R, Reddy KS, editors. Rheumatic fever. Washington, DC: American Registry of Pathology, Armed Forces Institute of Pathology; 1999. p. 217–34.
20. Aschoff L. The rheumatic nodules in the heart. Ann Rheum Dis 1939;1:161–6.
21. Saphir O. The Aschoff nodule. Am J Clin Pathol 1959;31:534–9.
22. Meira ZMA, Goulart EMA, Colosimo EA, et al. Long term follow up of rheumatic fever and predictors of severe rheumatic valvar disease in Brazilian children and adolescents. Heart 2005;91:1019–22.
23. Stollerman GH. Rheumatogenic and nephritogenic streptococci. Circulation 1971;43:915–21.
24. Ayoub EM, Taranta A, Bartley TD. Effect of valvular surgery on antibody to the group A streptococcal carbohydrate. Circulation 1974;50:144–50.
25. Fae KC, da Silva DD, Oshiro S, et al. Mimicry in recognition of cardiac myosin peptides by heart-intralesional T cell clones from rheumatic heart disease. J Immunol 2006;176:5662–70.

26. Robert S, Kosanke S, Dunn ST, et al. Pathogenic mechanisms in rheumatic carditis: focus on valvular endothelium. J Infect Dis 2001;183: 507–11.

27. Tandon R, Sharma M, Chandrashekhar Y, et al. Revisiting the pathogenesis of rheumatic fever and carditis. Nat Rev Cardiol 2013;10:171–7.

28. Narula J, Chopra PR, Talwar KK, et al. Does endomyocardial biopsy aid in the diagnosis of active rheumatic carditis? Circulation 1993;88:2198–205.

29. Gupta M, Lent RW, Kaplan EL, et al. Serum cardiac troponin-I in acute rheumatic fever. Am J Cardiol 2001;89:779–82.

30. Dinkla K, Rohde M, Jansen WT, et al. Rheumatic fever-associated Streptococcus pyogenes isolates aggregate collage. J Clin Invest 2003;111: 1905–12.

31. Dinkla K, Talay SR, Mörgelin M, et al. Crucial role of the CB3-region of collage IV in PARF-induced acute rheumatic fever. PLoS One 2009;3:e4666.

32. Cheadle W. Barbeian lectures on the various manifestations of the rheumatic state as exemplified in childhood and early life. Lancet 1889;133:821–7.

33. Bryant PA, Robins-Browne R, Carapetis JR, et al. Some of the people, some of the time: susceptibility to acute rheumatic fever. Circulation 2009;119: 742–53.

34. Engel ME, Stander R, Vogel J, et al. Genetic susceptibility to acute rheumatic fever: a systematic review and meta-analysis of twin studies. PLoS One 2011;6(9):e25426.

35. Zühlke L, Engel ME, Karthikeyan G, et al. Characteristics, complications, and gaps in evidence-based interventions in rheumatic heart disease: the Global Rheumatic Heart Disease Registry (the REMEDY study). Eur Heart J 2015;36:1115–22.

36. Jones criteria (revised) for guidance in the diagnosis of rheumatic fever. Circulation 1965;32: 664–8.

37. Guidelines for the diagnosis of rheumatic fever: Jones criteria, 1992 update. JAMA 1992;268: 2069–73.

38. Gewitz MH, Baltimore RS, Tani LY, et al. Revision of the Jones criteria for the diagnosis of acute rheumatic fever in the era of Doppler echocardiography: a scientific statement from the American Heart Association. Circulation 2015;131:1806–18.

39. Carapetis JR, Currie BJ. Rheumatic fever in a high incidence population: the importance of monoarthritis and low grade fever. Arch Dis Child 2001; 85:223–7.

40. Noonan S, Zurynski YA, Currie BJ, et al. A national prospective surveillance study of acute rheumatic fever in Australian children. Pediatr Infect Dis J 2013;32:e26–32.

41. Sanyal SK, Thapar MK, Ahmed SH, et al. The initial attack of acute rheumatic fever during childhood in North India: a prospective study of the clinical profile. Circulation 1974;49:7–12.

42. Harlan GA, Tani LY, Byington CL. Rheumatic fever presenting as monoarticular arthritis. Pediatr Infect Dis J 2006;25:743–6.

43. Tedeschi CG, Wagner BM. The problem of subclinical rheumatic carditis. Am J Med Sci 1956;231:382–8.

44. Feigenbaum H. Evolution of echocardiography. Circulation 1996;93:1321–7.

45. Vesey GL, Weidmeier SE, Ossmond GS, et al. Resurgence of acute rheumatic fever in the intermountain area of the United States. N Engl J Med 1987;316:421–7.

46. Folger GM, Hajar R, Robida A, et al. Occurrence of valvular heart disease in acute rheumatic fever without evident carditis: colour-flow Doppler identification. Br Heart J 1992;67:434–8.

47. Minich LL, Tani LY, Pagotto LT, et al. Doppler echocardiography distinguishes between physiologic and pathologic "silent" regurgitation in patients with rheumatic fever. Clin Cardiol 1997;20:924–6.

48. Wilson NJ, Neutze JM. Echocardiographic diagnosis of subclinical carditis in acute rheumatic fevers. Int J Cardiol 1995;50:1–6.

49. Marcus RH, Sareli P, Pocock WA, et al. Functional anatomy of severe mitral regurgitation in active rheumatic carditis. Am J Cardiol 1989;63:577–84.

50. Lembo NJ, Dell'Italia LJ, Crawford M, et al. Mitral valve prolapse in patients with prior rheumatic fever. Circulation 1988;77:830–6.

51. Tubridy-Clark M, Carapeti JR. Subclinical carditis in rheumatic fever: a systematic review. Int J Cardiol 2007;119:54–8.

52. Marijon E, Ou P, Celermajer DS, et al. Prevalence of rheumatic heart disease detected by echocardiographic screening. N Engl J Med 2007;37:470–6.

53. Marijon E, Celermajer DS, Tafflet M, et al. Rheumatic heart disease screening by echocardiography: the inadequacy of World Health Organization criteria for optimizing the diagnosis of subclinical disease. Circulation 2009;120:663–8.

54. Carapetis JR, Hardy M, Fakakovikaetau T, et al. Evaluation of a screening protocol using auscultation and portable echocardiography to detect asymptomatic rheumatic heart disease in Tongan schoolchildren. Nat Clin Pract Cardiovasc Med 2008;5:411–7.

55. Paar JA, Berrios NM, Rose JD, et al. Prevalence of rheumatic heart disease in children and young adults in Nicaragua. Am J Cardiol 2010;105: 1809–14.

56. Bhaya M, Panwar S, Beniwal R, et al. High prevalence of rheumatic heart disease detected by echocardiography in school children. Echocardiography 2010;27:448–53.

57. Remenyi B, Wilson N, Steer A, et al. World Heart Federation criteria for echocardiographic

diagnosis of rheumatic heart disease: an evidence based guideline. Nat Rev Cardiol 2012;9:297–309.

58. Bhaya M, Beniwal R, Panwar S, et al. Two years of follow-up validates the echocardiographic criteria for the diagnosis and screening of rheumatic heart disease in asympatomic populations. Echocardiography 2011;28:929–33.

59. Bacquelin R, Tafflet M, Rouchon B, et al. Echocardiography-based screening for rheumatic heart disease: what does borderline mean? Int J Cardiol 2016;203:1003–4.

60. Zühlke L, Engel ME, Lemmer CE, et al. The natural history of latent rheumatic heart disease in a 5 year follow-up study: a prospective observational study. BMC Cardiovasc Disord 2016;16:1.

61. Byass P, de Courten M, Graham WJ, et al. Reflections on the global burden of disease 2010 estimates. PLoS Med 2013;10:e1001477.

62. Engel ME, Haileamlak A, Zühlke L, et al. Prevalence of rheumatic heart disease in 4720 asymptomatic scholars from South Africa and Ethiopia. Heart 2015;101:1389–94.

63. Horton R. Ghana: defining the African challenge. Lancet 2001;358:2141–9.

64. Beaton A, Aliku T, Okello E, et al. The utility of hand-held echocardiography for early diagnosis of rheumatic heart disease. J Am Soc Echocardiogr 2014; 27(1):42–9.

65. Zühlke LJ, Steer AC. Estimates of the global burden of rheumatic heart disease. Glob Heart 2013;8:189–95.

66. Carapetis JR. Rheumatic heart disease in developing countries. N Engl J Med 2007;357:439–41.

67. Otto H, Sæther SG, Banteyrga L, et al. High prevalence of subclinical rheumatic heart disease in pregnant women in a developing country: an echocardiographic study. Echocardiography 2011;28: 1049–53.

68. Omurzakova NA, Yamano Y, Saatova GM, et al. High incidence of rheumatic fever and rheumatic heart disease in the republics of Central Asia. Int J Rheum Dis 2009;12:79–83.

69. Watkins D, Zuhlke L, Engel M, et al. Seven key actions to eradicate rheumatic heart disease in Africa: the Addis Ababa communique. Cardiovasc J Afr 2016;27:1–5.

70. Irlam J, Mayosi BM, Engel M, et al. Primary prevention of acute rheumatic fever and rheumatic heart disease with penicillin in South African children with pharyngitis: a cost-effectiveness analysis. Circ Cardiovasc Qual Outcomes 2013;6: 343–51.

71. Longenecker CT, Aliku T, Beaton A, et al. Treatment cascade quality metrics for children with latent rheumatic heart disease in Uganda. Glob Heart 2016;11:e119–20.

72. Tompkins DG, Boxerbaum B, Liebman J. Long-term prognosis of rheumatic fever patients receiving regular intramuscular benzathine penicillin. Circulation 1972;45:543–51.

73. Bland EF, Jones TD. Rheumatic fever and rheumatic heart disease: a twenty year report on 1000 patients followed since childhood. Circulation 1951;4:836–44.

74. McGlacken-Byrne SM, Parry HM, Currie PF, et al. Failure of oral penicillin as secondary prophylaxis for rheumatic heart disease: a lesion from a low-prevalence rheumatic fever region. BMJ Case Rep 2015;2015. pii:bcr2015212861.

75. Figueroa FE, Fernández MS, Valdes P, et al. Prospective comparison of clinical and echocardiographic diagnosis of rheumatic carditis: long-term follow-up of patients with subclinical disease. Heart 2001;85:407–10.

76. Karaaslan S, Demirören S, Oran B, et al. Criteria for judging the improvement in subclinical rheumatic valvulitis. Cardiol Young 2003;13:500–5.

77. Ozkutlu S, Hal   lioglu O, Ayabakam C. Evolution of subclinical valvular disease in patients with rheumatic fever. Cardiol Young 2003;13:495–9.

78. Saxena A, Ramakrishnan S, Roy A, et al. Prevalence and outcome of subclinical rheumatic heart disease in India: the RHEUMATIC (Rheumatic Heart Echo Utilisation and Monitoring Actuarial Trends in Indian Children) study. Heart 2011;97: 2018–22.

79. Remon M, Atkinson D, White A, et al. Are minor echocardiographic changes associated with an increased risk of acute rheumatic fever or progression to rheumatic heart disease? Int J Cardiol 2015;198:117–22.

80. Zuhlke L, Mayosi BM. Echocardiographic screening for subclinical rheumatic heart disease remains a research tool pending studies of impact on prognosis. Curr Cardiol Rep 2013;15:1–7.

81. Alkhalifa MS, Ibrahim SA, Osman SH. Pattern and severity of rheumatic valvular lesions in children in Khartoum, Sudan. East Mediterr Health J 2007; 14:1015–21.

82. Vasan RS, Shrivastava S, Vijayakumar M, et al. Echocardiographic evaluation of patients with acute rheumatic fever and rheumatic carditis. Circulation 1996;94:73–82.

83. Yuko-Jowl C, Bakari M. Echocardiographic patterns of juvenile rheumatic heart disease at the Kenyatta National Hospital, Nairobi. East Afr Med J 2005;82:514–9.

84. Waller BF, Howard J, Fess S. Pathology of mitral valve stenosis and pure mitral regurgitation—Part I. Clin Cardiol 1994;17:330–6.

85. Chockalingam A, Gnanavelu G, Elangovan S, et al. Clinical spectrum of chronic rheumatic heart disease in India. J Heart Valve Dis 2003;(12):577–81.

86. Sultan FA, Moustafa SE, Tajik J, et al. Rheumatic tricuspid valve disease: an evidenc-based systematic overview. J Heart Valve Dis 2010;19:374–82.

87. Sampaio RO, Grinberg M, Leite JJ, et al. Effect of enalapril on left ventricular diameters and exercise capacity in asymptomatic or mildly symptomatic patients with regurgitation secondary to mitral valve prolapse or rheumatic heart disease. Am J Cardiol 2005;96:117–21.

88. Gupta DK, Kapoor A, Garg N, et al. Beneficial effects of nicorandil versus enalapril in chronic rheumatic severe mitral regurgitation: six months follow up echocardiographic study. J Heart Valve Dis 2001;10:158–65.

89. Chockalingam A, Venkatesan S, Dorairajan S, et al. Safety and efficacy of enalapril in multivalvular heart disease with significant mitral stenosis: SCOPE MS. Angiology 2005;56:151–8.

90. Sharma J, Goel PK, Pandey CM, et al. Intermediate outcomes of rheumatic mitral stenosis post-balloon mitral valvotomy. Asian Cardiovasc Thorac Ann 2015;23:923–30.

91. Palacios IF, Sanchez PL, Harrell LC, et al. Which patients benefit from percutaneous mitral balloon valvuloplasty. Circulation 2002;105:1465–71.

92. Wilkins G, Weyman AE, Abascal V, et al. Percutaneous balloon dilatation of the mitral valve: an analysis of echocardiographic variables related to outcome and the mechanism of dilatation. Br Heart J 1988;60:299–308.

93. North RA, Sadler L, Stewart AW, et al. Long-term survival and valve-related complications in young women with cardiac valve replacements. Circulation 1999;99:2669–76.

94. Robinson O, Romain J-L, Wilentz J, et al. Effectiveness of a nurse-led mechanical valve anticoagulation program for rheumatic heart disease patients in Haiti. Glob Heart 2016;11:e64.

95. Manji I, Pastakia SD, Do AN, et al. Performance outcomes of a pharmacist-managed anticoagulation clinic in the rural, resource-constrained setting of Eldoret, Kenya. J Thromb Haemost 2011;9(11):2215–20. Available at: http://doi.org/10.1111/j.1538-7836.2011.04503.x.

96. Skoularigis J, Sinovich V, Joubert G, et al. Evaluation of the long-term results of mitral valve repair in 254 young patients with rheumatic mitral regurgitation. Circulation 1994;90:167–74.

97. Grossi EA, Galloway AC, Miller JS, et al. Valve repair versus replacement for mitral insufficiency: when is a mechanical valve still indicated? J Thorac Cardiovasc Surg 1998;115:389–94.

98. Chotivatanapong T, Lerdsomboo P, Sungkahapong V. Rheumatic mitral valve repair: experience of 221 cases from Central Chest Institute of Thailand. J Med Assoc Thai 2012;95:S51–7.

99. Yakub MA, Dillon J, Krishna Moorthy PS, et al. Is rheumatic aetiology a predictor of poor outcome in the current era of mitral valve repair? Contemporary long-term results of mitral valve repair in rheumatic heart disease. Eur J Cardiothorac Surg 2013;44:673–81.

100. Remenyi B, Webb R, Gentles T, et al. Improved long-term survival for rheumatic mitral valve repair compared to replacement in the young. World J Pediatr Congenit Heart Surg 2013;4:155–64.

101. Finucane K, Wilson N. Priorities in cardiac surgery for rheumatic heart disease. Glob Heart 2013;8:213–20.

102. Anthony J, Osman A, Sani MU. Valvular heart disease in pregnancy. Cardiovasc J Afr 2016;27:111–8.

103. Regitz-Zagrosek V, Lundqvist CB, Borghi C, et al. ESC Guidelines on the management of cardiovascular diseases during pregnancy. Eur Heart J 2011;32:3147–97.

104. Elkayam U, Goland S, Pieper PG, et al. High-risk cardiac disease in pregnancy. J Am Coll Cardiol 2016;68(4):396–410. Available at: http://doi.org/10.1016/j.jacc.2016.05.048.

105. Mocumbi AO, Sliwa K. Women's cardiovascular health in Africa. Heart 2012;98:450–5.

106. Kassebaum NJ, Bertozzi-Villa A, Coggeshall MS, et al. Global, regional, and national levels and causes of maternal mortality during 1990–2013: a systematic analysis for the Global Burden of Disease Study 2013. Lancet 2014;384:980–1004.

107. Soma-Pillay P, Seabe J, Sliwa K. The importance of cardiovascular pathology contributing to maternal death: confidential enquiry into maternal deaths in South Africa, 2011-2013. Cardiovasc J Afr 2016;27:60–5.

108. Zuhlke L, Engel ME, Nkepu S, et al. Evaluation of a focussed protocol for hand-held echocardiography and computer-assisted auscultation in detecting latent rheumatic heart disease in scholars. Cardiol Young 2016;26:1097–106.

109. Kwan GF, Bukhman AK, Miller AC, et al. A simplified echocardiographic strategy for heart failure diagnosis and management within an integrated noncommunicable disease clinic at district hospital level for sub-Saharan Africa. JACC Heart Fail 2013;1:230–6.

110. Colquhoun SM, Carapetis JR, Kado JH, et al. Pilot study of nurse-led rheumatic heart disease echocardiography screening in Fiji—a novel approach in a resource-poor setting. Cardiol Young 2013;23:546–52.

111. Engelman D, Kado JH, Reményi B, et al. Focused cardiac ultrasound screening for rheumatic heart disease by briefly trained health workers: a study of diagnostic accuracy. Lancet Glob Heal 2016;4:e386–94.

112. WHF. 2015. Available at: http://www.world-heart-federation.org/what-we-do/rheumatic-heart-disease-rhd/25x25/. Accessed July 1, 2016.

113. WHO. Global action plan for the prevention and control of non-communicable diseases, 2013-2020. Geneva (Switzerland): World Health Organization; 2012.

114. Kwan GF, Mayosi BM, Mocumbi AO, et al. Endemic cardiovascular diseases of the poorest billion. Circulation 2016;133:2561–75.

115. Bukhman G, Kidder A. Cardiovascular disease and global health equity: lessons from tuberculosis control then and now. Am J Public Health 2008; 98(1):44–54.

Index

Cardiol Clin 35 (2017) 181–184
http://dx.doi.org/10.1016/S0733-8651(16)30119-9
0733-8651/17

Printed and bound by CPI Group (UK) Ltd, Croydon, CR0 4YY

03/10/2024

01040385-0008